Architecture and Health Equity
in an Imperiled World

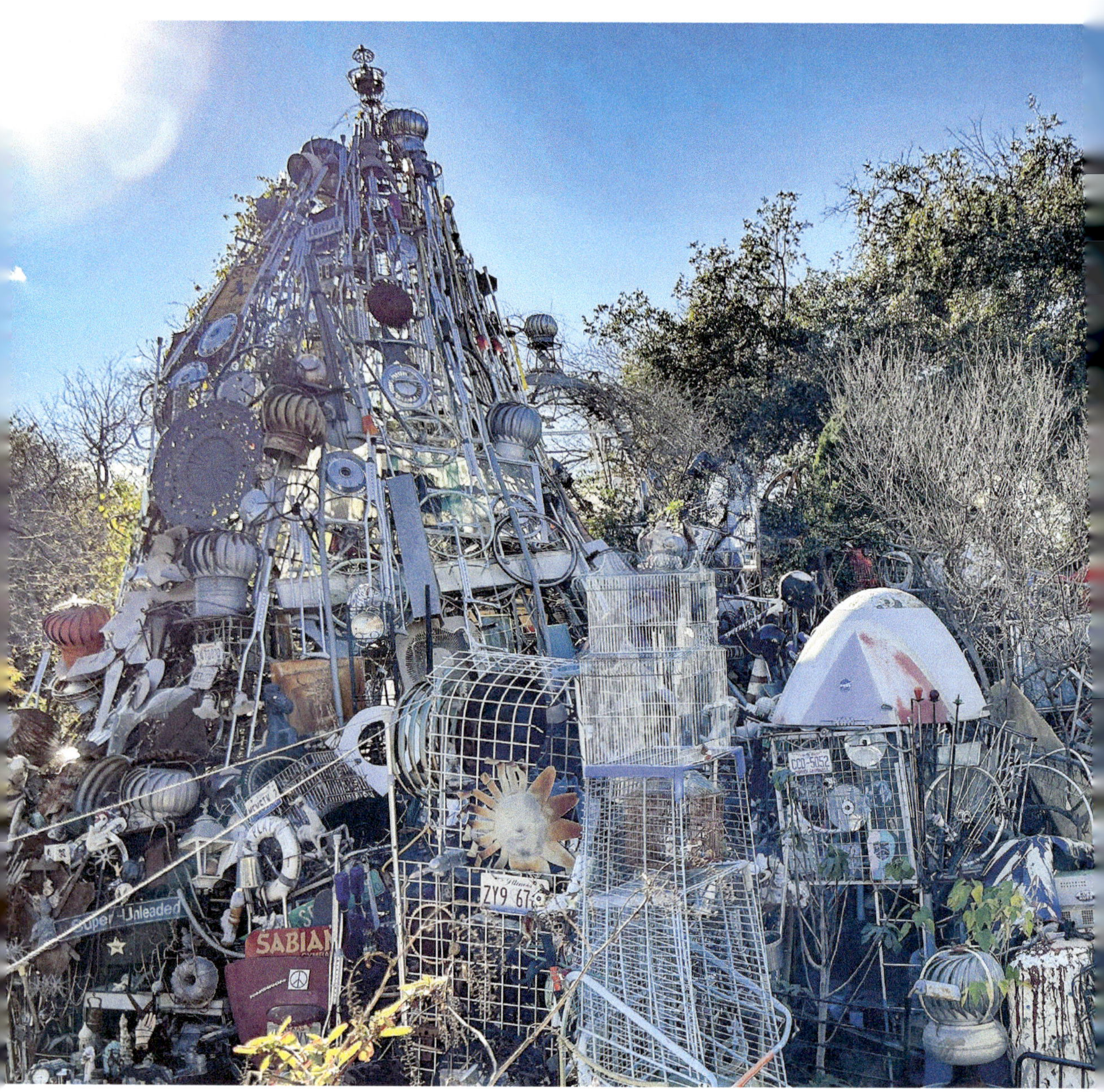

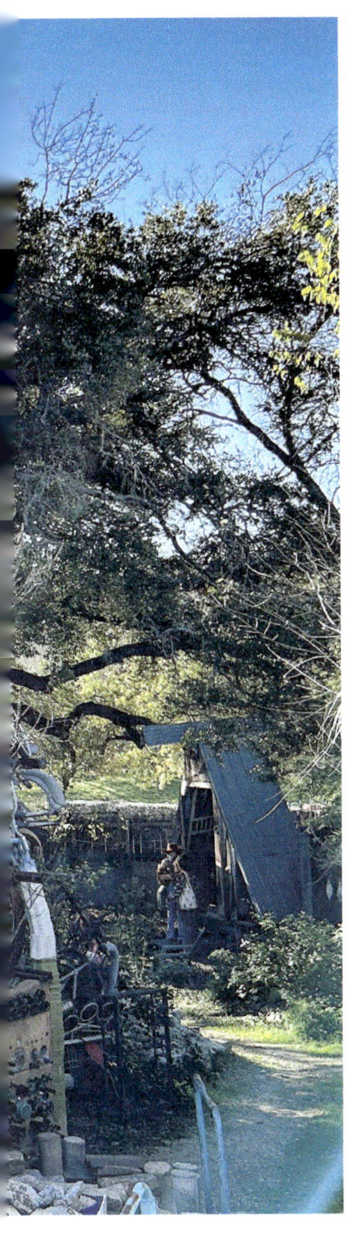

Architecture and Health Equity in an Imperiled World

Stephen Verderber

JOHNS HOPKINS UNIVERSITY PRESS

Baltimore

© 2025 Johns Hopkins University Press
All rights reserved. Published 2025
Printed in the United States of America on acid-free paper
9 8 7 6 5 4 3 2 1

Johns Hopkins University Press
2715 North Charles Street
Baltimore, Maryland 21218
www.press.jhu.edu

Library of Congress Cataloging-in-Publication Data is available.
A catalog record for this book is available from the British Library.

ISBN 978-1-4214-5250-0 (hardcover)
ISBN 978-1-4214-5251-7 (ebook)

*Special discounts are available for bulk purchases of this book. For more information,
please contact Special Sales at specialsales@jh.edu.*

EU GPSR Authorized Representative
LOGOS EUROPE, 9 rue Nicolas Poussin 17000, La Rochelle, France
Email: contact@logoseurope.eu

In memory of my devoted parents,

William Verderber (1924–1989) and
Helen Verderber (1924–2018)

Contents

Illustrations

Preface

The inspiration for this book was first instilled in 2005 and then reinforced in 2020. Each adverse event had a direct impact, both personally and professionally. The first, Hurricane Katrina, came roaring through New Orleans and the Gulf Coast region of the US in August 2005. To this day, this flood and wind event remains the costliest disaster in American history. My wife and our then-14-year-old daughter and 17-year-old son fled on the morning of August 28 to Houston with nothing more than the possessions we could hurriedly jam into our SUV. We left the family pets (two cockatiels, both of which somehow survived) in a bathtub, hoping the warning was a false alarm—not unlike what had occurred one year earlier, when we also evacuated the city. That dress rehearsal escape to Houston had alerted us to what could and later would happen. In 2005, a normally five-hour car trip to Houston took twelve hours that Sunday. In our Houston hotel room in the middle of night, we heard CNN's first report that New Orleans's federal levee system was falling apart. Floodwaters were rising across the city. Eighty percent of the city flooded, and our house was among the tens of thousands that were impacted. It would be three months before we slept again in our own beds.

Three days later we evacuated farther on—to Austin, Texas—again following the script from a year earlier. We lived in Austin in a rented house, having enrolled the kids at St. Stephen's Episcopal School. Meanwhile, I continued consulting with the State of Louisiana's Department of Health, while also struggling to reconnect with my academic colleagues at Tulane University, who suddenly and haphazardly had been scattered across the country like wayward leaves.

I became angered by the nearly nonexistent first-response abilities of the federal government in the disaster's aftermath. The silence was deafening in those initial days and weeks, while the need for emergency health care and housing support became acute. The miserable first-response showing by the Federal Emergency Management Agency, in particular, was maddening. Where were the architects? This would compel me to actively advocate thereafter for a new way of teaching architecture, emphasizing the importance of rapid-response architecture in the face of the planet's changing climate.

Returning to New Orleans full time in December 2005, I began to repair our damaged home, a process made all the more daunting by the paucity of reputable local contractors, increasing crime rates, governmental incompetence at all levels, and insurance company intransigence. Katrina inspired me to write the first book-length architectural examination of the possibilities of rapid-response architecture, *Innovations in Transportable Healthcare Architecture* (2016).

The second disaster event was the widespread upheaval caused by the coronavirus pandemic, which began in 2020. I had been granted a sabbatical from the University of Toronto for the first half of 2020. Kate Schwennsen, the head of the Clemson School of Architecture (where I had taught for six-and-a-half years before relocating to Toronto), offered me a residency at the university's magnificent Charles E. Daniel Center for Building Research and Urban Studies (known as "The Villa") in Genoa, Italy—a residency that would be abruptly halted six weeks in by the burgeoning public health crisis. This crisis was declared a global pandemic by the World Health Organization on March 11, 2020. The H1N1 pandemic originated in Wuhan, China, in late 2019, although the first major outbreak in Europe occurred in northern Italy, near Genoa, in early January 2020. With the world's attention now transfixed on this part of Italy, those of us at The Villa—Director Silvia Siboldi Carroll, support and teaching staff, and the twenty-four Clemson undergraduate architecture students who were in residency—carefully monitored the unfolding disaster in our midst. In the following days, lockdown travel restrictions were imposed across the European continent, and The Villa was closed down.

Everyone in residence was instructed to evacuate The Villa and leave Italy as soon as possible. Securing air flights and train reservations became an ordeal. Meanwhile, the parents of the students studying in Genoa were frantic, because everyone knew that the European epicenter was a little more than one hundred miles away. My partner, Pattie Willis, and I had just returned from a trip to Rome and Sicily the week before. Romans were getting restless, but the city was still functional. When we arrived in Sicily, the Italian prime minister issued televised travel warnings and encouraged everyone to wear an N95 mask for protection. Flying from Catania, in Sicily, back to Rome, the mood was completely different. Business establishments were shutting down everywhere, including in the Trastevere neighborhood, our base there. The stress was palpable as a quiet panic ensued. During those harried weeks, the basic thesis of this book was formulated.

In both the 2005 hurricane disaster and the COVID-19 pandemic, I was struck by how little effort was made to address the health needs of the poor and the medically underserved. With Katrina, the poor tended to reside in the lowest lying and, hence, most devastated neighborhoods. The city's entire health care infrastructure—hospitals, clinics, long-term care facilities, and home health services—was either severely damaged or destroyed. In the case of the pandemic, the poor and the medically underserved also tended to reside in health care deserts, with few public health resources—such as COVID-19 testing and treatment centers—that would have helped assuage the disease's transmission. Although both disasters were quite different in their scope and impact, the mitigation-related contributions of architects in each instance were inadequate at a time when the public health–assistance impulse among architects and architectural firms could clearly have been much more immediate and far more robust.

Chapter 1 therefore establishes the book's central thesis. Its three elements are (1) the climate crisis and its widespread impacts, now being experienced worldwide; (2) persistent health inequalities, which separate the haves from the have-nots and often lead to life-and-death outcomes; and (3) the supporting role of the built environment—specifically, architecture—which can either perpetuate or mitigate human health and wellness inequalities. When viewed as overlapping spheres, examining in-between covariances becomes important, which is what this book attempts to do. Throughout the pandemic, public health was placed in a glaring and often unfavorable spotlight, along with the supportive (or nonsupportive) role of the built environment. Successes, and dramatic failures, occurred in both spheres.

Chapter 2 briefly examines the historical role of architects (or its absence) in times of epidemics, focusing on five major epochs in the relationship between architecture and health. In each instance, I concentrate on the degree of functional support provided by the built environment, the role of public policymakers as responsive (or unresponsive) orchestrators of reactions to these crises, and the function of architecture as an intervention in controlling the spread of plagues and pandemics.

The coronavirus pandemic of 2020–2024 is the entire focus of chapter 3. It examines the role and efficacy of rapid-response architecture through unbuilt proposals, as well as the built work of architects in their attempts to address the urgent need for portable and fixed-site ambulatory testing facilities, laboratories, and inpatient quarantine treatment centers. I draw examples from numerous countries, culminating in the World Health Organization's Technical Science for Health Network's (Techne) INITIATE2 infectious disease treatment hospital prototype. I then comparatively assess these examples with respect to their salutogenic and biophilic design principles, as well as to public health and medical performance standards. The view here is that functional, health-equitable requirements are achievable, along with policies and resultant designs that also prioritize aesthetic, experiential, or psychological concerns.

Chapter 4 explores a reinterpretation and expansion of a historically rooted design strategy that I refer to as *theraserialization*—a strategic design concept applied here to health care architecture on an imperiled planet. This construct and its associated design strategies call for the dematerialization, or dismantling, of the physical barriers, actual walls, and limited visual connectivity that physically and perceptually isolate the interior from the exterior realm in hospitals and other building types devoted to the provision of health care. It is about visual transparency, openness, and a drawing together of the therapeutic affordances of nature and landscapes into the physical built environment. To a certain extent, this uses treatment principles dating from the ancient Greeks, later reprised in the tuberculosis sanitoriums of the late nineteenth and early twentieth centuries. The network of twenty-six contemporary Maggie's Centres is a tutorial of sorts in theraserialization and a new, health equity–inspired building type—the *nature immersion center*.

Equitable residential environments for medically underserved older persons are the focus of chapter 5. Globally, these individuals will be threatened more than ever before by health inequities, due to their residing in health care deserts—substandard living conditions that result in further health inequalities. I examine the plight of three particularly susceptible cohorts—unsheltered older persons; older persons with mental health disorders; and older persons with cognitive deficits, who are highly likely to fall into the first two categories—in light of the managed retreat initiatives that will be necessary in the coming years in the face of rising seas, drought, and wildfires, among other disasters. Fifty architecturally based planning and design considerations for long-term care built environments, institutional settings, and community-based settings are presented in an accompanying appendix. Particular attention is paid to the urgency of establishing essential, equitable, public health policies and architectural supports in response to the accelerating climate crisis.

Chapter 6 focuses on the specialized field of health care architecture and its relationship to public health. I reappraise sustainable and resilient design strategies through the philosophical lens of posthumanist social, cultural, and ecological concerns. *Posthumanism*—consideration of intersecting human, nonhuman, and technological worlds—is discussed as a means of moving beyond the splintering relationship between the humanities and what comes after them, known as the posthumanities. This expanding ideological movement is interdisciplinary in scope, with important contributions currently coming from the fields of geography, philosophy, the social sciences, gerontology, engineering, computer science, the fine arts, and (only very recently) the planning and design professions. Architecture has been strikingly slow to acknowledge the existence of this movement, with the specialized field of *architecture for health* still virtually tone deaf to its full ramifications and possibilities.

Chapter 7 examines some threads impacting the future of architecture for health, extending to 2050 and beyond. Eight themes are presented, each illustrated with examples. These themes are interdependent and are by no means meant to be constructed as all-inclusive or in any way finite. Prognosticating the future with respect to ecology and its ramifications for the built environment has been the subject of some excellent recent books, especially those focused on the climate crisis, including Jeff Goodell's *The Water Will Come: Rising Seas, Sinking Cities, and the Remaking of the Civilized World* (2017); David Wallace-Wells's *The Uninhabitable Earth: Life after Warming* (2019); and James Howard Kunstler's *Living in the Long Emergency: Global Crisis, the Failure of the Futurists, and the Early Adapters Who Are Showing Us the Way Forward* (2020 edition). The threads I examine include the reality that it makes little sense for university-based programs in urban and regional planning—in particular, architecture and landscape architecture—to fiddle with what *has been* while the world's needs change.

Built environment–induced health disparities are currently deepening across populations and locales, thereby amplifying human pain, suffering, geographic dislocation, and environmental degradation. The World Health Organization (WHO) defines *health inequities* as "systematic differences in health outcomes. Health inequities are differences in health status or in the distribution of health resources between different population groups, arising from the social conditions in which people are born, grow, live, work and age."* WHO views such conditions as unwarranted. They are reducible through local mitigation efforts, fostered by partnerships between government, private philanthropy, and nongovernmental organizations (NGOs), all working in concert with the private sector. Recent NGO reports published by WHO, the Urban Institute, and *The Lancet* have addressed the need to better leverage the potential of built environments for health to reduce the prevalence of these inequities at all scales of intervention—especially among economically disadvantaged groups and communities.

This is not meant to be yet another book that sounds the alarm about global warming. The scientific evidence is already abundant. For disbelievers, the United Nations provides a straightforward assessment of this threat to everyday life. Its Intergovernmental Panel on Climate Change concludes that we are to expect at least 3.2°F of warming, or about three times as much as the planet has experienced since the beginning of the Industrial Age.[†] As the ice sheets melt, major coastal zones will be inundated (including thousands of hospitals and other types of health care facilities). Hundreds of major cities and their surrounding low-lying regions worldwide will flood—with many becoming permanently submerged. In the eyes of informed decision-makers and laypersons, the twenty-first century may very well be the century from hell unless we act now. Adverse events are occurring faster—and often unexpectedly. Because of this, the entire topic can easily become incomprehensible, and even overwhelming. Without innovative planning, design mitigation policies, and action strategies, including responsibly designed built environments for health, the United Nations concludes that by 2100, Earth will likely experience an additional 4.5°F of warming.

Interdependencies between public health, catastrophes, persistent health inequities, and the potential within therapeutic architectural and environmental designs have been understudied. An effective response requires mitigating the inequities that are so often deeply rooted in the built environment. Because of this, the most vulnerable members of society need to be a major focus for public health professionals, architects, and allied design and planning professionals. Therefore, in this book I more

---

* World Health Organization (2018). "Health inequities and their causes." World Health Organization, 22 February. https://www.who.int/news-room/facts-in-pictures/detail/health-inequities-and-their-causes.

† Intergovernmental Panel on Climate Change (2018). *Special Report: Global Warming of 1.5° C.* New York: Cambridge University Press. https://www.ipcc.ch/sr15.

closely examine two particular types of catastrophes for their direct impacts on the built environment: supercharged adverse weather/sea level–rise events, and supercharged adverse public health events. There is a real threat that poor, medically underserved populations will not be privy to the therapeutic benefits of health-centric architecture and landscape design. This is why past as well as present trends are examined here in relation to these types of design to advance the public's health.

Acknowledgments

I greatly appreciated the opportunity to be Clemson University School of Architecture's Scholar-in-Residence in Italy in the first half of 2020. Many thanks for my being able to be based at the university's study-in-residence facility in Genoa, Italy. I am also grateful to the John H. Daniels Faculty of Architecture, Landscape, and Design at the University of Toronto for a sabbatical that enabled me to devote the needed time and energy to this project. The research reported in chapter 5 and in its accompanying appendix is the result of generous financial support provided by the Ontario Association of Architects, together with Jacobs Ltd. of Canada.

The Centre for Design + Health Innovation, which I founded in 2018 at the University of Toronto, provided my overall home base throughout the evolution of this book. Many thanks to my team of dedicated graduate and undergraduate research assistants, who worked diligently from start to finish—especially Damian Kercz, Shivathmikha Suresh Kumar, Lucas Siemucha, Catherine Dela Cruz, Darya Mishchenko, Erin Tostevin, and Gal Volovsky Fridman. Many thanks also to the students in the fall 2020 Architecture + Health Graduate Design Option Studio at the University of Toronto for their energy and commitment to the urgent design problem I challenged them with at a trying moment in the COVID-19 pandemic. Many thanks to Wendy and Jim Barney for providing me with the opportunity to write chapter 4 in Whistler, British Columbia, in January 2023, as well as the opportunity to complete the final edits of the manuscript in Whistler in January 2024.

Many thanks to the architectural firms who granted permission to reproduce their drawings and photographic images. I am especially indebted to all the Maggie's Centres I visited while in the United Kingdom in spring 2023, including in Oxford, Manchester, and Oldham, England. At each Maggie's Centre, I was able to participate, observe firsthand, and interview dedicated staff members, volunteers, and a number of patient-clients who, collectively, make these places among the planet's most compassionate and progressive health care architectural environments.

I am grateful for the support of academic colleagues and students during this project—and, for that matter, throughout my entire research and scholarship activities during my years at Clemson University (2007–2013) and, before that, at Tulane University (1985–2007). Their encouragement and insights have helped me delve deeper into the themes and subthemes that eventually shaped the core narrative of this book.

Earlier versions of certain ideas were introduced in some of my prior books: *Healthcare Architecture in an Era of Radical Transformation* (2000), *Compassion in Architecture: Evidence-Based Design for Health* (2005), *Innovations in Hospital Architecture* (2010), *Innovations in Transportable Healthcare Architecture* (2016), and *Innovations in Behavioural Health Architecture* (2018).

Above all, I continue to be inspired by my two children, Alexander and Elyssa Leigh Verderber, and my supportive partner, Patricia Ann Willis. And, finally, the image on the title page of the book is the Cathedral to Junk, in Austin, Texas, built by Vince Hannemann. He began work on it in 1988, when he was in his twenties. This iconic DIY labor of love in the backyard of a house on a residential street stands as a monument to our culture's hyperconsumerism and premature material obsolescence, with their harmful environmental impacts on the planet. It is a symbol both of despair and of hope that we humans will change our destructive habits.

Stephen Verderber
Toronto, January 2025

Architecture and Health Equity
in an Imperiled World

Part I

Coping with Catastrophe—Past and Present

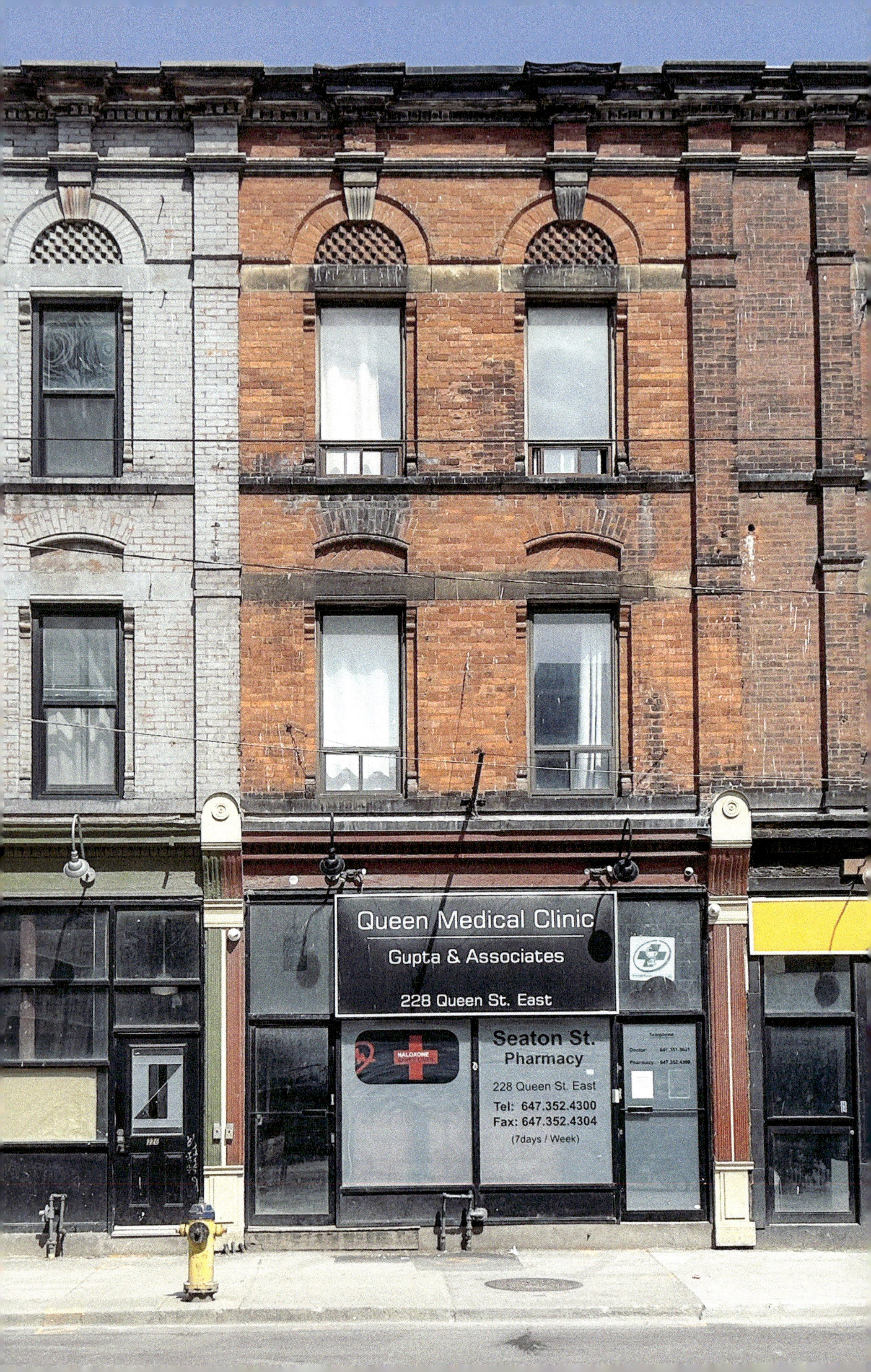

Queen Medical Clinic
Gupta & Associates
228 Queen St. East
Seaton St.
Pharmacy
228 Queen St. East
Tel: 647.352.4300
Fax: 647.352.4304
(7days / Week)
NALOXONE
Telephone
Doctor: 647.351.3621
Pharmacy: 647.352.4300

Introduction

The coronavirus pandemic of 2020–2024 recast public health and architecture in a new light. In the case of public health, for decades the tacit pact with society was if things were relatively under control and "quiet" on the public health front, then generally all was well. This assumption, however, was proved false. At the start of the twentieth century, the field of public health was more cohesive—and more ambitious—than its present bifurcated state. Then, a diverse coalition of physicians, scientists, industrialists, and social activists collectively viewed themselves as part of a larger social reform movement, one with the potential to be transformative. It was a coalition united by the goal of rectifying pervasive health inequities that continued to render certain populations especially susceptible to disease and death, due to unhealthful urban living conditions. In large part the coalition's efforts were devoted to rectifying the practice of haphazardly building cities and, more specifically, eradicating unsanitary housing and working conditions, rectifying the lack of green space for recreational activities, and remediating poor sanitation.[1] After decades of focused work, public health as a profession would succeed in lengthening average lifespans, controlling communicable diseases, and increasing health education. When COVID-19 reached North America, systemic disfunctionalities in this system were revealed. It was inadequate: understaffed agencies with meager budgets, due to funding reductions during the previous fifteen years; crumbling buildings;

Figure 1.1. Queen Street Medical Clinic, Toronto. Photo by Stephen Verderber.

and archaic equipment barely capable of coping with "normal" disease prevention interventions, let alone a fast-spreading, deadly respiratory virus.[2]

Had public health fallen victim to its relative success in controlling diseases up to then? Had its advancements in health promotion led to public complacency? Interestingly, throughout the twentieth century, the medical and public health professions had forged divergent paths, often advancing competing agendas, objectives, and methodologies. Medicine's triumphant scientific focus on the health of the individual—*personal health*—resulted too often in its marginalization of public health's broader interdisciplinary focus, which was *population health*. As public health professionals increasingly veered further from their earlier belief that social reforms were an absolutely essential part of disease prevention, it suppressed this stream of activity (fig. 1.1), and public health social advocates would move further away from medicine after the landmark discovery that infectious illnesses are caused by microbes, not adverse societal states. Germ theory offered a seductive new vision for redefining disease. As epidemiologists sought to identify the source of emerging infectious diseases, medically centric perspectives gradually became squarely focused on individual health versus everyday quality-of-life living conditions. The built environment was inadvertently sidelined as a potential cause of sickness and disease.[3] This paradigmatic shift dates from at least 1880 and provided public health with a license to be innovative in new ways.

Epidemiologists no longer felt compelled to deal with what, to them, were seemingly intractable Industrial Age expressions of age-old social problems, such as widespread urban poverty, inequity, racial segregation, and deeply rooted societal prejudices. They felt justified in freeing themselves from the role of social activists. It was now easier to focus on individual victims of disease and cure them, rather than concentrate on population health. Public health leaders in the early twentieth century went so far as to belittle their predecessors' efforts at social reforms, which they now viewed as inefficient, misguided, and archaic. Moreover, some leaders in the field dismissed the impressive achievements of the urban sanitarian movement in combating transmissible diseases, even though this movement had succeeded in fostering the construction of large-scale urban water systems in the late nineteenth and early twentieth centuries in hundreds of cities in North America cities and elsewhere in the world. The profession of public health migrated into laboratories at this point, as academically based researchers came to dominate what previously was a broader, more socially focused, multifaceted field.[4]

This new generation of epidemiologists defined public health in narrower and deliberately more scientific terms. Meanwhile, hospitals had become entrenched as the hub of the North American health care system, with biomedical investigation as its core research component, which became solidified after World War II. By the early 1950s, the social advocacy movement in public health was nearly completely extinguished. Empiricism, data collection, clinical diagnostic services, and disease tracing defining the field as it pulled away from its former allies in social and political arenas. In time this suppressed the field's visibility in the public's consciousness. Its sublimated position left it to continue onward in medicine's shadow, although with a diminished political power base. In most developed countries, one unfortunate outcome of this trend in recent decades has been poor health outcomes. The causes of pervasive health inequities came to be viewed mainly as a matter of personal health responsibility, rather than the collective responsibility of society.

By the end of the twentieth century, epidemiology in the US and many other parts of the world was nearly entirely detached from public health's grassroots social advocacy traditions. For example, rather than condemn the underlying social and cultural causes of drought and famine in Somalia, the focus now was to produce statistically driven reports, sponsored by the World Health Organization and the United Nations, on the number of people starving and dying, instead of on root societal determinants. Some signs of change were in the air, however. In the 1980s, the grassroots movement to eradicate HIV-AIDS had been fueled by social activists, and by 2000, a growing number of public health leaders were calling for a broad reappraisal of the entire field. This resulted in a new generation of social epidemiologists once again focused on the root social and cultural causes of health inequity—specifically, on the influences of systemic racism, poverty, and environmentally based determinants. In 2003, a landmark special issue of the *American Journal of Public Health* was devoted for the first time to the theme of "Health and the Built Environment," marking the profession's reawakened concern for broader consideration of expanded myriad potential causes of adverse health outcomes, as opposed to focusing almost solely on medical causes per se.[5] For architects and other environmental designers, would this signal reawaken social advocacy traditions of a century earlier? That publication coincided with renewed attention to the importance of urban design on individual and community health, and especially on the adverse consequences of suburban sprawl in relation to the troubling rise in chronic diseases, including type 2 diabetes, obesity, and heart disease. Would COVID-19 rejoin the on-again, off-again clinical and social advocacy traditions within public health? The medical science community, for its part, was continuing to straddle an unfortunate yet seemingly never-ending tug of war between politics (individualism must prevail above all else) and scientific reasoning (facts must prevail above all else).

In reality, the built environment played a major role in the pandemic, since social isolation was virtually impossible during lockdown if one had a front line job without paid sick leave, lived in overcrowded conditions, or had to use public transit. In this regard, the pandemic brought to light how hard it is for scientific inquiry and social imperatives to coexist in a climate where science implies objective reasoning and advocacy implies subjective reasoning, which is so susceptible to politicization. Precisely because of this, these streams of inquiry in medicine and public health should be of great interest to architects and allied professionals who seek health-promoting solutions through the planning and design of the built environment. This interest assumes, perhaps erroneously, that the underlying meaning of any profession whose members are licensed to practice by society should, across time, have evolved its own set of theoretical tenets and scientific discourses. These largely determine its relevance to society. In the case of architecture, its legal and jurisdictional mandates are to protect the public's *health*, *safety*, and *welfare*. To paraphrase, in the case of architecture, its societal charge includes a mandate to mitigate health inequities by addressing the needs of citizens exposed to unhealthful, physically unsafe built environments, including conditions pertaining to the unfolding climate crisis.

In the US, Canada, and many other federal jurisdictions, states and provinces are granted legal authority to self-govern registered architects. This agency and oversight embraces regulating its members' behaviors and activities related to the professional practice of architecture—that is, in protecting the public's health, safety, and welfare. The three intersecting elements in this relationship capture the codependences between health inequity, the health-promoting potential of environmental design, and the global climate crisis. These codependences and the overlapping space in between these spheres—human health and well-being, the quality of the built environment, and ecological health—constitute the primary focus and core thesis of this book (fig. 1.2).

Health equity is broadly seen as the ability of individuals and groups to possess a fair opportunity to reach their fullest health potential. This requires success in reducing threats to health. Causes of health inequities are by

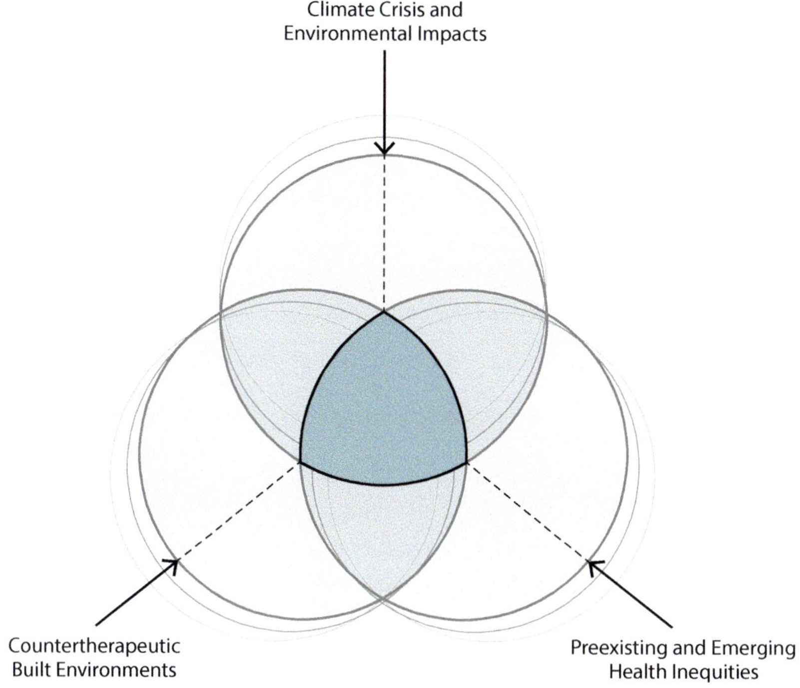

Figure 1.2. Triad of principal imperatives. Diagram by Stephen Verderber and Lucas Siemucha.

no means limited to income level, social status, race, gender, education, ageism, and attributes of the physical environment.[6] The term health equity itself is frequently used interchangeably with the term *health disparity*, the latter defined as the documentable differences in the quality of health and health care access across multiple populations. Inequality in this regard implies the occurrence of some form of social injustice, such as the "Cancer Alley" corridor of petrochemical industries and their adverse impacts on poor minority communities in South Louisiana, which the environmental justice movement and its underpinnings is attempting to remediate. The term *health inequity* is defined, for purposes of this discussion, as arising from unequal access to the social, economic, and racial justice determinants of health. This outcome may be caused by or result in less access to wealth and political influence for those individuals and communities consistently being deprived of opportunities to reach a state of relative healthfulness. Their worse health outcomes have been empirically linked to economic inequality. The prevailing consensus among environmental health experts is that the attainment of any reasonable level of health equity requires the judicious allocation of fiscal resources, improved *physical access to these resources*, and their equitable geographic distribution in direct proportion to unmet individual and community health needs.[7]

What is the difference between health equity and mere health equality? In the context of urban planning, architecture, and landscape architecture, it is about possessing more than mere equitable access to resources to improve health status. There is growing interest at this time in identifying health inequalities with respect to the role of the *quality of place* in neighborhoods and workplaces. This includes the sites where one socializes, worships, and obtains respite through engagements with nature and other forms of recreational activity at the local level and beyond. The term *place effects* refers to the health effects of variables that reveal the inner profundities of these places, not simply what they mean to the people who inhabit them. The two main types are collective and contextual place effects. A *collective effect* refers to aggregated group properties that exert an influence on health, over and above individual characteristics—for example, living in areas (and buildings) with a high proportion of people who possess common individual characteristics, such as age, social class, income, and race. A *contextual effect*, by contrast, refers to broader political, cultural, or institutional contexts (beyond buildings)—for example, the presence or absence of features intrinsic to places, such as infrastructural resources, economic policies at various levels of government, and existing social and public assistance programs. Place effects therefore consist of three steps, in ascending order of complexity. These involve not simply who you are in relation to where you are, but, rather, who you are depends on *where* you are.[8]

Putting any discussion of *design excellence* aside for the moment, the fact remains that professional architects design only 2–5 percent of all buildings constructed annually in North America.[9] Meanwhile, the United Nations expects the number of medically underserved persons worldwide to reach 2 billion by 2050, in a world with 9.7 billion persons.[10] A major tenet of the International Style of modern architecture, beginning with the social housing movement of the 1920s, was to use architecture as a tool to alleviate social inequities. This was a major focus of LeCorbusier and his contemporaries.[11] Ever since the counterculture movement in the 1960s, the public interest area of activity in architecture has endeavored to address unmet societal needs, mainly by continuing the tradition of affordable housing. Public interest architecture parallels and at times crosses over into the social advocacy stream of research and professional activity in public health. Unfortunately, with respect to affordable housing and related health concerns, too few professional architects in developed countries opt to stand in the eye of this storm. Yet only when someone steps away from the storm's eye do they realize its potential transformational power. In too many places, inadequate health care infrastructure, nonexistent or unaffordable housing, widespread health inequities, and life-threatening ecological dislocations continue. Fortunately, more architects are no longer remaining on the sidelines. They are beginning to react to the climate crisis. But, capitalism being what it is, most architects still work mainly for wealthy individuals, corporations, institutions, and governmental agencies who can afford to pay full professional fees and receive, in exchange, highly tailored professional services.

THE ANTHROPOCENE AND HEALTH INEQUALITY

The term *Anthropocene* was coined in 2000 by Paul J. Crutzen, an atmospheric chemist and Nobel laureate, as a means of communicating the transition from the relatively stable world of the Holocene to one in which humanity is now drawing the earth into a new, unstable, unsustainable state. This term, and what it denotes, immediately resonated and has since acquired broad, diverse interpretations across the sciences, humanities, and arts. Moreover, it is now being adopted by popular mass media. Its significance as a new, singular period in the earth's history (as geologically defined) was intimated by Crutzen and his colleagues, but without consideration of the complex technical and formal dimensions that typically surround newly proposed units of the geological time scale (GTS). At the International Geological Congress in 2016, the term Anthropocene was declared stratigraphically real and worthy of being defined at the epochal level. Research is currently underway to formally add the Anthropocene within the GTS, using protocols applied in the past to other GTS time units, such as the Pleistocene, Jurassic, and so on.[12]

Nature degradation is a primary theme throughout much of the recent ecocritical literature associated with the Anthropocene. This literature tends to focus on a form of environmentalism centered on independent narratives that are distinct from traditional, or mainstream, literary criticism narratives. It applies modes of ecocritical scholarship to literary criticism not commonly explored in this context and includes New Historicism, postcolonialism, deconstructionism, and feminist and Marxist theories—all being utilized to evaluate and acquire new insights into environmentalism as a movement in the twenty-first century. The work of writers —including Percy Bysshe Shelley, Upton Sinclair, Leslie Marmon Silko, and Susan Howe—has been reappraised through this ecocritical lens.[13] Buildings, places, cities, and natural landscapes are being widely reconceptualized as part of a single, complex, and often highly contradictory continuum of events and their associated impacts. Written works are similarly being contested, such as those by John Muir and Jane Addams; Aldo Leopold and William Faulkner; Robinson Jeffers and Theodore Dreiser; and Wendell Berry and Gwendolyn Brooks. In focusing on nineteenth- and twentieth-century writers, a main aim of this reassessment process is to establish a continuum within literature, centered on humans' timeless, interdependent relationship with the physical environment.[14]

Writers who extolled the virtues of nature and landscapes in the nineteenth and twentieth centuries are being reappraised.[15] These include Henry D. Thoreau, the father of American nature writing; John Burroughs, a schoolteacher and failed businessman who found his calling as a writer and elevated the nature essay to a beloved, respected literary form; and John Muir, founder of the Sierra Club, who celebrated the wilderness experience of the far western US as few before him had. These and other observers were making commentaries in an effort to extend society's moral responsibility to include due consideration of the well-being of all animals and plants. Rachel Carson, a scientist who raised the consciousness of the nation by revealing the catastrophic effects of human interventions on the earth's living systems, would publish *Silent Spring* in 1962. Edward Abbey, an outspoken environmental activist, charted the boundaries of ecological responsibility and sought to push them to political extremes. The question being collectively asked is, Will our descendants have the opportunity to experience forest and savanna landscapes, and will they to be able to experience the fullness of life immersed with thousands of interwoven and interdependent living species and inanimate things and places?[16] Then there is the larger question, Is the decline of the human species our greatest current threat, or is it the extinction of the planet itself? Themes of mass species extinction and the climate crisis are at the center of many recent films, including *Avatar 1* (2009) and *Avatar 2* (2022), as well as in the work of posthumanists. The latter represent an interdisciplinary movement consisting of theorists and practitioners who see the human species as the main source of our problem, as well as the potential means of turning around the earth's current period of rapid decline and its associated adverse impacts on human health and health equity.[17]

Edward Burtynsky, the renowned landscape photographer, writes:

> Our planet has borne witness to five great extinction events, and these have been prompted by a variety of causes: a colossal meteoric impact, massive volcanic eruptions, and oceanic cyanobacteria activity that generated a deadly toxicity in the atmosphere. These were the naturally occurring phenomena governing life's ebb and flow. Now it is becoming clear that humankind, with its population explosion, industry, and technology, has in a very short period of time also become an agent of immense global change. Arguably, we are on the cusp of becoming (if not already) the perpetrators of a sixth major extinction event, affected by a magnitude of forces as powerful as any naturally occurring global catastrophe, one caused solely by the activity of a single species: us. . . . Between 1900 and 2000, the increase in world population was three times greater than during the entire previous history of humankind—a quadruple increase from 1.5 to 6.1 billion people in just one hundred years . . . with (proportionally) countless more living in abject poverty and helplessness than those few with seemingly unassailable comfort, wealth, and power.[18]

The Anthropocene's physical record consists of myriad indelible human-caused intrusions made on the planet. Burtynsky was a pioneer in the visual documentation of these highly disturbing yet aesthetically breathtaking views from the air of the immense damage being inflicted. Beginning with his earliest photographs in the 1980s, he has concentrated on strip mining, oil refineries, suburban sprawl, and hyperurbanism, among other landscape-loss themes. His and his colleagues' visual documentary work is drawing much-needed attention to the widespread deleterious impacts being imposed on the planet. The use of photography to convey the scale of this environmental destruction has functioned to make it more vivid and purposeful by focusing on the act of revelation.

The global health care industrial complex contributes significantly to these adverse impacts. It is an energy- and resource-intensive sector within society, as well as a producer of large volumes of solid and liquid wastes and air pollutants. The health care industrial complex has a profoundly large ecological footprint, yet at the same time—paradoxically—it has an ethical duty to cause no harm.[19] Because of this, it should stand apart as a leader in the transition to a healthier future on planet Earth. In terms of the planning, design, and construction of the built environment, the concept of a "green" health care system has only emerged in the past two decades, led by global advocacy organizations, including Healthcare Without Harm, the Worldwide Fund for Nature, Greenpeace, Ocean Conservancy, and the Living Planet Index. The focus of these organizations has been five-fold: (1) energy conservation; (2) pollution prevention; (3) resource and species conservation and solid waste reduction; (4) improved indoor air quality and patient safety, and (5) environmentally responsible facility design and management.

The specialized area within the North American profession of architecture known as *architecture for health* awoke two decades ago to the gravity of this looming crisis. "Sustainable health care" architecture and "net-zero architecture" has been its near-singular focus, however, versus any more-thorough examination of deeper contributing forces. As things now stand, the former will not be enough. A lack of research on the shortcomings of the very popular certification program known as Leadership through Energy Efficient Environmental Design, or LEED, run by the US Green Building Council, is glaring. Built environments for health in the Anthropocene deserve and will require far more research on the human impacts of what is designed and constructed, given that buildings account for nearly 40 percent of all carbon emissions, with the production of concrete alone accounting for 8 percent annually.[20] The quest for a "sustainable" or "resilient" architecture for health with respect to hospitals and allied building types alone is important, but it ultimately is an insufficient response in the climate crisis in the face of rampant deforestation, expanding periods of drought, the depletion of fresh water, flash flood events, increasingly massive wildfires, species die-offs, sea level rises, and continued urban overdevelopment.[21]

In the Anthropocene, the die-off of animal species is but one prominent example of human thoughtlessness. From great white sharks to Bengal tigers, top predators are sleek, fast, and surgically precise in their actions. They are consummate specialists, drawing exactly what they need from the environment while maintaining an ecological balance in the process. Enter humans, who grasp at anything and everything within reach if it can be monetized. A recently published study of humans as global predators has revealed some hard numbers, divulging a rapacity that staggers the imagination.[22] Humans collectively prey on about 15,000 wild vertebrate species, or roughly one-third of all species on the planet. Domestic livestock were not included in the study, although the pet trade alone accounts for more than half all hunted species on land. Whether those in such categories are eaten or not, all uses lead to the same result—removing these species and their genetic diversity from their longstanding ecosystems. Overall, 40 percent of the 47,000 species included in this study were classified as endangered, further underscoring the unsustainability of human over-harvests of wildlife. This undermines supposed globally agreed-to species conservation goals.[23] The increasingly well-documented record of human destructiveness portends an unwelcome future for all living creatures. This is among the greatest challenges we face in the twenty-first century. How do we live together in a socially just, harmonious, ecologically sustainable way? Wealthy nations, as well as those that aspire to this standard of living, will have to establish conservation and restoration policies if any meaning-ful degree of true ecological and human health, or *eco-humanist equity*, is to be achieved. This means we will all have to adapt our ways of life to the new normal by consuming less, wasting less, and doing much less harm to the earth, because the adverse environmental feedbacks occurring now are already directly exacerbating the system's ability to address the unmet health care needs of society.[24]

BLACK SWANS AND CASCADING CALAMITIES

In 2020, humanity was confronted with four crises at once—medical, eco-nomic, social, and climate-related—causing far-reaching public health, financial, and geopolitical reverberations. In times of uncertainty, individ-uals and communities suffering from health inequities are least equipped to effectively cope. When a coastal community is faced with a rising sea level, those intrinsic predilections that draw us toward nature can quickly morph into fear and uncertainty, causing information overload and people turning off their reaction to the stressor.[25] In the pandemic, places that once were accessible suddenly were inaccessible, due to lockdowns. When previously interesting places to visit—such as vibrant urban cen-ters or, conversely, tranquil beaches and shorelines—become sources of environmental stress, it is a warning sign.[26] In describing the double hit of the COVID-19 pandemic and the economic downturn that almost immedi-ately occurred with it, the term *Black Swans* was being used describe the calamitous situation many municipalities faced. Such events possess the power to change the course of a society. In defining a Black Swan event, Nassim Nicholas Taleb writes:

> First, it [a Black Swan] is an *outlier*, as it lies outside the realm of regular
> expectations because nothing in the past can convincingly point to its
> possibility. Second, it carries an extreme impact. Third, in spite of its out-
> lier status, human nature makes us concoct explanations for its occur-
> rence *after* the fact . . . a rarity [that is] retrospectively predictable. Black
> Swans explain almost everything in our world, from the success of ideas
> and religions, to the dynamics of historical events, to elements of our
> own personal lives . . . but we tend to act as if they do not exist! . . . Ask
> a portfolio manager for a definition of "risk" and you will often be given
> assurances that *exclude* any real possibility of a Black Swan.[27]

Black Swan logic, however, considers what we don't know as being far more relevant than what we do know. Taleb describes the underappreci-ated behind-the-scenes sectors in society, whose efforts to help mitigate or guide the course of a disaster remain unnoticed before a Black Swan event, such as what transpired on 9/11 in New York City in 2001. These disaster preparedness and mitigation specialists are not seen as heroes, because widespread media outlets are directed to the first responders. Normative reality becomes irrelevant as rare but suddenly consequential shocks and jumps that occur rapidly seize our collective attention. Statistically speak-ing, the bell curve of normativity ignores these large, sudden deviations, as it cannot handle them, yet the laws of statistical probability make us blindly confident that we are somehow capable of taming environmental and public health uncertainties. Two twenty-first-century catastrophes—Hurricane Katrina (2005) and the coronavirus pandemic (2020–2024)—were both Black Swan events. Katrina was portrayed as a rare, unexpected environmental weather disaster, resulting in more than 1,800 deaths. To most, the pandemic was also seen as a rare and unexpected public health crisis. The widely held view was that both events were incomprehensibly unexpected, relative to their scope and actual destructive impact, when reassessed after the fact.

Both were transformative. In 2005's Katrina episode, the US Army Corps of Engineers' hurricane protection system was proved, in retrospect, to be highly faulty, as it failed in twenty-three locations in New Orleans. It was a system in name only and, long after the fact, was reinforced and rebuilt at a federal taxpayer cost of $14.5 billion (USD). In spring 2020, New Orleans was once again impacted by cascading catastrophes while con-currently caught in the deadly COVID-19 pandemic. An unusually massive rainfall event resulted in widespread urban flooding—a public health emergency exacerbated by a climate crisis emergency.[28] For both Katrina and the pandemic, critics and media pundits opined on how society had been caught off guard—unaware, unprepared, and unable to immediately switch to a Plan B to maintain the status quo.[29] In response, landscape architects and other architects have generated climate-resiliency schemes featuring bioswales, rain gardens, retention ponds, earth berms, levees, seawall barriers, and even oyster beds—all presented in reports to public officials for review and implementation. Such mitigation strategies are useful, but they come with a big *if* in terms of whether there will be enough money to build them.[30]

Meanwhile, by April 2020, four months into the COVID-19 pandemic, the level of recorded carbon dioxide emissions globally had fallen by 30–40 percent in many countries and cities. For the first time, this was visible, tangle proof of humans' ability to dramatically reduce greenhouse gas emissions. Between 1980 and 2018, major disasters in the US alone have cost more than $1 billion (USD), having risen from six per year to thirteen (i.e., mega-storms, massive floods, mega-wildfires). Federal disaster relief in the US is currently split between 17 agencies and 300 mandated compliance programs. The response to Superstorm Sandy in 2012 involved twelve states, dozens of cities, and hundreds of local utility companies, transportation agencies, and governmental offices, with each responsible for capturing its due slice of the fiscal disaster relief pie. The pandemic further underscored a failed labyrinth of uncoordinated federal disaster response efforts.[31]

Bureaucracies appear uniquely ill suited to cope with catastrophe, and a single Black Swan can sow chaos across all levels of government simultaneously. Despite years of warnings and countless consultants' reports, leaders at all levels of government continue to underappreciate the urgent need to fix their dysfunctional disaster preparedness systems. Of course, spending funds to prepare for a disaster that may or may not arrive lacks built-in political cachet, unlike tax cuts, a new road, or a new branch library, although such preparations are a direct investment the public cannot afford to avoid. Every dollar spent preparing for a catastrophe saves roughly $6 (USD) in relief aid.[32] Up to 80 percent of the damage caused by Hurricane Katrina could have been prevented with stricter, stronger, preemptive minimum construction standards in local and state building codes. Since wealthy nations are now also experiencing the dislocating effects of the crisis, it can no longer be dismissed as a geocentric phenomenon confined to developing countries. The floods that struck in Germany and Belgium in

2021, the mega-wildfires in the western part of the US and across Canada in 2023, and the intensifying hurricanes along the US Gulf and Atlantic coasts are finally attracting genuine, widespread attention in the popular media.[33]

A disaster event, Black Swan or otherwise, does not simply go on hiatus or become suspended in time, simply because a public health emergency is simultaneously occurring.[34] Many communities in the US with significant, unmet health care needs that experienced the adverse socioeconomic consequences of COVID-19 had been weighted down for generations by the inequitable brunt of fossil fuel pollution, or simply by being located near these toxic places. Unsurprisingly, African Americans compose the major percentage of those adversely impacted. If you are Black or Latino, and especially if you are poor, you are predisposed to these effects.[35] In terms of architecture and public health, outpatient clinics, community hospitals, specialized infection control hospitals, long-term care facilities, urban medical centers, mobile vehicular health care units, post-disaster transitional housing communities, and testing laboratories tend to not be located in places that allow direct access by the above-mentioned groups. With any infrastructural network being only as strong as its weakest link, medically underserved locales have traditionally been out of sight, out of mind.

COMPASSION AND BUILT ENVIRONMENTS FOR HEALTH

The built environment can be a source of physical and emotional stress, pain, fear, and even death. A well-known theory in the field of environmental psychology—*functionalist-evolutionary theory*—is premised on inherent, chronic uncertainty in the physical environments in which humans evolved across the millennia. In extreme situations, individuals and populations were (and continue to be) forced to cope with physical environmental uncertainty to survive. This shaped our acute multisensory faculties, including our visual depth perception and acute auditory and olfactory senses. We developed an ability to predict events and likely successful outcomes from them before they occurred. Today, these physical and predictive cognitive abilities bear directly on our health and well-being.[36] Our physical and cognitive competencies determine behavioral outcomes, including stability (or instability), equilibrium (or disequilibrium), and the degree of personal control (or lack of control) within a physical setting. The ability (or inability) to predict future likely outcomes is of paramount importance. *Behavioral reactivity* is the term often used to describe the type of human response to conditions posed by a given physical setting. In environmental psychology, coping with an uncertain or unpredictable situation is referred to as *cognitive restructuring*, a process that enables an individual to deal with a particularly pressing physical setting, such as learning to accept something for what it is, versus what it should or can be. In general, a physical setting may exert a low, moderate, or high degree of *environmental press*, a relationship most frequently represented as a single continuum from low to high. Correspondingly, an individual's personal competency and autonomy within that setting (also frequently represented as a continuum) is able to be assessed as low, moderate, or high. Any physical setting can be multidimensionally examined as such, including its meaning and aesthetics; patterns-of-use factors; maintenance and upkeep factors; and environmental comfort/discomfort factors, including temperature, air quality, infection control measures, and overall functionality.

The core premise of functionalist-evolutionary theory is that humans crave and strive to process useful environmental information, with the effective cognitive patterning of multisensory information allowing one to discern foreground from background; colors; inanimate and animate objects; and extreme environmental conditions, such as excessive heat threats and rising tides. Our homeostatic efforts to reduce physical and cognitive uncertainty are being challenged in the current climate crisis and will require ever-more-adroit abilities to take in and make sense of incoming stimuli. Humans process information for its legibility, coherence, complexity, and uniqueness, making a decision to obtain help in times of need. This has a direct bearing on our access to health care. Highly preferred buildings and places generally draw us toward them, without causing an undue threat of stress or harm. A closer examination of the triangulated space at the heart of the aforementioned triad of primary concern is illustrated in figure 1.2. This further reveals the essential role of compassion for other humans' well-being, as well as for the health of the ecological environment. Here, its broader expression—compassionism—concerns policymaking and subsequent planning in the design and management of built environments for health. Thus *compassionism* can be defined as efforts to eliminate chronic and emerging health inequities through the provision of therapeutic built environments and ecologically positive interventions to mitigate the adverse impacts of the climate crisis. These concerns are diagrammed in figure 1.3, where four quadrants are identified vis-à-vis biaxial continuums. The arc in the upper right quadrant expresses a highly propitious health outcome condition, where compassion exists for the medically underserved as a combined function of satisfactory access to health care resources in therapeutically and ecologically supportive physical settings. These constructs are defined as follows:

1. *Discompassion versus Compassion*: This low-to-high metric refers to the degree of compassion exhibited by health care provider organizations and the architects, interior designers, engineers, and planning professionals commissioned to design and construct human health-centric built environments that are also ecologically compassionate. This is fundamental in attaining health equality in the face of devastating diseases, epidemics, global wars, totalitarian rulers, famine, apartheid, genocide, and catastrophic natural disasters. Despite all these challenges, the human spirit prevails, and it is through acts of compassion that societies endure and advance. In discompassionate times, the opposite occurs when architecture functions as a direct physical manifestation of a society's normative values, helping to render us incapable of uplifting our health or nurturing our psyche. Its most brutal expressions include hellish prisons and the dehumanizing, architecturally discompassionate insane asylums built from the seventeenth through early twentieth centuries in North America and elsewhere.

2. *Individual versus Community*: This low-to-high metric measures the well-being of an individual versus the well-being of the community to which one belongs. Personal freedoms and personal autonomy are of utmost importance. The great mask-wearing debate during COVID-19 personified the classic public health conundrum of placing the well-being of all over the personal autonomy of the few. As for the built environment, hundreds of hastily arranged COVID-19 infection control infirmaries and quarantine housing facilities were quickly built worldwide, with architects and their governmental and philanthropic clients seeking to achieve some measure of both health equality and equity for the infected individual—plus, by extension, protecting the health of the broader community. Unfortunately, due to the failure of providers to make proper disaster preparedness plans, thousands of inhospitable, generally countertherapeutic facilities were set up ad hoc, such as in parking lots and sports facilities, with their users subjected to a dehumanizing psychological and physical experience.

3. *Low versus High Health Status*: This low-to-high metric centers on human health-equity outcomes and healthfulness. Low health status denotes discompassion and often manifests in a poor-quality architectural environment. Conversely, high health status denotes significant compassion, conveyed though architecturally humane and ecologically restorative health-centricity. Supportive care settings express the normative values of their creators and builders, where one client will value a high-quality architectural health care physical setting, whereas another will accept only the bare-bones minimum. In the latter case, the client may justify a lack of investment by instead putting additional resources into better staffing ratios and longer hours of operation, telling the architect, "We don't need a Taj Mahal." Often the outcomes of such tradeoffs are difficult to quantify, although they do have ripple effects. For instance, a well-designed examination room allows oft-needed supplies to be kept at hand, enabling the caregiver(s) to remain in the room without always needing to go down the corridor to retrieve supplies, thus interrupting the flow of care.

4. *Political Disempowerment versus Empowerment*: This fourth low-to-high metric addresses the function of health equity relative to political empowerment. Health inequality and political inequality go hand in hand, with the same applying to economic inequality. The presence of high-quality health education interventions—programs to inform individuals of their care and treatment options—in medically underserved communities is often viewed as an essential component. But having access to diagnosis and treatment is only one metric in assessing the political empowerment of health care recipients (and their caregivers, for that matter). Educate them on the attributes of ecologically restorative built environments for health care, provide the necessary number of such facilities, and locate them in the right places to make them as geographically accessible as possible. Medically underserved communities in health care deserts serve no one's interests, politically or otherwise, unless the aim is repression. For example, the deployment of portable vehicular clinics to underserved locales on a rotating basis is a public health policy that can aid tremendously in eradicating health care deserts—a strategy discussed further in chapter 3.

Disasters and catastrophes highlight how public health specialists and those who plan and design these built environments are susceptible, by default, to professional biases, possibly limiting the effectiveness of their responses. These include the following:

- The *availability bias trap*, which is a predilection to base critical decisions on information already readily available in our memory, rather than on new evidence-based knowledge.
- The *hindsight bias trap*, which causes humans to attach higher probabilities to events after they have occurred versus before they occur.
- The *inductive reasoning trap*, which leads humans to formulate general rules of ethical conduct and subsequent actions on the basis of insufficient information.
- The *fallacy of disjunctive behavior trap*, a condition that causes humans to overestimate the probability that a given disaster event will actually occur, while, at the same time, these professionals paradoxically tend to underestimate the probability of other disaster events occurring.
- The *confirmation bias trap*, which inclines humans to look for confirmation of one's initial hypothesis, rather than to search out countervailing evidence that may disprove its existence.
- The *contamination effect trap*, where irrelevant but proximate prior information is allowed to influence current decision-making.
- The *affect heuristic trap*, where preconceived value judgments are allowed to interfere with the assessment of cost/benefit tradeoffs.
- The *scope neglect trap*, which prevents humans from proportionately adjusting what should be sacrificed to mitigate adverse event outcomes of a higher order of magnitude.
- The *overconfidence in calibration trap*, which leads these professionals to underestimate the confidence intervals within which their estimates would be accurate, resulting in the conflation of "best case" outcome scenarios with most probable outcome scenarios.
- The *bystander apathy trap*, which inclines these professionals to abdicate their individual responsibility when confronted with group-think normative social behavior.[37]

Cognitive dissonance is an additional construct to help understand how public health specialists and those who plan and design the built environment rationalize and act regarding health emergencies. This term is generally defined as the psychological disconnect associated with a decision that does not correlate with the underlying evidence and often manifests in an expert saying one thing in public and something completely different in private.[38] How might our comprehension of disasters and catastrophes evolve beyond these rather unsophisticated interpretations of them, particularly when they go from being eminently anticipated, on the one hand (i.e., predicted), to being interpreted, on the other hand, as Black Swans (i.e., a huge surprise), and then to being misinterpreted as extraordinarily vast (i.e., incomprehensible) events in scope and magnitude? An inability to adroitly anticipate this interpretive shift from adverse event predictability to Black Swan–status events underscores a central dilemma and perhaps explains why widely predicted disaster occurrences are often treated as entirely *new* events by the mass media. The shift from a Black Swan to an incomprehensible event, however, is the difference between a disaster that kills a great many people at one locale and another that has much wider and deeper consequences geographically, such as an unexpectedly intense global heat wave.

Despite society's gradually increasing understanding and acceptance of catastrophes, such as the climate crisis and global pandemics, in reality most such events are localized and are relatively contained geographically. There is an intrinsic fractal structure embedded in a catastrophe, resulting in a high-rise apartment building's collapse being interpreted as a microcosm of a much larger potential disaster, such as the collapse of fifty high-rise apartment towers in a single city. Meanwhile, typical architects and their firms, capitalistic at their core, continue to focus on wealthy private clients and prominent taxpayer-funded governmental ones. In the climate crisis, will this emphasis in architecture pivot from mainly serving the rich and influential to including the poor and the medically underserved? Thankfully, through improved education, public health professionals and architects can be trained to anticipate, pinpoint, and address the scope and magnitude of future catastrophes and their local impacts. Neill Ferguson addresses this think globally, act locally conundrum:

> Even the largest earthquake is not felt all over the world. Even the
> biggest wars are not in fact fought in every country. The world wars
> were notable for their compression in terms of space as well as time
> . . . [while] most of the world's landmass experiences little to no fighting
> at all. What matters is, first, whether or not a disaster strikes a densely

populated part of the earth and, second, if the death and destruction in and around the epicenter has repercussions further afield. In the case of a large volcano, the smoke and ash emitted can spread far and wide, profoundly affecting the climate on other continents. In short, their most important feature is whether or not there is contagion—that is, some way of propagating the initial shock thorough ecologically based biological networks together with the social networks of humanity.[39]

Complexity is a term widely used by natural scientists and computer scientists to make sense of a wide range of dissimilar environmental feedback systems, including through artificial intelligence (AI), fractal geometry, and computer modeling of, for instance, the biological structure of a rainforest. This research seeks to identify analogs between natural ecological systems and artificial, or human-induced, ones. These complex systems are often nonlinear and capable of generating miniscule disruptions that are indiscernible or impossible to predict *a priori*, yet small inputs can induce phenomenally amplified, unanticipated outcomes or effects elsewhere. The history of catastrophe is this intersection between natural ecological and human-created complexities. The line can be exceptionally blurry when attempting to distinguish a naturally induced adverse event from a human-derived one.[40] Public health catastrophes, as they intersect with the history of cities and architecture, are therefore often about unforeseen and poorly managed disaster events. Each disaster event in recorded history has been complex and contradictory, with no two being alike—the confluence of a natural and a human-induced *network* of input-outcome failures. These inputs-outputs continue to prematurely restrict humans' disaster-preparedness thought processes and subsequent actions. To paraphrase Ferguson, in public health and corresponding architectural emergencies, such as COVID-19, practicable cause-effect *response networks* should ideally possess these six disaster-preparedness attributes:

1. A given network is not an isolated entity, and its elements are transferrable to other networks.
2. Networks that are similar in structure and content gravitate toward one another.
3. Even weak connections within and between networks can possess deep affordances and resonance.
4. A network's internal structural strength directly correlates with its value and applicability.

5. A network must be fully capable of acting predictably (and unpredictably) at all times.
6. Networks seek to mesh with other networks, propagating and reproducing to ensure their continued survival and relevancy.

Public health and architecture intersect with contagious disease mitigation in a fluid interplay, continually shifting between myriad network typologies (including pathogens from insect and animal carriers) and historically persistent health and social inequities embedded in buildings and the larger built environment. Unfortunately, network-based responses on the part of architects have often been feeble, disconnected from more comprehensive response networks operating in real time and space. The COVID-19 pandemic awoke architects and allied environmental planning and design professionals to the criticality of intermodal networking: a continuous process that, of necessity, must constantly tear down and conceptually redefine itself. Its aim is to eradicate these persistent, historically rooted social inequities, as well as new ones that are being created by the climate crisis. Each individual professional and professional organization has a responsibility to equitably serve *all members of society*—not just the powerful and the privileged.

Catastrophes, not unlike world wars and massive global financial crises, are history's great interrupters and intruders. Whether human-induced or naturally occurring, whether prophesized or striking like a bolt out of the blue, each event provides moments of opportunity, although positive results can only happen if this possibility for improved preparedness is, in fact, seized as an occasion for revelation, self-reflection, reassessment, and education. Unfortunately, a catastrophe such as a hurricane or severe drought divides its direct victims into three disparate groups: the prematurely dead; the lucky survivors; and the permanently transformed, having been wounded or traumatized in some specific manner. A catastrophe separates the fragile, the most vulnerable, from the more resilient. Human progress itself is the leading progenitor of transmissible diseases and pandemics. This has always been the case and will likely continue to be so. Cities and buildings function as transmitters during adverse events and facilitate unfortunate consequences for their inhabitants. In the Anthropocene, the built environment cries out for compassion, ecological planning, design excellence, and construction in a way that promotes health equity for all. Will the rainforests be destroyed in the name of so-called *human progress*? Will the atmosphere become so polluted with carbon emissions that our imperiled planet reaches the point of no return? The four baseline constructs presented here represent an attempt to capture key determinants of health inequality at the heart of the triad of primary concern represented in figure 1.2 and elaborated on in figure 1.3.[41]

This triad can be further extrapolated to inform a quasi-structural diagram of rapid-response, public health–focused architecture for health (fig. 1.4). Its three tiers represent contextual determinants, covariances, and outcome determinants. Baseline determinants along the bottom of the diagram consist of political, technological, access-to-care, and cultural factors affecting the tiers of this vertically oriented diagrammatic representation. Two diagonal vectors—one representing the importance of therapeutic, health-promoting built environments, and the other, the importance of maximizing individual and community health and well-being—have a potentially positive influence in reducing inequitable health outcomes. The lower tier addresses the importance of assessing overall purpose and functional appropriateness, the value of theory, the importance of place and context in the design response, and the need to identify key prior case study precedents that are of value in responding to the design task at hand.

These determinants of built form directly influence the upper tier, which represents the essential role of the design response and its resilience in the face of increasingly extreme pressures exerted on it by the climate crisis. Design excellence transcends mere sustainability, insofar as the building or place will consume a minimum amount of nonrenewable energy and, thus, contribute to broader ecological *restoration* (discussed at length in chapter 4). Therefore, answers to the challenge of cascading Black Swans must become a top priority. The responses of public health specialists and architects must do better than the thousands of gyms, warehouses, sports stadiums, parking lots, parks, convention centers, and military facilities that were randomly pressed into service worldwide, virtually overnight, as COVID-19 testing and infection control quarantine centers. Individuals and populations particularly susceptible to being short shrifted include:

- medically underserved victims of pandemics and other public health emergencies who lack access to appropriate diagnostic and treatment services, due to residing in health care deserts (chapters 2 and 3),
- medically underserved persons in need of physical and psychological restorative health care, accessed by reengaging with the timeless, therapeutic affordances inherent in nature and landscapes (chapter 4 and appendix A),

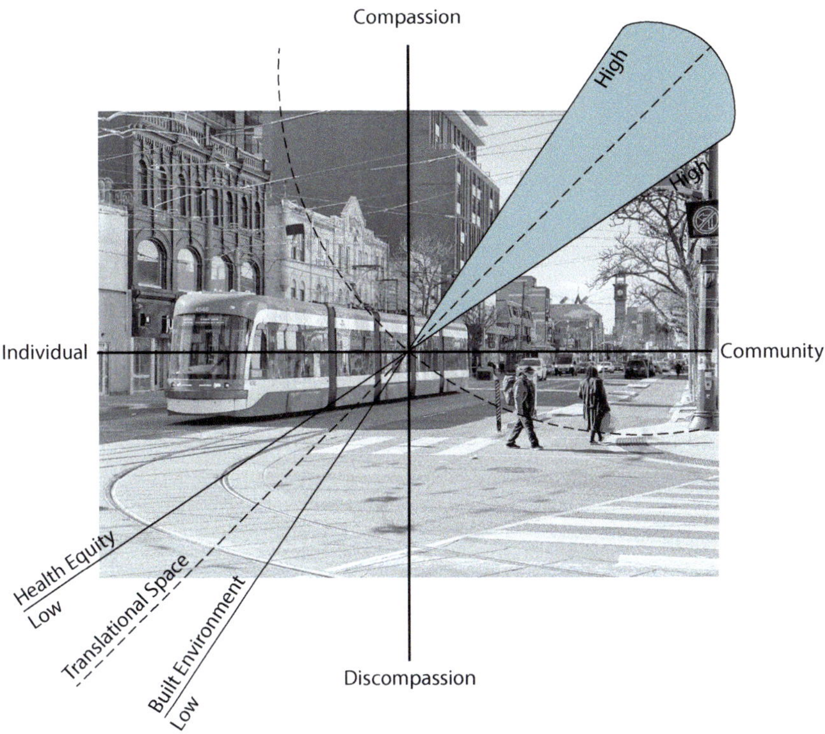

Figure 1.3. Dimensions of health equity in the built environment. Diagram by Stephen Verderber and Lucas Siemucha.

- medically underserved older persons at risk of being relegated to substandard housing in the climate crisis, due to age discrimination and society's general indifference to their health care needs or quality of life (chapter 5 and appendix B),
- the role of posthumanism as an alternative paradigm in the ongoing effort to ameliorate persistent health inequities in the built environment in the Anthropocene (chapter 6), and
- the role and function of future events and trends likely to determine the prospects of public health and its relationship to built environments for health promotion in the Anthropocene (chapter 7).

In the coming years, many endangered communities globally will need to move to safer locations. In the US, an entire Indigenous community in far southern Louisiana is in the process of being relocated to higher ground fifty miles north, in the first managed retreat initiative of its kind in the US, costing nearly $800 million (USD).[42] Recent visionary architectural proposals include floating buildings and even utopian schemes, transforming entire cities in China and elsewhere into literal sponges in response to rising seas.[43] With buildings now capable of floating above seawater, this and related innovative schemes are being announced on an almost weekly basis, such as an adapted three-level barge, currently the largest floating office building in the world, now moored in Rotterdam's harbor in The Netherlands. The client, the Global Center on Adaptation (GCA), is a nonprofit that advises countries, cities, and institutions on long-term mitigating architectural strategies in coastal zones and other waterfront communities. The GCA itself opted for its new headquarters to demonstrate the possibilities of proactive, climate-responsive architecture.[44]

In the Anthropocene, posthumanist perspectives and strategies will, of necessity, rise to the forefront in importance. *Anthropos* means "human," although by itself this word is meaningless. Anthropos does not merely imply humanism per se. The word Anthropocene prompts a reassessment of what it means to be human on this planet, because it is clear we cannot return to some fabled ideal of traditional humanism, with our species indisputably at the center of the universe. In June 2014, the *Oxford English Dictionary* added "Anthropocene," defining it as "the era of geological time during which human activity is considered to be the dominant influence on the environment, climate and ecology of the earth."[45] At the very least, public health, architecture, and allied planning and design disciplines deserve to be reexamined through the lens of an interdisciplinary posthumanism—with our species decoupled from the restrictions of egocentric Western biases. It just might offer a new moral equivalency, with full, ethical due consideration and respect for the agency and unspoken "voices" that emanate from all forms and varieties of living species, ecologies, and inanimate "things" in an imperiled world.

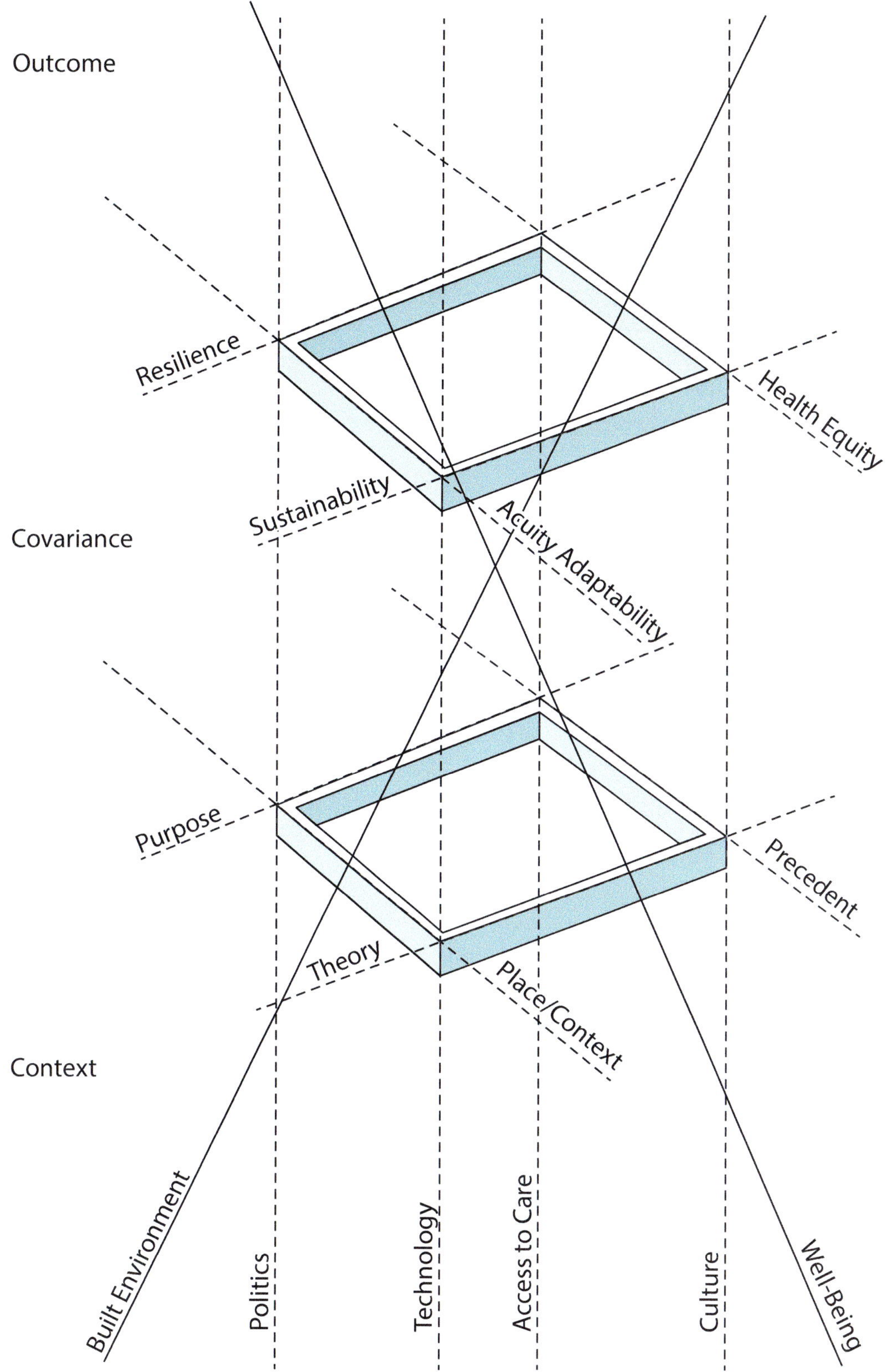

Figure 1.4. Determinants of well-being in the built environment. Diagram by Stephen Verderber and Lucas Siemucha.

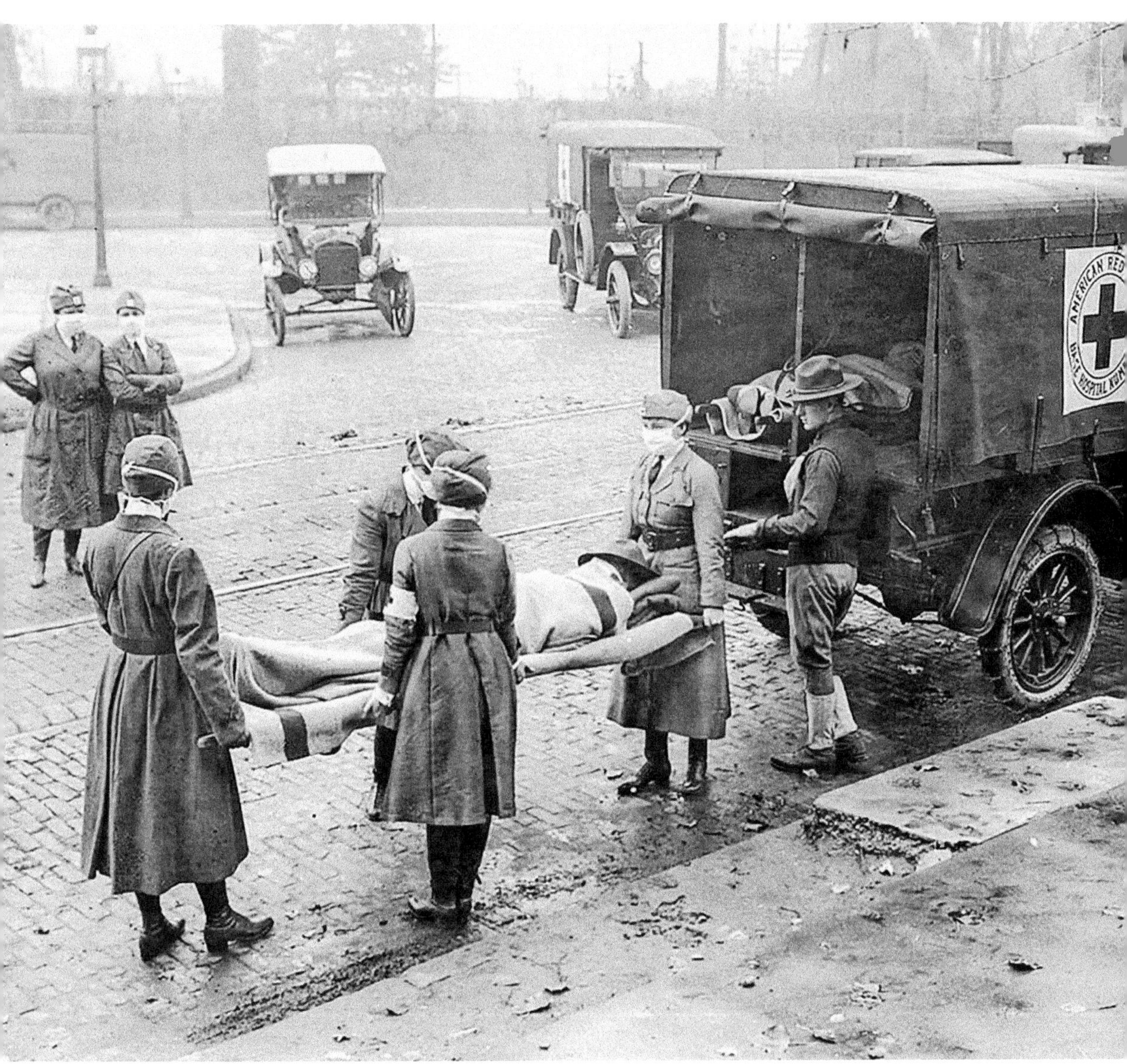

Figure 2.1. Spanish Flu pandemic, 1918–1920. In the public domain.

Chapter 2

Pandemical Architecture for Health

Complexities and Contradictions in History

The recollective knowledge of horrible events periodically intrudes into the public consciousness but is rarely retained for long.[1]

Judith L. Herman

For centuries, hospitals have been constructed with the aims of caring for the ill and finding out how to most effectively isolate contagious from non-infectious patients. In the architectural and urban history of public health disasters and catastrophes, however, architectural historians have devoted surprisingly little attention to any of this. The following discussion is an attempt to trace some key events in this history. Emphasis is placed on the intersection of infectious diseases and pandemics with urbanism, architecture, nature, and landscapes, in light of the reality that *progress itself is a disease-causing agent*. Diseases, including HIV-AIDS and COVID-19, are first and foremost a consequence of human advancement. Populations migrated into rainforests, crisscrossed oceans, scaled the heights of mountains, and, in the process, exposed virtually all corners of the globe to previously isolated, unknown, often deadly viruses. The recent, incredibly fast-moving Ebola pandemic is one such example, as it exposed unsuspecting communities and regions to a new, exotic pathogen. Human progress breeds disease—and has always done so. This reality is at the heart of the following discussion. Cities and buildings, as well as nature and landscapes, have always played a role in fostering or, in some cases, mitigating the adverse health outcomes brought about by foreseen as well as unforeseen disasters and catastrophes (fig. 2.1).

Any attempt to chronologically trace historical events along a reconstructed timeline is subject to imprecision, because transformative events and their outcomes occurred in complex and contradictory ways. Nonetheless, certain landmarks along these various intersections lend themselves to a certain degree of examination through major epochs in the theory and history of health and the built environment. These epochs, to date, are the Ancient, Medieval, Renaissance, Nightingale, Modern Megahospital, and Meta-Healthscapes epochs.[2] The first five provide the structural framework for this chapter, while the Meta-Healthscape epoch (epoch 6) is discussed in detail in chapter 7. The epidemiological historian Kenneth F. Kiple cautions that no framework of this type, however, is foolproof, meant to be inclusive, or otherwise construed as definitive:

> Disease is not a human invention. Rather, it is a biological process as old as life itself. Humans, unlike their predecessors at the top of the food chain, have not been content simply to live on and off of the planet. For at least the last 400,000 years and especially the last 10,000, they have diligently labored to rearrange it. We call such rearranging "progress" . . . [but] at times progress seems a kind of Russian roulette that sooner or later will impose the ultimate penalty on us for undoing nature without knowing what we are doing, such as forests being transformed into farms and farms transformed into urban and industrial sprawl. . . . Moving epidemiologically to the opposite side of the "forest to urban and industrial sprawl" paradigm, progress has placed most of us in the developed world squarely in the midst of a cancer epidemic . . . and a major cause of cancer is the ultraviolet component of sunlight, now increasing in intensity due to atmospheric pollution.[3]

THE ANCIENT WORLD (EPOCH 1)

Synopsis: The end of the Ice Age coincided with the impetus to explore beyond the Bering Straits, and this fostered the Agrarian

Revolution. At the dawn of the Neolithic Revolution, human populations began to concentrate themselves in denser physical conditions. This resulted in the domestication of livestock in growing urban center barnyards, located in close proximity to the dwelling. The shield that once protected hunter-gatherers from exposure to zoonotic diseases was now endangered. Sedentary agriculture focused on a single crop, requiring an unprecedented amount of human labor. Birthrates soared, and as the population of villages expanded, so did the probability of hosting contagious diseases. From earliest times, caves had functioned as a refuge for the care and treatment of the sick and dying. In early Neolithic settlements, a sick house was set aside in the village to care for the ill, as it was an acceptable practice to separate these individuals from the mainstream community. In ancient Greece, the Middle East, and Asia, treatments were frequently based on wellness care, including the use of water and exposure to natural vegetation and fresh air for their restorative properties. The earliest known hospitals were in Iraq, Iran, Egypt, and Turkey. Early hospitals in the Middle East and in Asian urban centers were more advanced, in comparison with their European counterparts. Greek healing centers were known as religious (sacred) Asclepiad. Later, the Romans introduced the secular valetudinarium (military hospital) and the ubiquitous public bath complexes that were constructed across their empire. Health inequalities centered on social and racial discrimination of the poor, with the wealthy classes being able to barter or otherwise purchase higher quality health care.

Builders' primary focus: *Wealthy and powerful private donors and government.*

Predominant building types: *Huts, caves, and, later, private and public-funded healing centers for military and civilian uses.*[4]

Sickness and Sedentism

The earliest hunter-gatherers congregated in small isolated bands, frequently relocating, and seldom remaining in one place long enough to pollute the water, generate a significant amount of solid waste, or attract disease-transmitting insects and animals. These small bands avoided contagious diseases, particularly illnesses (such as measles and influenza) caused by microparasites. In time, human populations would begin to function as hosts, with most diseases originating from domesticated animals that provided humans with eggs, milk, and meat. The earliest parasites that managed to thrive in humans were mainly microorganisms (i.e., intestinal worms, lice, fleas), continually adapting as human settlements migrated across diverse landscapes and climates. Humans were also susceptible to parasites transmitted through wild animal hosts: leptospirosis, fever, brucellosis, salmonellosis, tularemia, malaria, and yellow fever. Notably, hunter-gatherer communities did not acquire the nutritional deficiency diseases that would later appear in more-domesticated, sedentary communities. The DNA of hunter-gatherers indicates their protein intake surpassed that of all succeeding generations, up to the late twentieth century.

> Humans and their domestic animals lived check to jowl fouling the water
> they drank and the soil. . . . Squalid conditions of the villages offered a
> paradise to . . . rats, mice, ticks, flies and mosquitos that became adept
> at spreading one or more diseases, incubating as pathogens ricocheting
> back and forth between animals and their owners. Human diet deterio-
> rated rapidly as a concentration on tending and consuming a single crop
> robbed bodies of important nutrients and, consequently, of the ability to
> resist disease.[5]

The Neolithic Revolution, in terms of human health, was regressive, transforming agrarian populations into shorter, less physically robust farmers, and, later, into urban dwellers—prime targets for contagious disease.

Ancient Greece and Rome

The Athenian historian and general Thucydides (460–400 BC) recorded perhaps the earliest account of a bona fide *epidemic*. The war between Athens and Sparta, as he described it in the opening chapter of his *History of the Peloponnesian War* (during 431–404 BC) was prolonged and intense. But the war itself was only one of numerous disasters to befall ancient Greece. There were earthquakes, droughts, and famine, followed by deadly plague. Of all the calamities that affected Athens, the plague, which struck in the war's second year (430 BC), was regarded as the worst. It originated in Ethiopia, spread through Egypt to the port of Piraeus, and from there to Athens. Athens was highly vulnerable, because the Athenians had retreated behind their fortified city walls, intending to wage a largely naval war. The arrival of the plague transformed this walled-in city into a death trap, causing one-quarter of the urban population to perish.[6]

At the Asklepieion in Pergamon (fourth century BC) in ancient Greece, therapeutic treatment regimens were routinely prescribed.[7] For example, treatments for a tuberculosis (TB) patient might consist of horseback riding, heliotherapy, reading, and relaxation—all outdoor activities. The attending caregiver-therapist was well versed in the restorative benefits of engagement with nature, a main form of treatment. A detailed description of the Asklepieion was provided by Aelius Aristides (117–185 AD).

In contrast to the five ancient Greek city-states and Athens at the time of Pericles, Rome in the second century AD was a vastly more populous, complex society, and, as such, was much more vulnerable to plague. At its height, the Roman Empire encompassed nearly 70 million subjects, perhaps one-quarter of all humans alive at the time. Niall Ferguson writes:

> Already highly susceptible to gastrointestinal infections and malaria, the Romans appear to have suffered the first major smallpox epidemic in the winter of 165–166 AD during the reign of Marcus Aurelius (161–180 AD). The Romans believed they had brought the plague upon themselves by sacking the temple of Apollo at Seleucia during their war against the Parthians; in reality, returning soldiers may have brought the disease with them, or the plague may have accompanied slaves imported from Africa. . . . Plague persisted until around 192 [AD]. . . . It was a later, recurring pandemic that would be seen as the death blow to the Roman Empire: the Plague of Justinian.[8]

It was customary in Imperial Rome to send those affected with lung ailments on a sea voyage, often to Sicily or Egypt. Cicero (106–43 BC), gravely ill with tuberculosis, coughing and spewing blood until he became emaciated, undertook voyages to Greece and Asia in 80 BC He would return to Rome, entirely cured, two years later. For centuries, it was assumed that disease was the result of bad heredity, with little to be done to save its victims except through convalescence in a dry, warmer climate, accompanied by a far less stressful daily regimen. Balmy air and sunny skies, it was thought, were elixirs, with the therapeutic power to arrest the destruction of lung tissue and the sapping of physical strength that caused the infected to die.[9]

CONTAGIOUS DISEASE IN THE MIDDLE AGES (EPOCH 2)

Synopsis: Whenever a medieval city was stricken by plague, that city was rapidly closed off physically, with fortified walls and guarded gates, to prevent further contagion. In Europe, urban residents were confined to their homes and required to appear at their windows during daily rounds (inspections), to ensure all household occupants were present and accounted for. Hastily built wooden canals led from the residential districts to a common street for the transportation of supplies—and bodies. Christian religious orders provided care through networks of monastic chapel-ward infirmaries, many with cross-ward plans, isolating infectious disease patients in these hellish back areas. The Middle Eastern medical center mosque hospitals in Cairo and Baghdad continued to be more advanced than their European counterparts. Across Europe, bloodletting was used to treat an assortment of ailments, diseases, and sicknesses. Later, the antecedents of modern scientific surgical procedures would be introduced as medicinal alternatives to commonplace treatments. The Catholic Church placed a singular focus on faith in healing, although its infirmaries were equally hellish from sanitary and infection-control standpoints. Faith supposedly guaranteed redemption and salvation, because recovery rarely occurred. Greek and Roman antecedents with respect to the therapeutic affordances of nature were forgotten. Fortifications were built to protect these early medical centers from attack in uncertain times. An excellent example from the period is St. Gall's chapel-ward hospital (ninth century AD) in Switzerland. New building types—the insane asylum and leper colony—would emerge as repositories for the mentally ill and social outcasts.

Builders' primary focus: Wealthy and powerful benefactors, religious orders, and, later, secular (public) organizations.

Predominant building types: Monastic chapel-ward infirmaries, hospices, edge-of-town and rural leper colonies, public plague hospitals, and early insane asylums.[10]

From the Neolithic Revolution to the fall of Ancient Rome, humankind remained highly vulnerable to the destructive waves of contagious diseases. Today, we share some sixty-six diseases with dogs, fifty with cattle, forty-six with sheep and goats, forty-two with pigs, thirty-five with horses, and twenty-six with poultry. During the Middle Ages, pathogens drawn together by close transactions between humans and animals caused both the rapid growth of trade and commerce and the mutation of diseases—at times evolving into ravaging plagues and pandemics. Then, as now, disease transmissibility has required dense human settlements and the physical movement of individuals from place to place.

The Plague of Justinian

The cause of this epidemic can be traced to numerous accounts, including that of Byzantine-era historian Procopius of Caesarea (500–565 AD) who, in his *History of the Wars*, described in detail its course and its destruction. Bishop Gregory of Tours (538–594 AD) described how it surged across Western Europe, ricocheting around the Mediterranean.[11] The Plague of Justinian (542–543 AD) is cited as the root of a pandemic that lasted until the middle of the eighth century. Procopius traced the origin of the pandemic to Egypt and trade routes with India, with *Rattius rattus* migrating westward from South Asia. Although the Romans had established extensive trade and travel routes across the Eurasian landmass, the pandemic itself first spread via merchant ships.[12] The first cycle of bubonic plague was nearly as catastrophic as that of the Black Death—the name bestowed on the second cycle of this pandemic eight centuries later. In Constantinople, at its peak the pandemic killed 10,000 persons every day. It depopulated entire towns across the Mediterranean region, extending from Italy to France to the North African coast, as well as also reaching England. Overall, nearly 100 million people died during the two centuries of the first pandemical cycle. It is generally assumed that the first wave killed at least 25 percent of the population in the territory that formerly was part of the Roman Empire, and the Black Death would later kill another 25–50 percent of the communities it infected throughout Europe and the Middle East (fig. 2.2). The inhabitants of rural villages were affected the least, whereas inhabitants of densely populated port cities were the most severely impacted, as these were places where rodent populations were constantly a threat, due to the burgeoning merchant shipping trade.

Bubonic Plague (the Black Death)

By 1340, Europe was a quixotic patchwork of kingdoms, principalities, duchies, bishoprics, and numerous semiautonomous city-states. This plague attacked in multiple waves. In England, after the initial outbreak, a second wave arrived in 1361–1362, followed by a third in 1369, and a fourth in 1375. In Italy, around a hundred towns were completely depopulated, and many bigger cities lost large percentages of their population. The massive mortality rate is credited with the rise of an entirely new labor system, which would supplant the feudal system. In addition, the open sewers of the burgeoning villages and cities of medieval Europe were rife with disease-transmitting rodents and insects. And, increasingly, children were afflicted by new diseases, including measles and smallpox. The word *plague* is based on the Latin *plaga*, meaning a strike or blow causing a wound. Until the bubonic plague in the 1330s and 1340s, plagues were believed to be caused by acts of God, either as punishment for sin or as "His" plan for the end of the world. The Black Death changed everything in this regard, because the focus now turned to the plight of its victims.

During the fourteenth century, bubonic plague returned at least four times to most Mediterranean urban centers. In Firenze (Florence), with a prior population of approximately 100,000, 100–200 deaths occurred daily through the late spring, when suddenly 400–1,000 died every day. The term *quarantine* was coined in Venice at this time. Italian cities were forced to institute a "health passport" to certify travelers' plague-free status before embarking/disembarking on ships. This measure was taken to lessen the burdens of temporary quarantine confinement. In larger cities, the local board of health quickly grew in importance and was soon given authority to enforce the controlled isolation of the sick, as well as manage medical services, philanthropy, burial of the dead, and record keeping.[13] By the end of the Middle Ages, urban-based governmental agencies would spawn the rise of the modern bureaucratic state. In London, the Great Fire of 1666 killed infected rats, inadvertently cleansing the city of a virulent wave of the bubonic plague, while rendering over 85 percent of the city's population homeless.

Urbanization also contributed to the rise in leprosy in the Middle Ages. Medieval societies stigmatized lepers as well as epileptics. There are two types of leprosy. One produces the *leper*, the archetypal societal outcast. The other is a disease caused by infection with *Mycobacterium leprae*, today referred to as Hansen's disease. The need to castigate the afflicted—labeled *outsiders*—remains a fundamental cause of health inequalities to this day. In Leviticus (a book of codes and laws dating from around 1000 BC), the focus was on the lepers themselves, with a need to expel these "unclean" persons and then ritually cleanse contaminants from their dwellings.[14] As the Catholic Church continued to proselytize the message

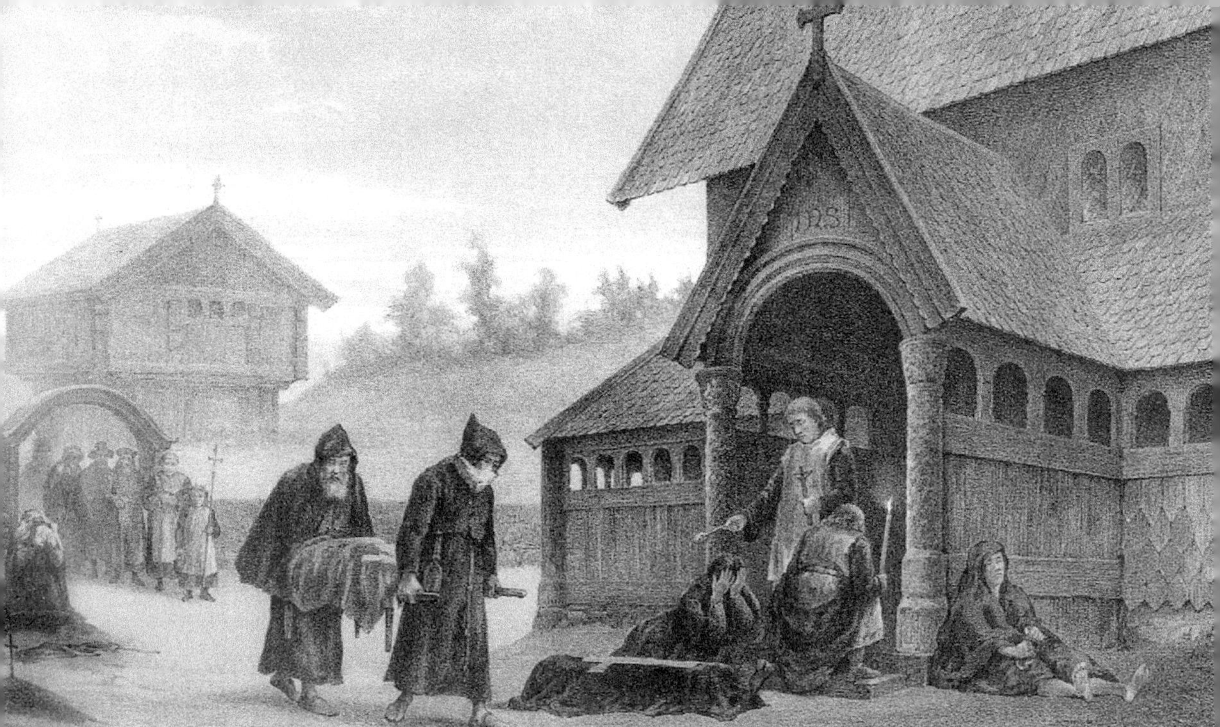

Figure 2.2. The Black Death of 1349 killed two-thirds of Norway's population. Courtesy of Mary Evans Picture Gallery, London, UK.

of Christianity, biblical portrayals of leprosy were powerfully rooted in sin and disease, reinforcing the message of the redemptive power of Christ in the salvation of the afflicted. Medieval churches, shrines, and monasteries were built on or near pre-Christian healing sites, and holy places of worship further reinforced this message.

To summarize, in the Middle Ages, Catholic missionaries proselytized the unconverted, while the wealthy sought to buy or barter their way out of exposure to disease, remaining in isolation in their castles and villas, far from the masses. The first plague hospitals, leprosaria, and lazarettos were built, and sections of chapel-ward monastic infirmaries were converted to house plague victims. The autonomous plague hospitals, leprosaria, and lazarettos built beyond the fortified walls of a city functioned as health care facilities for the diseased and medically underserved.

CONTAGIOUS DISEASE IN THE RENAISSANCE (EPOCH 3)

Synopsis: Hospitals in the Renaissance were conceived to principally emulate the ornate palaces of the period. Public hospitals emerged as a successor to donor (bequeathed) hospitals. The advent of humanism placed "man" (humans) as the focal center, with a reawakened concern for the inner profundities of human anatomy. Vast plague hospitals were constructed, such as the Ospedale Maggiore di Milano in Italy, founded by Duke Francesco Sforza and opened in 1456. It was designed by three architects: Filarete, Francesco Maria Richini, and Donato Bramante. Soon it would fall victim to chronic underfunding and dreadful sanitary conditions. Scientifically based medical education and medical practices independently emerged at this time. The Italian Renaissance was dominated by an emphasis on classical antiquity and the idealization of classical thought in matters of governance. The abbot (today's CEO equivalent) of a medieval monastic infirmary hospital gave way to the hospital superintendent, supported by a growing army of specialists throughout the hospital. For the insane, opulent palace-hospital institutions were erected, such as Bethlehem (Bedlam) Hospital in London, UK, in 1676. Its stately external facade projected a noble outer face to the public, while inside it was hell on earth for its many hundreds of "patient-inmates." The private isolation room first appeared as a separate room, adjacent to the main chapel-ward, and was used mainly for the rich—since, throughout history, the wealthy could buy privacy and spatial isolation from the masses. Meanwhile, the lower classes were subject to immense, unkempt, disease-ridden open wards and, later, overcrowded outpatient clinics. These trends were incisively examined by French philosopher Michel Foucault in The Birth of the Clinic.[15] *The immense chapels of monastic hospitals gradually diminished in scale within palace hospitals, yet they were still visually prominent at the center of strictly symmetrical floor plans and exterior facades. A prime example is the palace hospital (1576–1585) in Wurtzburg, Germany. The straitjacket was invented at St. Thomas Hospital in London in the eighteenth century, while engagement with nature and landscapes was dismissed as a therapeutic or restorative treatment for the sick and diseased. Notable exceptions were the strictly picturesque broad lawns, placed behind large brick or stone walls, setting an institution apart from its urban context. Panoptical insane asylums and prisons first appeared at this time, including the Glasgow Lunatic Asylum (1801–1810).*

Architects' primary focus: *Wealthy private benefactors and religious organizations.*

Predominant building types*: Hospitals, hospices, edge-of-town lep-rosaria, rural leper colonies, and specialty plague hospitals.*

Beginning in the Renaissance, local public health boards established non-pharmaceutical interventions long before they properly understood the true nature of any contagious disease. Recurrent plague outbreaks led cities to establish five policies to limit its transmission: (1) border lockdowns and travel bans, with marine and land quarantines to keep the disease out; (2) social distancing, in the form of bans on all gatherings; (3) burials of the dead in special pits, with destruction of their personal belongings and, sometimes, their dwellings; (4) legally enforced lockdowns; and (5) confinement of the infected to pest houses, lazarettos, and private dwellings. Individuals' health status was monitored vis-à-vis bills of health, to certify that the arriving ship or overland caravan was not plague ridden.[16]

Typhoid and influenza spread via unsanitary conditions in densely populated cities and villages in Europe and elsewhere. At the time, the *filth theory of disease* was adhered to by leading physicians. The correlation appeared obvious: with the Industrial Revolution fostering urbanism, more and more people crowded into increasingly filthy urban centers, frequently living adjacent to factories. Ancient means of sanitation were soon overwhelmed by this rapid population growth, spawning intestinal diseases such as typhoid, pneumonia, smallpox, erysipelas, and tuberculosis. It was argued at the time that the foul air sickened people—a condition attributed to unsanitary streets filled with manure, dead animal carcasses, garbage, fecal material, and the corpses of diseased citizens removed from severely overcrowded dwellings. It would soon be proved, however, that typhoid did not arise from unsanitary filth per se—it was a contagious disease.[17]

Influenza is a zoonotic disease that humans episodically cross-transmitted with domesticated animals, such as pigs and fowl. It manifests in regions where animal domestication has existed the longest in recorded history. But humans also share this disease with undomesticated bird species. It is generally assumed that influenza spread via international trade routes during the late Middle Ages, resulting in three pandemical waves in Europe in the sixteenth century: 1510, 1557, and 1580. The last of these pandemics traveled from the Mediterranean to the Baltic region in four months. By the seventeenth century, relatively few influenza pandemics were occurring in Europe. Nonetheless, lethal regional outbreaks did continue to occur. In the eighteenth century, deadly influenza reemerged, due to increasing urbanization; the continued proliferation of agriculture;

animal domestication, with livestock often kept in dense urban centers; and increased international trade. At least three and as many as five pandemical flu outbreaks occurred in Europe in the eighteenth century. The worst was in 1781–1782, having originated in Asia. It soon swept through Europe, and then to the Americas and Africa.[18]

Emergence of the Isolation Room

Beginning at this time, contagious patients were increasingly housed in smaller isolation back wards and private rooms, as opposed to large open wards. These rooms housed from one to as many as twenty beds. They were reserved for lepers, the violent insane, plague victims, the superannuated, and the rich. The last two categories of patients were not diseased, but rather were characterized by social class, dictating the type of care and accommodations the upper echelons would expect to receive if one was not able to be cared for at home. Toward the end of the Middle Ages, it was not uncommon for persons of economic means to prepay to ensure that they would have a place to stay for the remainder of one's life. In time, entire buildings were inequitably constructed for this purpose—often at the expense of the poor and the disenfranchised. In some cases, the main level would house a large open ward, with the second level housing private and semiprivate rooms for the contagious sick, and the third level containing private rooms for pensioners.[19] In the case of the leprosarium of St. George in Stettin (Szczecin), Poland, in the sixteenth century, a central dominating church was surrounded on three sides by a cloistered courtyard (fig. 2.3). It was built immediately beyond the city's walls; separated by a moat, walls, and guarded gate; and sited on the main road into town, so passersby could leave donations in the alms box without ever making direct contact with the compound's ostracized occupants. This and many other leper compounds would grow in size to become autonomous colonies. A chapel was nearly always a key architectural part of these colonies, and residential living quarters were spartan, usually with dirt floors.

The Lazaretto

Leprosy was a dreaded, disfiguring disease, but plagues would strike suddenly, killing entire neighborhoods and even entire towns. The local *lazaretto* (from the Italian *lazaret*) was invented at this time—an isolation hospital principally for screening and quarantining maritime travelers. Lazarettos

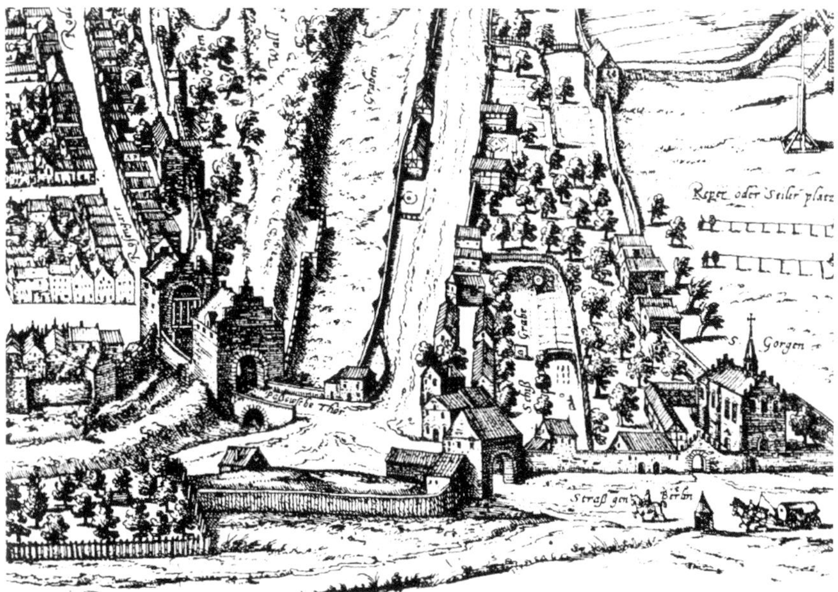

Figure 2.3. Leprosarium of St. George, Stettin (Szczecin), Poland, sixteenth century. Courtesy of Institute for the History of Medicine and Pharmacy, Christian Albrecht University of Kiel, Germany.

were built to sequester persons who were either infected or suspected of being infected with leprosy or plague. The earliest lazarettos were ships housing the infected, permanently docked at anchor. Later, isolated island complexes were built near the city, or a single building was constructed on the mainland, far from the city center. A leper colony administrated by a Christian religious order was often called a *lazar house*, after the parable of Lazarus the beggar. The initial proposal for the lazaretto in Milan, Italy, called for 200 small structures, one per patient, scattered across a large donated site. The built version (1488) comprised 288 contiguous cells around an octagonal church. It was a four-sided, almost square enclosure, built beyond the city's fortified walls and surrounded by a moat, a ring road, and a canal. This one-level structure had small rooms, connected by a continuous vaulted colonnade that allowed air circulation. There were only two entry points, each heavily guarded. The chapel was open air, so every patient could view the altar from their window.

During peak outbreaks, lazarettos housed as many as 16,000 contagious disease victims, and in overflow conditions, the remainder occupied makeshift tents and huts erected in the complex's massive courtyard. In structures without this space for overflow beds, as many as forty patients would be crammed into each permanent room. Patients and supplies were transported on crude wooden pushcarts, and makeshift mattresses of straw were placed literally everywhere, including throughout the lengthy open-air arcades. Paths were carved out among this sea of humanity in the vast courtyard to maintain the essential flow of people and supplies. Somewhat paradoxically, in non-plague periods, these institutions were nearly empty, although during peak outbreaks, they were never large enough. Lazarettos required significant capital expenditures to maintain them, regardless of whether they were overcrowded or virtually empty.[20]

In 1592, during a plague outbreak, a lazaretto made of wood huts was built on Manoel Island, Malta, in the Mediterranean. It was demolished in 1593, after the disease had subsided. In 1643, Grandmaster Lascaris built a permanent lazaretto on the same site, to control the periodic influx of plague and cholera victims arriving on merchant ships. The continued efforts of the Order of Saint John to develop this island into a first-rate infectious disease treatment hospital succeeded, in relative terms. It was extensively employed during a subsequent plague outbreak in 1813, and again during a cholera outbreak in 1865. In 1855–1856, it was also used during the Crimean War (see below) as a military hospital for British, Italian, and French troops. This complex was expanded over time. It closed in 1929, although the original building still stands. Figure 2.4 depicts this structure in 1906, viewed from the bastions of Valletta. It was surrounded by a high wall, to prevent the infected "inmates" from escaping. There were six cemeteries nearby, but only one remains today. The site is currently being redeveloped and restored for commercial and residential uses (fig. 2.5).[21]

With an ever-increasing need for the construction of public health facilities to isolate the contagiously diseased, in 1634 Malachias Geiger proposed a facility for a plague hospital (unbuilt). A moat of running river water surrounded the entire fortification, turning it into an island, thus isolating it from the healthy population on the shore. The wide arcade arches allowed an octagonal chapel in the central court to be seen from the window in every patient's room. Each room had a privy, emptying into the moat. Thirty-two rooms, each housing three beds, were on the two long sides of a rectangular courtyard. Along the two shorter sides of the courtyard, rooms twice that size, each housing a single bed, were designated for the wealthier classes. The compound could only be entered by two footbridges, which could be lowered or drawn up.[22]

Architecturally, the public health plague hospitals of the period were neoclassical in their exterior appearance, with near-absolute symmetry. The

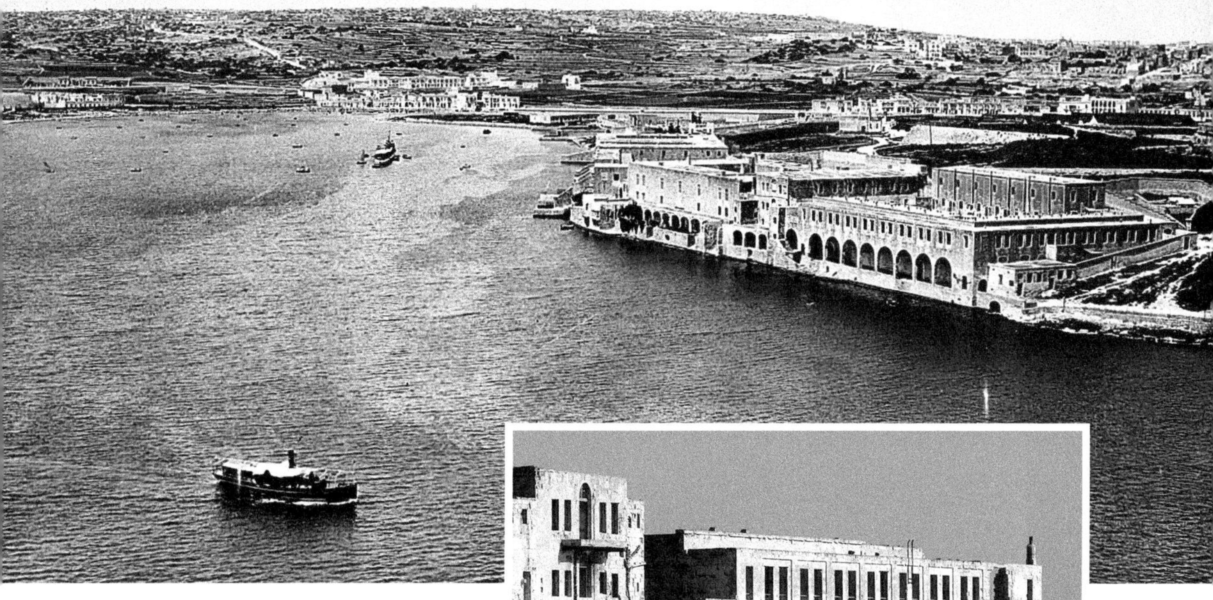

Figure 2.4. *(above)* Lazaretto, Manoel Island, Malta, 1906. Courtesy of P. Djajkovski / Galea Debono, *Times of Malta*.

Figure 2.5. *(right)* Lazaretto, Manoel Island, Malta, 2020. Courtesy of P. Djajkovski / Galea Debono, *Times of Malta*.

prototype for Geiger's proposal was Milan's infamous lazaretto, the afore-mentioned plague hospital affiliated with the Ospedale Maggiore. Another facility, the one-level Pest House (1635–1644) in Leiden, The Netherlands, featured a square exterior courtyard surrounded by eight large open wards, each housing thirty-one beds arrayed along the outer perimeter wall, sur-rounded by a moat with guarded footbridges. This appears to be a common architectural solution for plague institutions: large open wards, as well as a number of small private rooms. During peak outbreaks, the open courtyard space in the center became filled with additional patients—a common prac-tice by this time (fig. 2.6).[23] Europeans came to expect the bubonic plague's periodic return. In response, they ramped up quarantine and isolation pol-icies, while also continuing to construct specialized public health facilities, with the aim of improving early detection. In 1720, a plague reached Mar-seilles, France, due to a breakdown in that city's quarantine system. When each merchant ship arrived at its port, some passengers were able to bribe the public health officials to avoid being confined in the local quarantine facility. As a result, a new wave of death commenced, killing more than 50,000 out of a total population of about 100,000. By that fall, bodies were being piled up in public squares. News of the catastrophe in Marseille quickly spread throughout Europe:

> All maritime commerce ceased and quarantine mandates were imposed
> on the city and surrounding region. Non-Europeans were viewed as
> such a public health threat that the Austrian-Hungarian Empire built
> a 1,500-mile-long cordon sanitaire that stretched overland from the
> Balkans to north of the Danube River, with guard houses so closely sited
> the guards could stay in visual contact with one another. . . . The guards
> were not looking for rats or fleas so the investment did little to stop
> the spread of plague. Trade routes redirected through central Russia
> brought plague to St. Petersburg and Moscow in 1770–71, an epidemic
> as devastating as that of Marseilles a half-century earlier.[24]

A painting from 1721 depicts the main town square in front of Marseille's Town Hall, filled with both desperate citizens in various states of near-death and despair and those attempting to flee the stricken city (fig. 2.7).

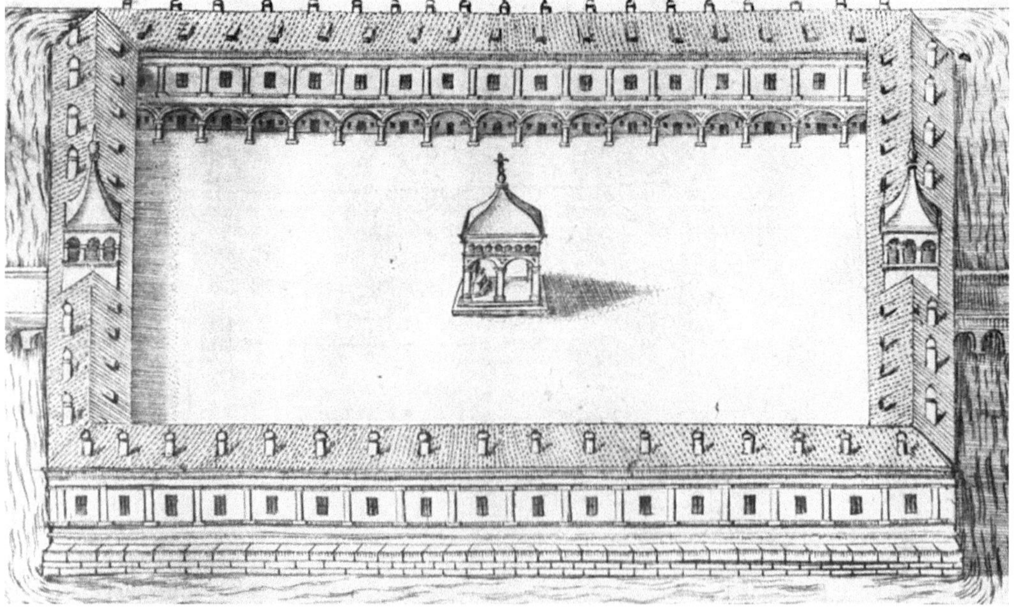

Figure 2.6. Engraving of the Pest House (1635–1644) in Leiden, The Netherlands. In Dieter Jetter, "Zur Typologie des Pesthauses," *Sudhoffs Archiv für Geschichte der Medizin und der Naturwissenschaften*, September 1963.

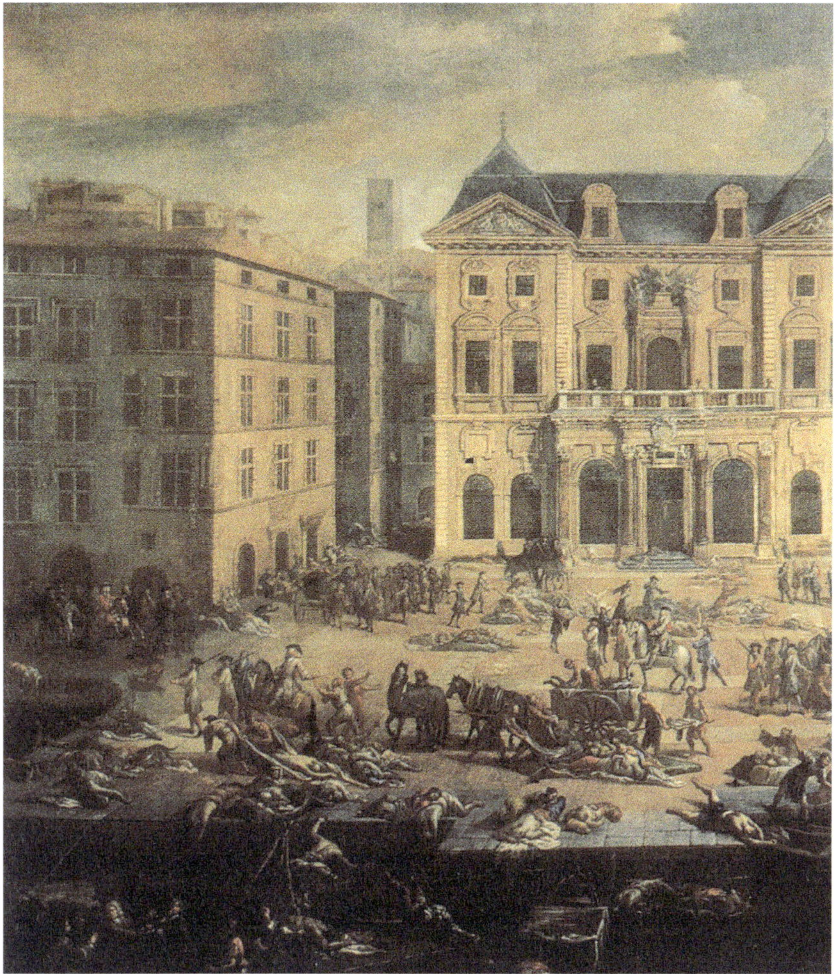

Figure 2.7. View of the Town Hall, Marseille, France, during the plague of 1721. Painting by Michel Serre (1658–1753). Reproduced by permission of Musée des Beaux-Arts, Marseille, France / Bridgeman Images.

Architect Luigi Vanvitelli designed and built an architecturally elaborate lazaretto (1733–1743) in Ancona, Italy. It was commissioned by Lorenzo Corsini (1652–1740), later to become Pope Clement XII (1730–1740). The first stone for the quarantine hospital of the Port of Ancona was laid in 1737. Ancona served Italy in its trade with the Balkans and the eastern Mediterranean region. The architect had carefully studied the lazarettos built at Leghor, Genoa, and Venice (all in Italy) before designing the one in Ancona (figs. 2.8 and 2.9).[25] Vanvitelli designed an austere pentagon, surrounded on all sides by sea, distant from the shore, with a formidable wall and batture, reminiscent of a military fortress. The parti transitions from the pentagon to a circle at the center of the large, open, central courtyard. A domed chapel is at the center (fig. 2.10). All quarantined persons were able to hear Mass from the small window in their dormitory cell. The facility's raised floor was pierced by a series of drainage manholes, allowing the dead to be dropped directly below into the sea.

In 1787, Pope Carlos III ordered the construction of a lazaretto on the Felipet Peninsula, off the Spanish coast, at the entrance to the Port of Mahón in the Mediterranean. In the eighteenth century, Spain became especially threatened by plague and yellow fever. This complex was configured similarly to those in Ancona and elsewhere: built offshore, formidable, with a central courtyard, and looking like a fortress with its high walls and narrow, restrictive entry portal. Two cemeteries were on-site.[26] Renaissance-period plague would disappear from Europe by the end of the seventeenth century, as there were only two widespread epidemics after 1670. These final episodes, however, were nearly as deadly as the earlier Black Death. It remains impossible to precisely determine the extent to which the design of cities or individual buildings directly contributed to this reduction in death and misery. The decline in pandemical outbreaks in Europe by this time has generally been attributed to a reduction in the infected rodent and flea populations that traveled aboard merchant ships, plus improved fumigation efforts both on land and at sea.

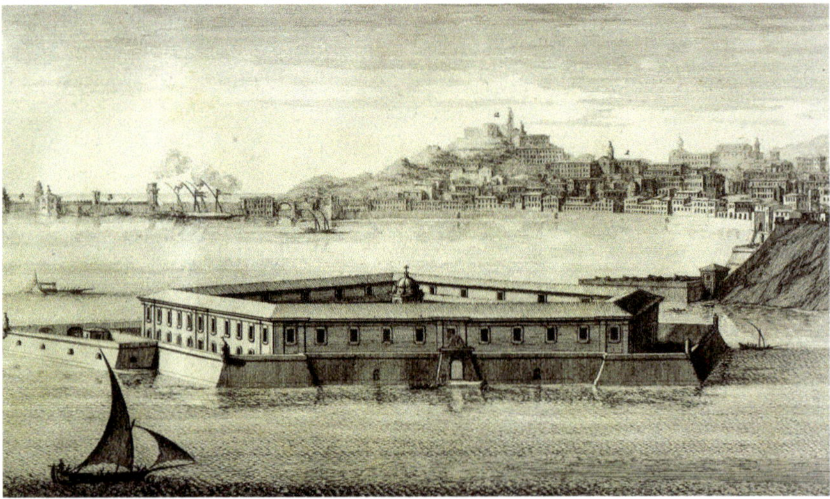

Figure 2.8. Engraving (1739) of the Lazaretto at Ancona (now Italy), built in 1733–1743. Building architect: Luigi Vanvitelli. Courtesy of Biblioteca nazionale Marciana, Venice, Italy.

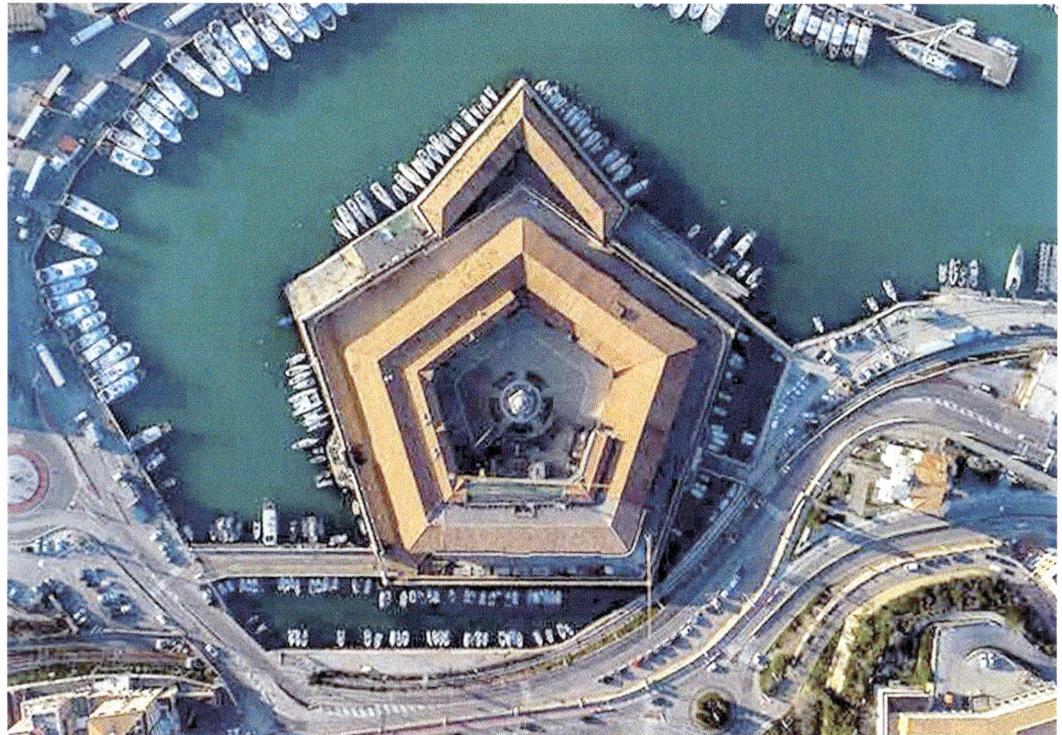

Figure 2.9. Ariel view of the Lazaretto at Ancona (now Italy). Courtesy of Stefano Crialesi / Galea Debono, *Times of Malta*.

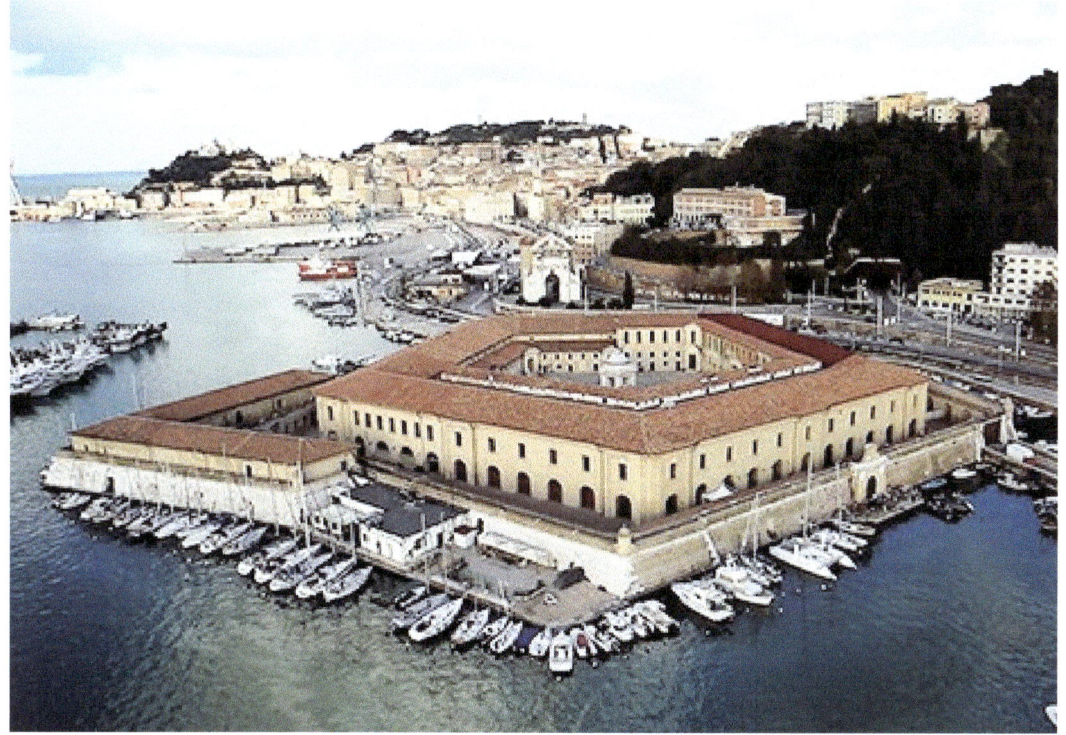

Figure 2.10. The Lazaretto at Ancona (now Italy). Courtesy of Stefano Crialesi / Galea Debono, *Times of Malta*.

CONTAGIOUS DISEASE IN THE NIGHTINGALE ERA (EPOCH 4)

Synopsis: Modern medical principles were translated into architectural form, beginning in the mid-nineteenth century and accelerated in the pioneering work of Florence Nightingale (1820–1910). She was an English social reformer, statistician, and the founder of the modern nursing profession. She perfected what is known internationally as the Nightingale open ward hospital. Later on, adaptations of her precepts on building forms and hygiene, and the therapeutic role of nature and landscapes in the healing process, would be incorporated in high-rise Nightingale hospitals up to 1940. During British colonialization, political pressures at home in England had brought immense pressure on the military to provide effective health care for injured soldiers fighting in far-off conquests across the Empire. Nightingale is generally considered the first modern medical facility planner. A close precursor had opened nearly ten years earlier, however: the Lariboisière Hospital (1846–1853) in Paris, one of several pavilion hospitals built after the second cholera pandemic (1832) to reflect new hygienic best practices. After her successes on the front lines of the Crimean War in Turkey (1855–56), Nightingale authored Notes on Nursing *(1858) and* Notes on Hospitals *(1859). Meanwhile, I. K. Brunel's prefabricated acute care and infectious disease hospital was built at Renkioi, Turkey, concurrent with Nightingale's extraordinary work at the converted barracks hospital at Scutari (a district in Istanbul, Turkey).*[27] *This off-site prefabricated hospital (built in the UK) was shipped to Renkioi. It consisted of two rows of one-level prefab wards, built of wood, arrayed along dual-circulation spines. In the American Civil War (1861–1865) and during the North American Indian Wars, the US military constructed many tent field hospitals, influenced by Nightingale. Parallel to the work of Nightingale, in the late nineteenth and early twentieth centuries, many tuberculosis sanitoriums were built in Europe and elsewhere, constructed in the International Style of modern architecture. These institutions embrace the therapeutic potential of nature and landscapes.*

Architects' primary focus: Wealthy private benefactors, religious organizations, public health agencies, hospitals, and tertiary medical centers.

Predominant building types: TB sanitoriums, secular wellness retreat-spas, religious-affiliated wellness retreat-spas, and public health contagious disease hospitals.

Plague outbreaks, less frequent by the mid-nineteenth century, continued nonetheless, attributed to the construction of railroad networks, larger sea vessels, and new overland trade routes made possible by improved roads. In China, local governments continued to contend with plague outbreaks in trading cities, which had been occurring since the Qing Dynasty (1636–1911). Rats were once again the source, and their transmutability had a deleterious impact on the emerging trade centers of Southeast Asia. Western response to a virulent plague in India in the late 1890s resulted in the burning of victims' clothing, mass quarantine edicts, funeral pyres, and the razing of many entire shantytowns. Meanwhile, plague had spread throughout the Pacific Rim, extending to Australia and San Francisco by 1900. In San Francisco, public health authorities forced over 20,000 Asian immigrants into quarantine encampments in the city's Chinatown district. By 1900, most regions of the world had been adversely impacted, and plague transmission would continue in the twentieth century, albeit on a lesser scale—in certain ways, mirroring prior disease transmission patterns.[28]

In Europe, plague-associated racism, discrimination, and profound health inequalities had persisted since the Middle Ages, manifesting in anti-Semitic pogroms and purges of the socially unwanted, including gypsies. In North America, plague-associated discrimination occurred against Asians, Indigenous populations, African American communities, and poor immigrant communities. International cooperation was nonexistent until the convening of the first International Sanitary Commission, which met in Paris in July 1851, although the representatives of the twelve participating countries could not agree on standard quarantine measures for dealing with cholera, yellow fever, and the plague. Leprosy persisted widely throughout the nineteenth century. In 1865, Hawaii's colonial government purchased land for permanently quarantining lepers on the volcanic island of Molokai, hemmed in on three sides by the sea and on the fourth by mountains.[29] By 1900 the US had established leper colonies on the islands of Culion and Cebu in the Philippines and, a decade later, in rural Carville, Louisiana, ten miles south of Baton Rouge, on the site of a former plantation on the east bank of the Mississippi River.[30] The colony at Carville was a wholly self-sufficient campus, not unlike the rural insane asylums of the period. This campus featured farmland, barns, livestock, various workshops, and congregate dwellings in pavilions housing up to ten families each, separated by landscaped courtyards. The complex also featured a chapel and a community center housing a bowling alley and general grocery store. The grounds and agricultural land at Carville were extensive.

The US Columbia River Quarantine Station was opened in 1899 (it closed in 1938) in Naselle, Washington. This complex was established when the US Congress mandated health inspections of all incoming ships, to prevent the spread of infectious disease. The complex consisted of numerous one-level wood frame structures, including dormitories, with other buildings housing permanent on-site support staff and administrators. During its first year of operation, the station screened 6,120 people arriving on 97 sailing vessels and 35 steamships. By the 1920s, the number of immigrants coming from Asia had fallen precipitously, due to restrictive immigration laws plus new fumigation methods, thus reducing the need for the station.[31]

Yellow Fever, Dengue Fever, and Typhus

Until 1900, little definitive knowledge existed concerning how diseases were transmitted inside hospitals. One such disease, typhus—first identified in 1546 by the father of epidemiology, Girolamo Fracastoro (1478–1553)—had been variously referred to as war fever, ship fever, jail fever, and camp fever. It spread rapidly in hospitals among those patients in large open wards. A high transmissibility rate was compounded by the fact that specific contagious diseases were still difficult to isolate.[32] Nightingale, while a proponent of open wards, recognized the importance of isolation, with some entire wards devoted to the highly contagious. She advocated for sanitary conditions in hospitals and patients' direct visual contact with nature, including windows with apertures reaching up to ceilings high above the patient's bed, yet with low sill heights, so the bedridden could feel connected with the outdoors, sunlight, and fresh air. Her influence significantly declined after 1945, although most urban hospitals in the Americas and Europe still operated their open-plan Nightingale wards, supplemented with isolation rooms and small open-plan isolation wards. Steel frames, curtain wall construction, the newly invented Otis elevator, and electricity allowed these structures to rise to twenty floors and higher. A prime US example of a late Nightingale high-rise hospital is Charity Hospital (1938) in New Orleans.

Tuberculosis

This disease has a long history of causing pain, suffering, and death. Its rise was attributed to the densely populated inner urban, gritty cities of the Industrial Revolution. TB was viewed as a disease of the poor and the working class, the unsanitary, and the medically underserved. In the West and elsewhere, and particularly for the upper classes and the wealthy, fresh air, proper nutrition, and restorative respite away from the city were the principal methods of treatment. Therapeutic natural settings were built for the affluent who wished to escape the ills of the city. Later, when publicly built and operated centers appeared, middle-class individuals and some members of the working class were also sent away from the city for treatment. Patients would be confined to a sanitorium for months or even years. The sanitarium hospital method of public health treatment for TB was little impacted by advancements in germ theory, with the exception of a newfound emphasis on the mitigation of bacteria-laden phlegm, or sputum. In London, the Royal Chest Hospital was founded in 1814, the Brompton Hospital for Consumption in 1841, and the City of London Hospital for Diseases of the Chest in 1848. Yet these institutions were all designed and built as conventional hospitals. The first documented example in the UK of an institution specifically designed for the open-air treatment of TB patients was the Royal Sea Bathing Infirmary for Scrofula, founded in 1791 by Dr. John Coakley Lettsom (1744–1815), a Quaker physician based in London. He had been convinced of the medicinal amenity of fresh sea air because, as he observed, local fishermen did not suffer from such respiratory ailments.[33]

In Europe, numerous TB sanitoriums were built in the late nineteenth and early twentieth centuries in mountainous locales, where patients in residency could attain rest and solace in bed and by sitting on broad, open-air balconies and landscaped terraces. The Swiss Alps, at Davos, where a resort had existed since 1841, emerged as an ideal locale to inhale therapeutically "pure air." This rediscovered mode of treatment (although the ancient Greeks and Romans had known it long ago) was enthusiastically expressed in a guidebook extolling the virtues, architectural and otherwise, of Davos, published in 1880.[34] Because this place and others like it were so successful, in 1907 a new, expanded TB facility, the Queen Alexandria Sanitorium, opened in Davos, designed entirely without neoclassical ornamentation. This new state-of-the-art hospital-retreat expressed the emerging modernist attitude toward the treatment of this highly transmissible disease. The facility was designed by Otto Pfleghard and Max Haefeli, with engineer Robert Maillart. The physician-architect was becoming a quasi-bacteriologist, and these physicians, with a deep interest in architecture, generated design principles out of the figurative laboratory scrutiny of disease-causing microbes. It is arguable that the practice of architecture itself became bacterially driven. By this time, microbes were both the literal and the metaphorical basis of a new style of architecture and urbanism.

Modern architecture represented this new style, with bright, transparent spaces to promote visual hygiene. The white surfaces and forms of modern architecture were incorporated unambiguously in such structures, to highlight their cleanliness. These sanitoriums were gently sited on mountainsides, in forests, beside lakes, and on coasts, with row upon row of terraces angled toward the sun to heal fragile bodies. This reductionism and its unfettered functionality directly challenged the then-prevailing neoclassical aesthetic in architecture. It is as if the discipline had taken the cure, with TB sanitoriums modernizing architecture itself. Their deep-set sun terraces served as crucial medical instruments, with the entire building ultimately functioning as a heliotherapy device. Even the beds were suspended in metal frames, to enable them to be rotated up to a steep angle, aligned to allow the maximum benefits of heliotherapeutics.[35]

Inside, everything was being rethought and redesigned to promote maximum visual openness and healthfulness—furniture, equipment, door handles, window treatments, wall and floor surfaces, ceilings, lighting—all in support of the belief that pollution-free temperate climates and nature were the best treatments for TB. This view would persist well into the mid-twentieth century. In the US, sanitoriums were built on seashores and in the mountains, in the deserts of the American Southwest and in the Adirondacks, remote from large urban industrial centers. This was the era when the American wilderness became fashionable as a place to vacation and obtain respite from urban ills. The success of heliotherapy and ultraviolet ray therapy demonstrated that lungs respond well to sustained therapeutic exposure to the natural environment.[36] By the 1950s, North Carolina's public health board was granted legal authority to commit a diagnosed TB patient to prison if that person refused a period of residency at the state-run sanitorium, located in the mountains of western North Carolina near Asheville—a reprise of the legal authority bestowed on public health tribunals centuries earlier.

Architecturally, the most famous sanitorium of the twentieth century was Alvar Aalto's Paimio Sanitorium (1929–1932), built near Helsinki, Finland. It fused the new modernist ideology and aesthetic with the timeless therapeutic affordances of nature and landscape immersion. The hospital's slender residential wings rose up above the landscape, and its broad roof terraces on each level functioned as open-air treatment sites. This institution's remoteness from the city similar to its medieval precursors.[37] Paimio continues to receive well-deserved praise for its visionary fusion of modernism with best public health and medical health practices, many of which dated from ancient Greece. By the 1950s, observers extolled the therapeutic powers of nature and landscapes:

> Sanitorium life is a reaction against the stuffy, overheated hospital rooms of bygone days. Patients now take in outdoor treatment whatever the weather. Wide open windows and curative outdoor balconies . . . [and] wrapping oneself in blankets is an essential part of the cure, almost a ritual. Like any new drug, fresh air is taken in with a vengeance along with rest and exercise. . . . It is a healthy, restful, peaceful life . . . making the sanitorium a haven for the tuberculosis patient. It is an atmosphere that Shelley experienced, and expressed in the poem "Euganean Hills":

> *Soft sunshine and the sound*
> *Of old forests echoing round*
> *And the light and smell divine*
> *Of all the flowers that breathe and shine:*
> *We may live so happy there,*
> *That the spirits of the air,*
> *Envying us, may even entice*
> *To our healing paradise*
> *The polluting multitude.*[38]

By the late twentieth century, tuberculosis was closely associated with persons and populations suffering from health inequities—the poor and the medically underserved—along with ineffective or nonexistent local public health care agencies. Then, and to this day, the medically underserved remain prone to contracting TB, despite the availability of a new generation of antibiotics. Antibiotic-resistant strains of TB keep emerging, however, rendering a fully reliable, effective vaccine an elusive goal (fig. 2.11).

The Spanish Flu Pandemic of 1918–1920

In the nineteenth century, three major influenza pandemics occurred: in 1830–1831, 1833, and again in 1889–1890. In the case of the third pandemic, known as the Russian flu, millions of deaths occurred in Europe, the

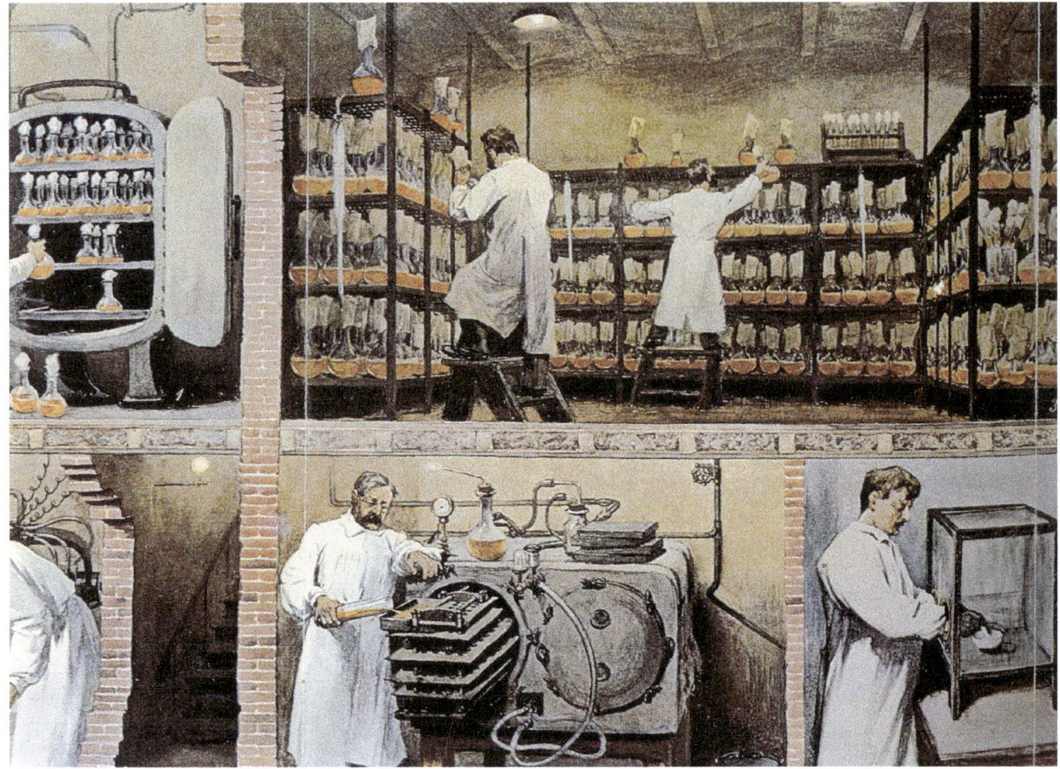

Figure 2.11. Laboratory preparing tuberculosis serum in Marburg, Germany, showing the various stages of the process. Painting by Fritz Gebeke, 1906. Courtesy of akg-images, London, UK.

Americas, New Zealand, and Australia. During the Boer War in South Africa, every infectious disease patient's bed was provided with a mosquito net (fig. 2.12). Nonetheless, the global influenza outbreak that began in 1918 claimed the lives of as many as 30 million worldwide. By contrast, deaths from all causes sustained by the armies that fought in WW I (1914–1918) were estimated at 8.5 million. In early 1918 a wave of an unusual strain of H1N1 influenza appeared, most likely having originated in the US. By that fall, a tidal wave of contagion commenced, followed by a third wave in winter 1918–1919. This pandemic had gestated in the crowded conditions of military camps in the US and the trenches of the Western Front in Europe during WW I. The virus traveled with military personnel from camp to camp at the height of America's military involvement. At its most virulent peak, the virus had sickened 20–40 percent of all enlisted US Army and Navy personnel. Moreover, this pandemic inadvertently diverted urgently need resources away from essential combat-theatre medical support and equipment.[39]

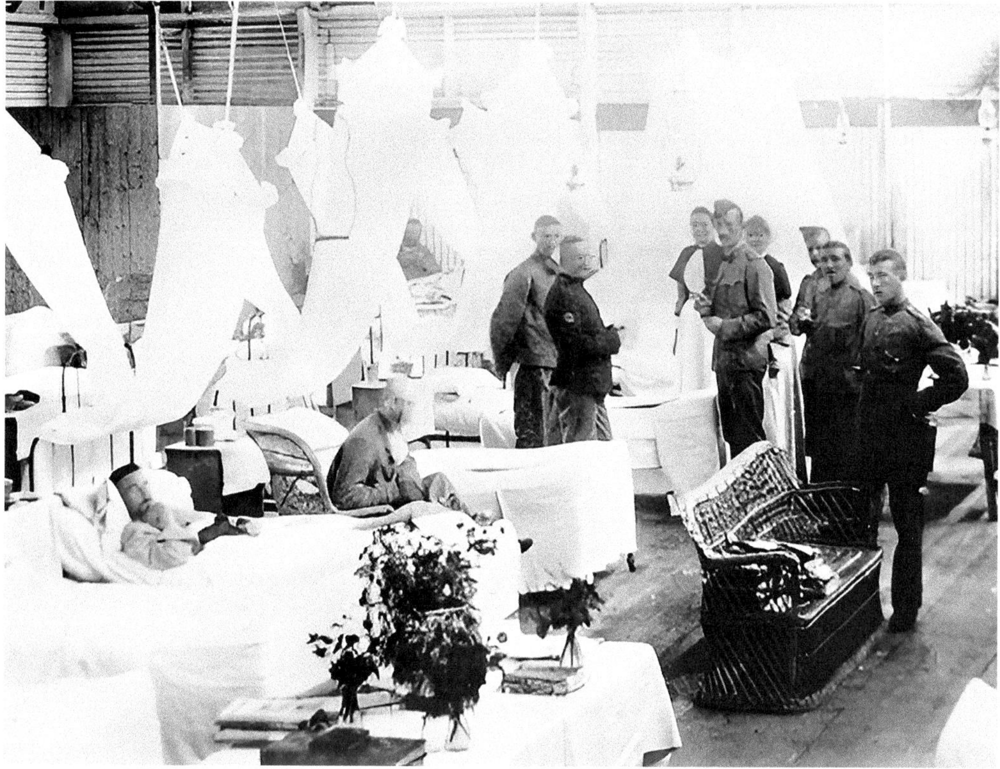

Figure 2.12. Australian Army field hospital in South Africa during the Boer War. Note the mosquito netting over patients' beds. Courtesy of Australian War Memorial, Campbell, Canberra, Australia.

Memories of traumatic events such as wars and destructive pandemics are notoriously vivid and inaccurate, yet fragmentary recollections often provide the most valuable information available concerning the nature of events such as this.[40] Remembering forgetfully perhaps accounts for the subsequent historical disengagement from this pandemic, as well as why so little was written in its aftermath or about the role of the architectural environment.[41]

Erich Remarque, in the classic WW I novel *All Quiet on the Western Front,* noted the hazardous interdependency between influenza outbreaks and troop unreadiness in combat theatres: "We have almost grown accustomed to it; war is a cause of death like cancer and tuberculosis, like influenza and dysentery. . . . Shells, gas clouds, and flotillas of tanks—shattering, corroding, death. Dysentery, influenza, typhus—scalding, choking, death."[42] The military's public relations focus was to highlight ongoing military operations and maintain troop readiness during the period when the Spanish flu outbreak raged most intensely. Did this suppression of attention correspond with the need to not provide the enemy with any information that could be used against their opponents in combat operations? Regardless, no new medical facility types were specifically developed in response to this pandemic. On this point, Alfred F. Crosby prophesized the global coronavirus pandemic that would occur twenty-three years later: "Our ability to predict where the next dangerous H1N1 flu strain will appear is enormously complicated by the fact that we share and exchange flu viruses with domesticated mammals, birds, and wild creatures. . . . The next influenza pandemic may hit us from, for instance, China, where people and pigs live in contiguity in thousands of villages, and where new strains may be spawning all the time."[43]

Epidemiological historians often compare the Spanish flu pandemic to the fourteenth-century bubonic plague. Both public health catastrophes came to be characterized, post-event, by a near-identical type of cultural amnesia in the annals of history.[44] Meanwhile, efforts were well underway by this time to address public health in cities and towns. The Garden City movement—a direct reaction to contagious disease—began with Ebenezer Howard's 1898 book, *To-morrow: A Peaceful Path to Real Reform*, republished in 1902 as *Garden Cities of To-morrow*. While its focus was on the therapeutic benefits of urban gardens, Howard sought to alleviate urban unhealthfulness by envisioning a network of new towns with socially integrated populations and mixed land uses.[45]

By 1900 in the UK, land-use zoning laws had been enacted in support of medical and epidemiological efforts to mitigate future public health crises. In 1908, France enacted its first Law for the Public Health Protection. Frederick Law Olmsted, the pioneering American landscape architect who is considered the father of the urban-park-as-nature-refuge movement, believed that urban parks were of equal public health and aesthetic benefits to the residents of increasingly dense, polluted cities. Public health agencies in many jurisdictions globally soon enacted similar single-land-use zoning ordinances. Often these provisos misinterpreted Howard's initial precepts, as the new zoning laws usually resulted in a patchwork quilt of low-density developments that, in the following decades, would come to dominate automobile-dependent, aesthetically characterless urban sprawl in many parts of the world, with its harmful public health consequences continuing well into the twenty-first century.[46]

CONTAGIOUS DISEASE IN THE MODERN
MEGAHOSPITAL ERA (EPOCH 5)

Synopsis: In architecture, after 1945 the International Style dominated hospital aesthetics and functionality. In the post–World War I period, health care facility planning emerged as a distinct professional specialization, due to the growing complexities inherent in the hospital-as-machine for healing. Large urban medical centers became the epicenter of the health care universe. Hospitals were constantly playing catch-up to the latest technological advancements in diagnoses and treatments within a constantly changing health care industry. The utopian megahospitals of this period symbolized the apotheosis of a near-total faith in technology—with a hospital running the risk of being branded as architecturally dysfunctional on opening day, due to the accelerated rate of medical technological change. McMaster's Medical Centre (1968–1972) in Hamilton, Ontario, symbolized the apotheosis of this bigger-is-better movement in interstitial hospitals.[47] The interstitial movement would run out of currency by 1990 in North America and elsewhere, due to its 40 percent higher initial construction cost. Instead, smaller hospitals were built, often expressing local vernacular styles and traditions as part of the new postmodern aesthetic sensibility in architecture. Architecturally, these health care facilities rejected the austere minimalism of the International Style—a style dating from the 1920s.[48]

Architects' primary focus: Large institutional clients and private benefactors.

Predominant building types: Large urban medical centers, suburban community hospitals, and long-term care nursing institutions, with a correspondingly decreased focus on TB sanitoriums and state-run residential psychiatric institutions. Now the emphasis was on networks of primary care and specialized community-based ambulatory care clinics in local settings, and on the emerging hospice movement—a building type that symbolized a complete rejection of the modern hospital.[49]

Interestingly, architectural literature on the history of the twentieth-century, high-tech, International Style hospital makes scarce mention of the intersection of architecture and pandemics. Until 1938 and the beginning of WW II, the Nightingale open ward continued (by and large) to drive the functional planning of hospitals. By the 1920s, specialized freestanding hospitals had been built to specifically treat contagious disease patients. In the US, more than thirty infectious disease hospitals were in operation in the mid-1930s. But by the mid-1950s, most of these institutions had closed (with the exception of the few remaining TB sanitoriums). A dismissal of the therapeutic value of nature and landscapes in the treatment of infectious diseases would have lasting consequences, as would become apparent in the COVID-19 pandemic decades later.[50] After 1945, the intensive care unit became the widely accepted standard as the most effective way to treat the extremely ill. The emphasis was now increasingly on pharmaceutical intervention (antibiotics) and advanced medical technology (ventilators), versus the autonomous infectious disease hospital's prior emphasis on non-pharmaceutically based physical separation, isolation, and a greater degree of communality with nature and landscapes.[51]

A generation of new suburban hospitals were constructed at the urban periphery, connected to the urban core by newly built superhighways. Longtime urban residents in many cities in North America mass-migrated to the booming suburbs. This post–World War II migration left behind the poor and the medically underserved—populations who often experienced greater social and racial discrimination. In North America and in many other places, the neighborhoods where these older hospitals had been located witnessed economic disinvestment after WW II, as new capital investment was diverted elsewhere. In the 1946–2000 period, this, combined with a wave of impressive and even transformative medical science developments, made architecture more subservient than perhaps ever before. With medical science expanding unabated, so did hospitals. To provide some overview of these complex and contradictory developments in history, a chronological timeline of key developmental events in the intersection between architecture, public health, and urban health is represented in a three-part diagram (fig. 2.13). The first five associated epochs (of six overall, to date—see chapter 7) are represented in these diagrams. Landmark events are cited as occurring along a space-time continuum, beginning with the Ancient epoch to the present. These five epochs cover various significant events, including the coronavirus pandemic. An emerging sixth epoch in the Anthropocene—the Meta-Healthscape—and its associated diagrammatic timeline is discussed at length in chapter 7.

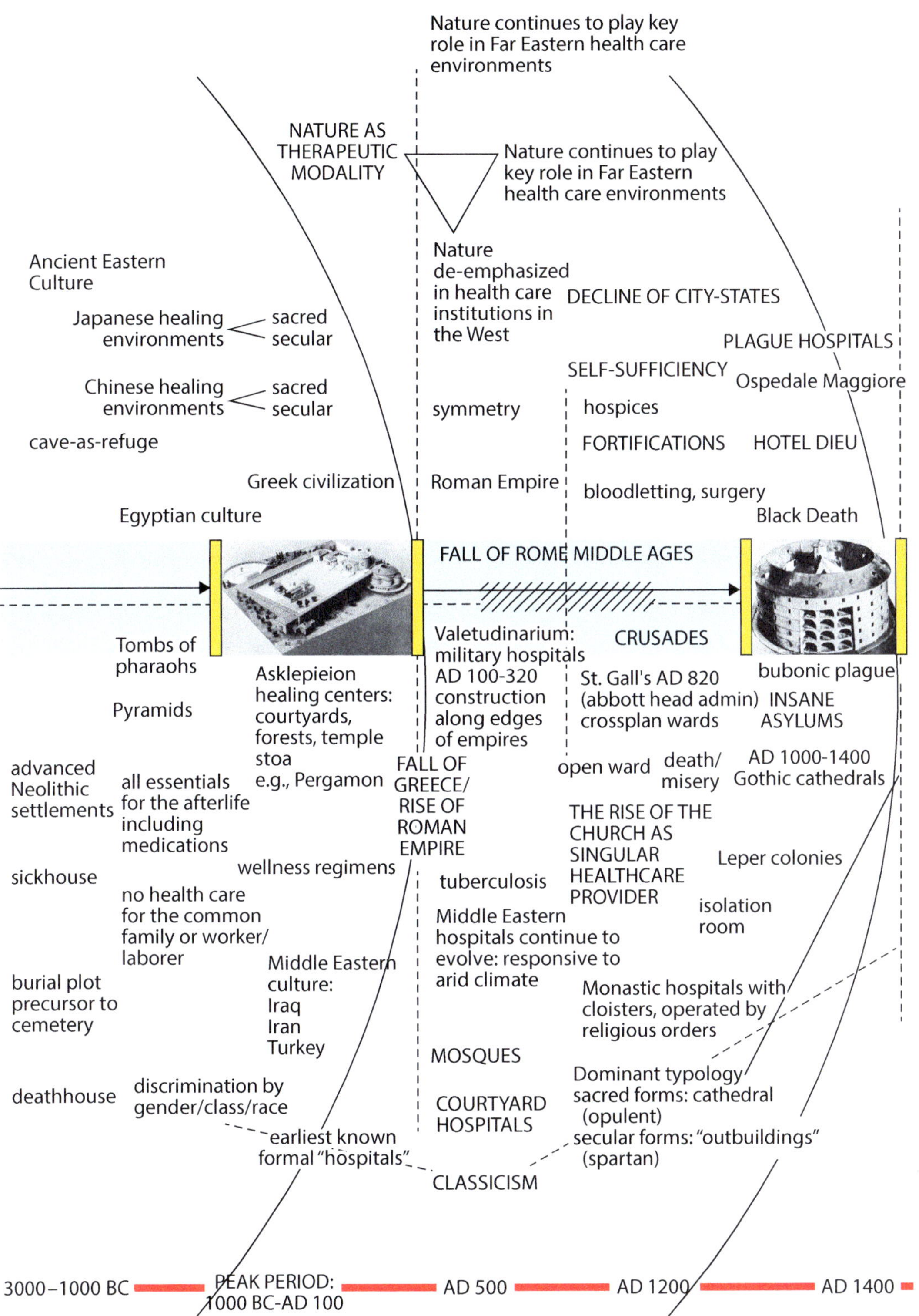

Figure 2.13a. Landmark developments in the history of architecture and health (epochs 1–5). Diagrams by Stephen Verderber.

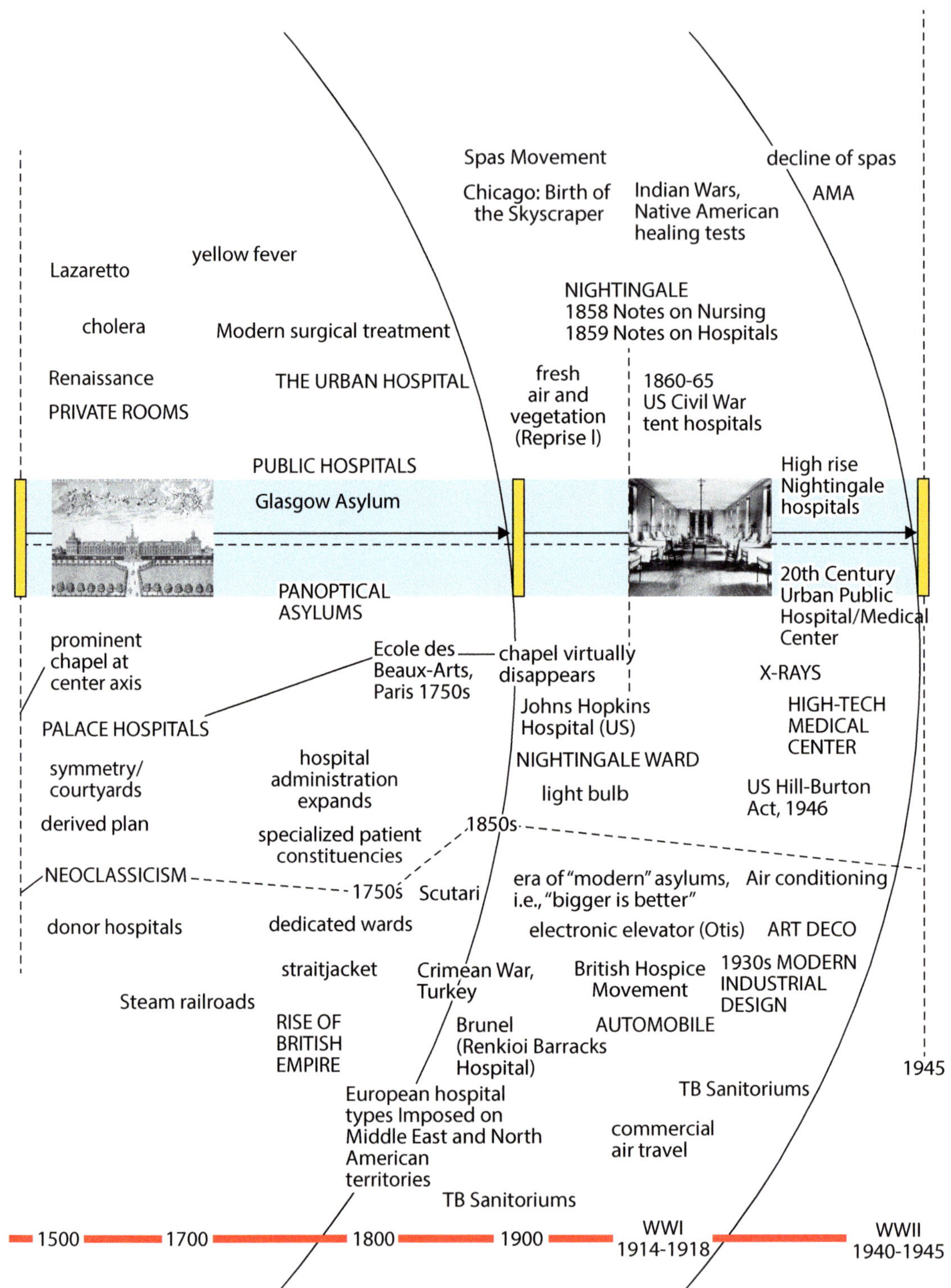

Figure 2.13b. Landmark developments in the history of architecture and health (epochs 1–5). Diagrams by Stephen Verderber.

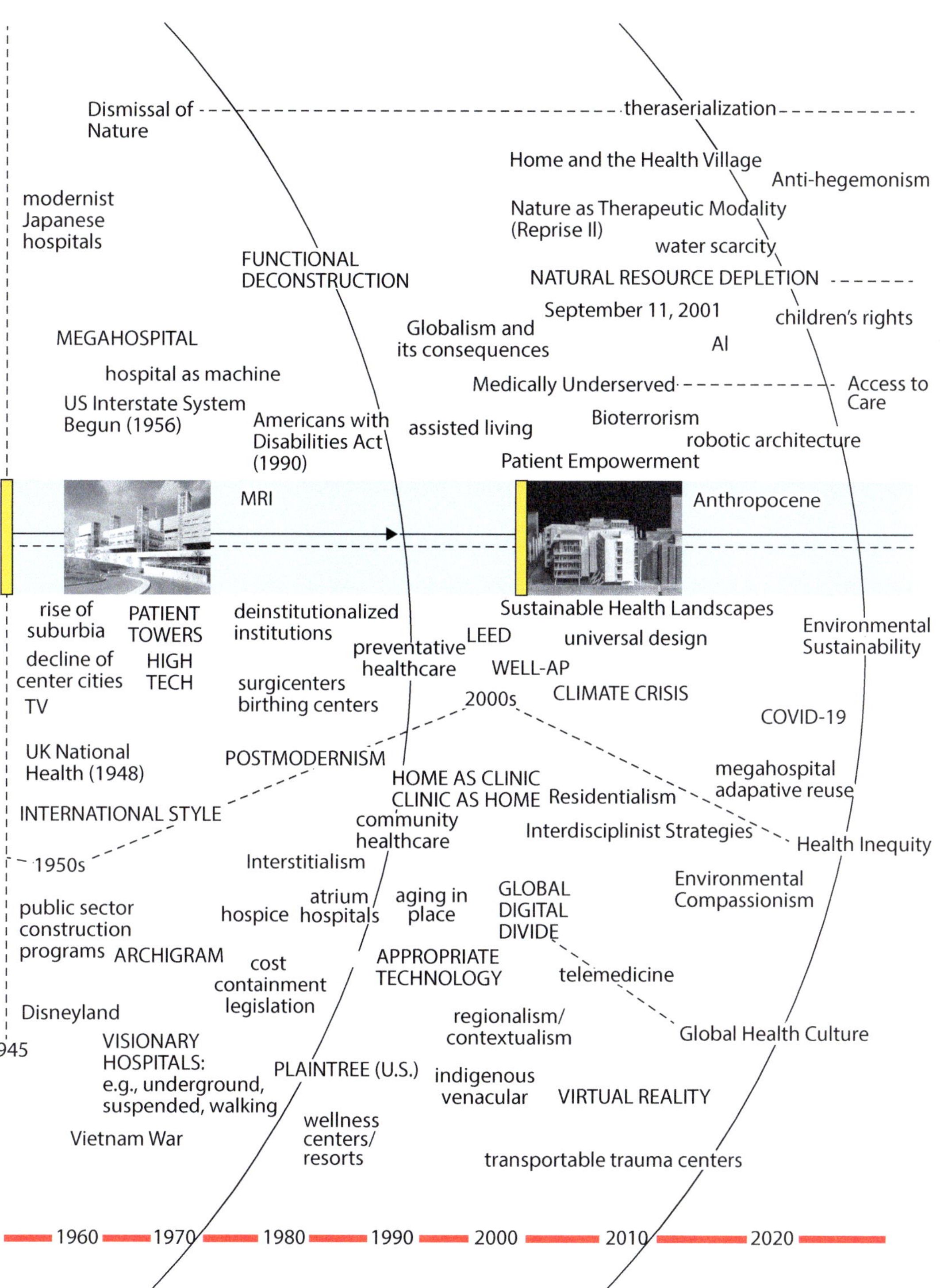

Figure 2.13c. Landmark developments in the history of architecture and health (epochs 1–5). Diagrams by Stephen Verderber.

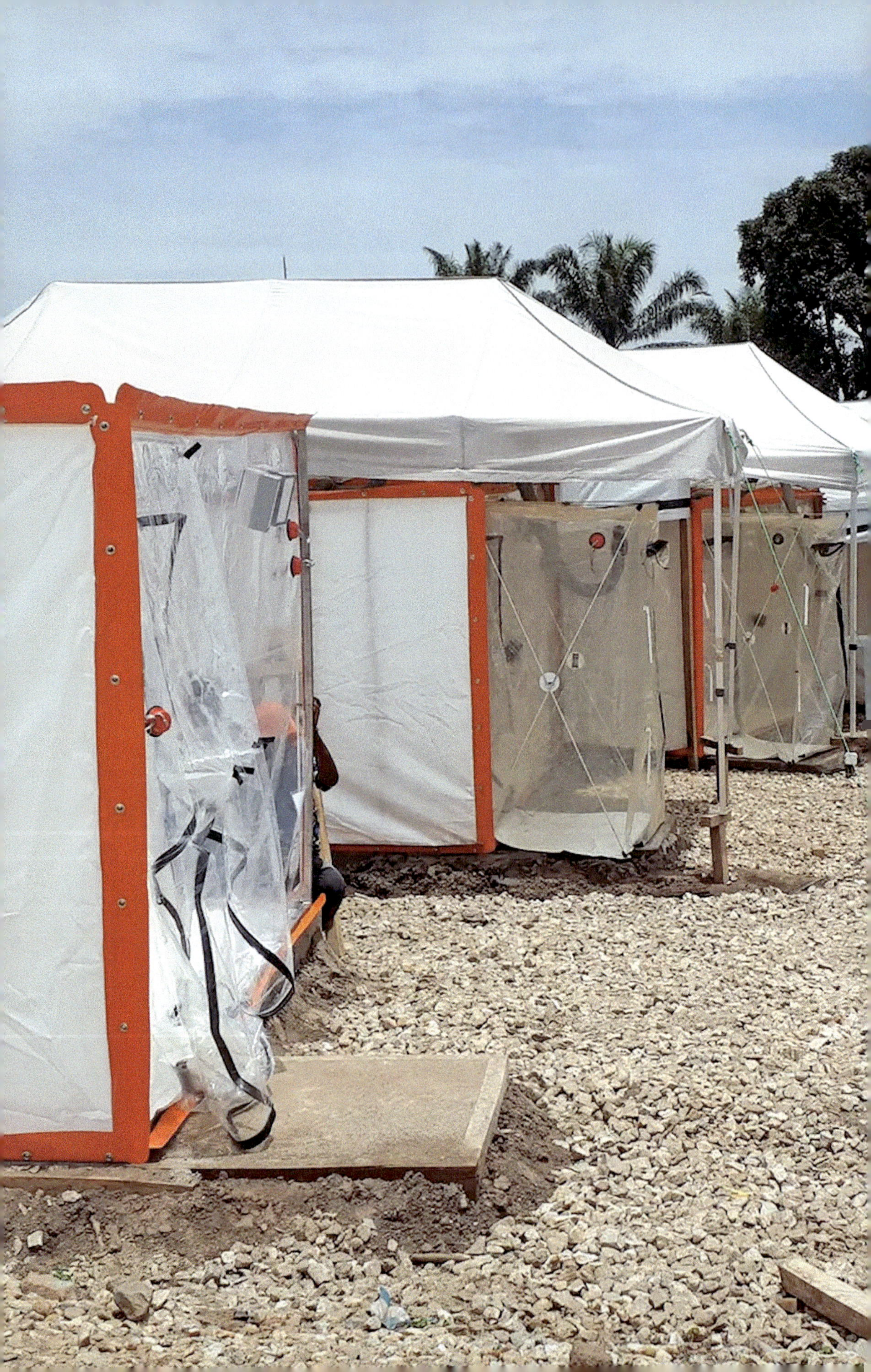

Chapter 3

Pandemical Architecture for Health

COVID-19

INTRODUCTION

Throughout history, pandemics and plagues have led to mandated lockdowns and quarantine measures. During the recent Ebola outbreak in West Africa (2014–2016), nations imposed near-total lockdowns in an attempt to thwart widespread contagion. Some stricken communities became so fearful of their local hospital that they assiduously avoided contact with it, resulting in hospital abandonment.[1] Similarly, the COVID-19 pandemic caused widespread dislocation, pain, and suffering, to a degree rivaling the Spanish flu pandemic (1918–1920) a century earlier. The latter event infected nearly 500 million people—nearly one-third of the world's population—in four waves, with a death toll estimated at between 20 and 50 million. It ranks among the deadliest pandemics in recorded history. The coronavirus pandemic resulted in 704 million cases and over 7 million deaths, as of April 2024.[2] Early on, proactive governments—such as in Israel, Italy, and New York City—sprang into rapid-response mode. The Chaim Sheba Medical

Figure 3.1. ALIMA Cube installation, West Africa, during the Ebola outbreak, 2020. Courtesy of ALIMA (Alliance for International Medical Action).

Center at Tel HaShomer in the greater Tel Aviv area quickly set up an underground forty-five-bed COVID-19 intensive care unit (ICU) surge hospital in its parking deck in just seventy-two hours.[3] In Spain, two expansive halls of Barcelona's Olympic Vall d'Hebrón municipal sports center were repurposed into a temporary 132-bed surge hospital, and the city later set up two additional temporary surge hospitals, both in repurposed sports arenas.[4] In Guayaquil, Ecuador, however, the health care system completely collapsed. At the height of an outbreak there in early 2020, bodies were crudely being wrapped in plastic and placed at curbside to await initial transfer to a municipal sports stadium and then to the central morgue.[5]

Since the 1960s, the movement in architecture known as public interest (PI) architecture has strived to ameliorate shelter and health care inequities. Much PI work has happened ad hoc, with services donated by individual architects and architectural firms on a pro bono basis. A vast percentage of this community-based work had not received the attention it deserved, and this insufficient recognition persists. For most architects, this has been a missed opportunity, with relatively few professional architects and firms in wealthy countries devoting any real percentage of their time and expertise to demonstrably standing in the eye of this storm—that is, lending their expertise in responding to public health emergencies and other disasters. First responders require immediate assistance, and rapidly deployable temporary structures for housing and other uses could have made a difference. But, capitalism being what it is, most architects still work mainly for wealthy individuals, corporations, institutions, and governmental entities—all of whom are able to pay full professional fees and, in exchange, expect to receive highly tailored professional services. This fee-for-service modus operandi has been antithetical to the PI movement in architecture. Professional architects design only 2–5 percent of all buildings constructed annually in North America.[6] Meanwhile, the United Nations expects the number of medically underserved persons worldwide to reach 2 billion by 2050, in a world with 9.7 billion.[7] The disruptions attributed to COVID-19 caused economic displacement, with many of those who were impacted tumbling into unsustainable emergency shelter conditions. COVID-19 opened the door for PI architecture to be part of the solution. Unfortunately, the reality is that engineers continued to dominate the provision of portable facilities for health care throughout the pandemic (fig. 3.1)—with architects still too often relegated to the sidelines, mainly for being labeled as poor first responders.[8]

Public health specialists and health care organizations, by contrast, must function as effective first responders, often in a matter of hours and days, not months or years. Nonetheless, the need was great for well-designed modular prefabricated tents, containerized structures, hybrid configurations, and pop-up testing/treatment facilities to help mitigate disease transmission rates and the geographic dispersion of the coronavirus. The structures that did appear were often bare-bones types, typically erected in medical center parking lots and diverse, remote, often random installation sites. They were commissioned as pop-up COVID-19 testing sites, laboratories, immunization units, and 24/7 ICU surge facilities, including in the aforementioned convention centers, gymnasiums, and some vacant big box stores. Against this backdrop the aim of this chapter is to present the following:

- *Typological Overview*: To review the four basic modular prefabricated building types: redeployable walk-up/drive-up outdoor pop-up testing and laboratory container-based units (type 1); nomadic testing and immunization units (type 2); pop-up units installed in repurposed host structures (type 3); and hybrid 24/7 autonomous infectious disease treatment facilities (type 4). Many are lift-pack systems, meaning they are manufactured off-site and transported to the field via truck, rail, air, ship, or some combination thereof. These can be freestanding structures or ones erected within repurposed host buildings.
- *Salutogenic and Biophilic Amenities*: To examine this architectural typology vis-à-vis certain pertinent salutogenic and biophilic design principles—that is, indoor-outdoor visual connections, personal privacy, and patient (and staff) dignity, in accord with sociocultural and political narratives, together with the degree to which this typology expresses Vitruvian precepts of commodity, firmness, and delight. Both unbuilt and built proposals are reviewed.
- *Field Deployment Protocols*: To describe, from public health policy, medical, and facility-commissioning perspectives, the facility-related staffing and operational issues required to successfully deploy and put into field operation rapid-response facilities in disaster strike zones in diverse geographic and cultural contexts. Basic administrative, medical protocol, and deployment challenges are briefly outlined.

ARCHITECTURE AND PREFABRICATION

Why premanufactured buildings for health care? An influential book written twenty years ago by two Philadelphia architects, Stephen Kieran and James Timberlake, presented an alternate paradigm for a more socially and ecologically responsible ideological approach to the practice of architecture. In *Refabricating Architecture*, they extolled the virtues of off-site prefabrication in the twenty-first century.[9] They argued that in the past, craftsmanship had been the commonly accepted cultural wellspring of all manufactured commodities within a society, but that today, machines have widely supplanted the function of traditional handcrafting. Pioneering twentieth-century architects had pursued a brand of utopianism made implicit in machine-based production processes. But their oft-failed experiments today serve as a cautionary tale of idealism overrun by a host of counterintuitive forces. As the construction industry consolidated in the 1960s and 1970s, repeated failures were made in off-site prefab components, particularly with respect to then-emerging, just-in-time manufacturing platforms.

As Kieran and Timberlake pointed out, the global automotive industry is currently dominated by integrated production platforms. In epicenters of modular platform manufacturing, like this one, individual components are completed in diverse geographic locales and then fitted together in one place in the final stage of the assembly process. In the auto industry, design and production teams are formed at the very outset to design and procure each independent module. All modular components are preassembled off-site, with every part—down to each screw—defined and controlled by a 3D-process template that details all functions and installation procedures. Pretesting occurs iteratively, and quality control gates exist at all stages, requiring certification before construction can advance to the next stage. This results in excellent quality control, more construction options, less production time, and a lower final cost for the finished product. Every autonomous module arrives complete and ready to be installed. Why can't this approach work with rapid-response architecture for health? The most obvious impediment remains the construction industry itself.

Currently, the final product for most buildings only emerges at the end of an excessively protracted traditional construction process—virtually the same way structures have been built for hundreds of years. And this is how many construction industry labor unions want it to remain.[10] It seems logical to extend this auto industry reasoning to health care architecture, particularly in the context of the climate crisis and persistent health inequities, even through a significant percentage of the North American construction industry, as represented by its powerful unions, continues to be "threatened" by off-site, prefab, modular manufactured construction. This resistance to change in the face of shifting external realities is rooted in its perceived threat to hundreds of thousands of conventional construction jobs. Interestingly, against this backdrop, in the early months of the COVID-19 pandemic, numerous prefab modular architectural proposals were published online by architectural design teams based in various parts of the world. These originated from developed as well as less-developed countries and collectively represented all four of the prefab modular facility types described above. A subset of twenty of these proposals, both unbuilt and built, from the first twelve months of the COVID-19 pandemic is presented below.

Autonomous Walk-Up Units (Type 1)

COVID-19 Mobile Unit

This unbuilt modular unit, designed by the firm M-RAD, based in Santa Monica, California (US), is essentially a trailer pulled by another vehicle (fig. 3.2). It is fabricated in lightweight steel and depicted here in a salmon hue, with the option to imprint patterns and textures on its outer panels. It features three testing stations, each with a window with a circular pass-through portal. An outward-projecting panel affords a modicum of privacy, serving as a personal distancing device. Three nurses would staff this unit. A portable lift allows an individual in a wheelchair to be elevated to standing height to administer a COVID-19 nasal swab test (CNST). This prototype, however, is not equipped for on-board immunizations. The unit, as shown, is deployable throughout Los Angeles, including in such well-known settings as the Santa Monica Pier, along Beverly Hills' Rodeo Drive, and on the sidewalk of Hollywood's Walk of Fame. At night, this installation is dependent on external (streetlight) illumination.[11] It is almost as if one is walking up casually to order a hot dog and fries, not unlike the famous Tail O' the Pup hot dog stand, an iconic commercial vernacular fixture in Los Angeles since the 1930s.

Prefab COVID-19 Test Center

This 20-foot custom-built intermodal shipping container (fig. 3.3)—designed by Grimshaw Architects with SG Block and Osang Healthcare (US)—features a bank of solar panels on the roof; the panels are installed on-site. It has eight walk-up testing stations, with an A/B/C/D footprint (four on each side

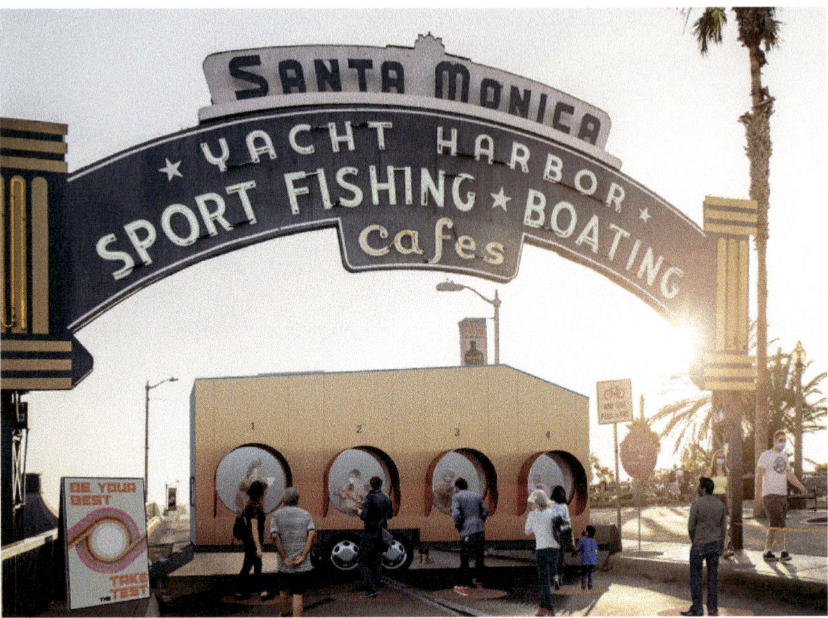

Figure 3.2. COVID-19 Mobile Unit, unbuilt proposal, United States, 2020. Courtesy of M-Rad Architecture, Inc., Los Angeles, California.

of the container unit). A window with a circular opening is provided for administering CNSTs. The testing stations are partially shielded from one another by personal distancing panels. The overall white color of these containers contrasts with their color-accented banding. Additional panels can be installed as rooftop sunscreens. One end of the unit has a sign-in / point-of-contact window, with a staff entrance provided on the opposite end. Staff members housed inside would seem to be rather cramped for space, with little room for medical equipment, including personal protective equipment (PPE), administrative workspace/desks, or storage space for patient specimens. A roof vent ensures the unit's continuous negative air pressurization. This unit sits slightly above the ground. The unit depicted here does not appear equipped to provide immunizations within the container.[12]

Citizen Care Pod

This built prototype—developed by WZMH Architects, PCL Construction, Insight Enterprises, and Microsoft, with Parkin Architects, in the firm's Toronto and Vancouver offices (Canada)—is based on a standard modular intermodal shipping container (fig. 3.4). The white-and-blue exterior provides a backdrop for the International Red Cross logo (readily visible). It is adaptable to various site contexts and functional needs, is reconfigurable, and can be quickly installed on an open site. Its multiple testing stations are somewhat separated from one another by projecting diagonal personal-distancing panels, with identifying testing station numbers. An external clip-on HVAC unit maintains negative air pressurization. Six design options are shown on the firm's home page: (1) with and without solar roof panels; (2) with "outboard" walk-up testing stations; (3) with an inset outer wall panel, presumably to protect patients from the elements; (4) with a drive-up window for testing and another with a pass-through portal for CNSTs; (5) as a single-occupancy "phone booth," where the patient stands outside; and (6) as a double or triple-length hybrid installation for testing and immunizations, combined with an on-board laboratory. The Citizen Care Pod appears adaptable to diverse site and climate installation contexts.[13] An additional option shown on the firm's home page is an elevated step-up unit, similar to the installation depicted here at Vancouver International Airport in British Columbia.

Vehicular Nomadic Units (Type 2)

School Bus Mobile Unit

This is a conventional school bus converted into a rolling COVID-19 testing and immunization unit (fig. 3.5). This relatively inexpensive concept—developed by Perkins & Will, Schmidt Hammer Lassen, and the ARUP Group (US)—calls for repurposing a fleet of conventional school buses, then sending them out to school sites throughout the hinterland. This bus-as-clinic is rapidly deployable to serve medically underserved communities, which is perhaps its main advantage, together with being self-powered. A fleet of repurposed buses can be expanded by simply adding more units to the network. The driver doubles as the first point of contact, and technicians scan patients' barcode data and then administer CNSTs through a plastic protective membrane barrier/window. The extracted specimen may be processed in the on-board lab, with the COVID-19 test result quickly recorded via barcode technology and entered into a central database. The interior of the bus is subdivided into three compartments: (1) administration and registration, (2) testing and laboratory, and (3) staff work / PPE storage zone. Outside, a pull-out canvas tent projecting from the vehicle protects patients from the elements, with tables and chairs set up beneath, functioning as an "outdoor room," including staging areas for waiting and testing/immunization.[14]

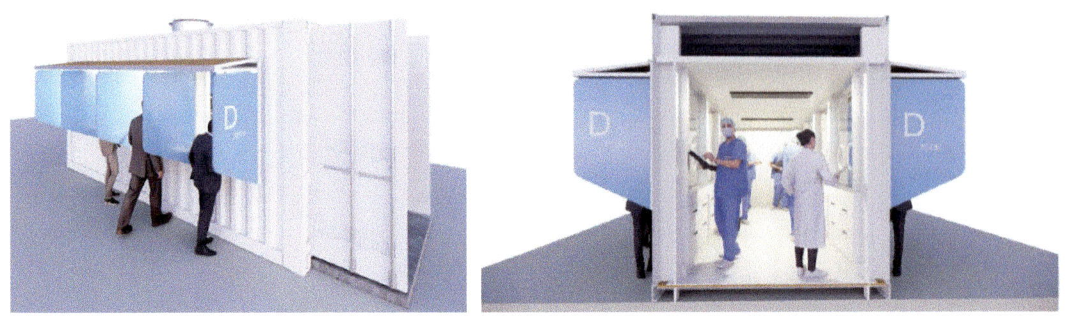

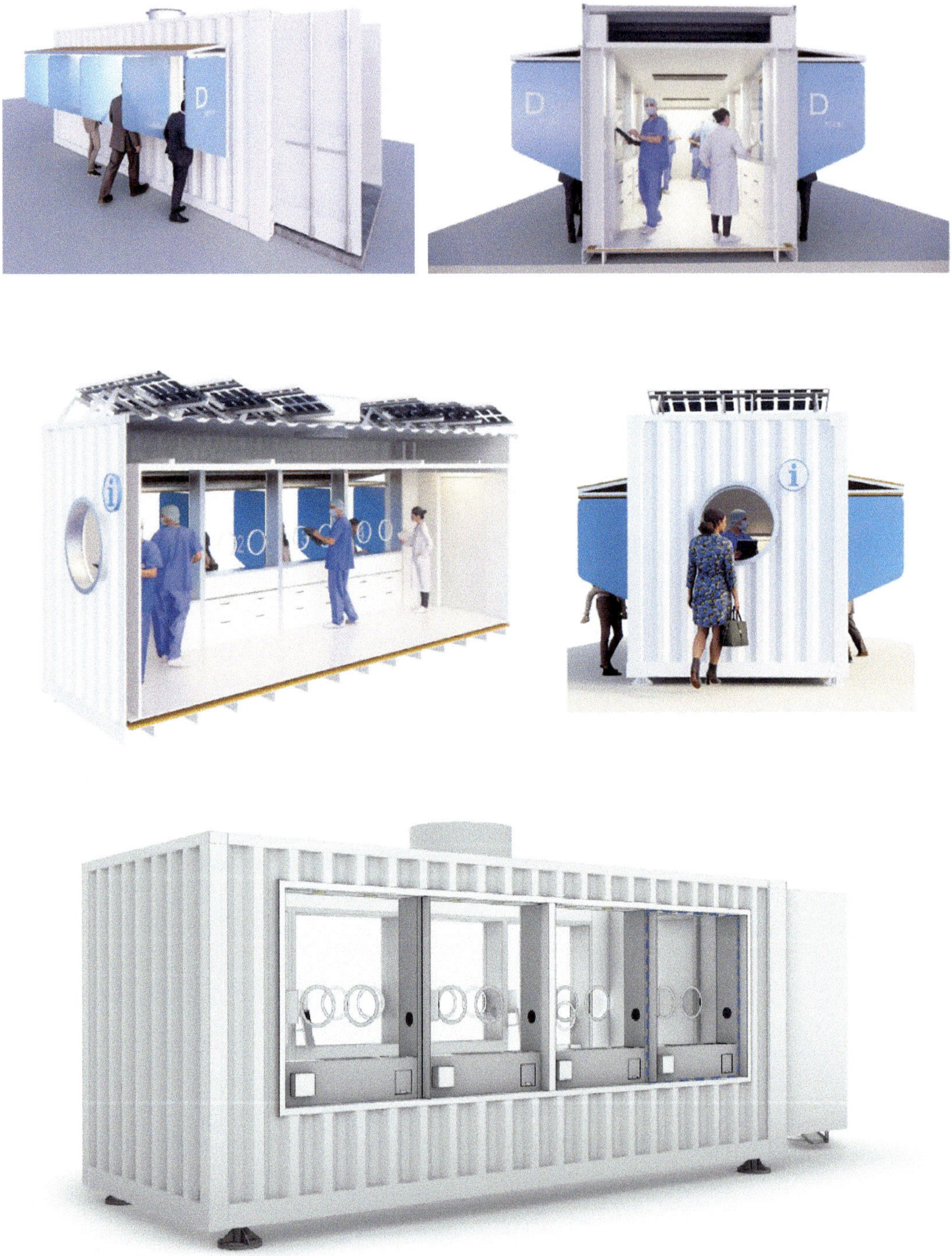

Figure 3.3. Prefab COVID-19 Test Center prototype, United States, 2020. Courtesy of Grimshaw Architects, London, UK.

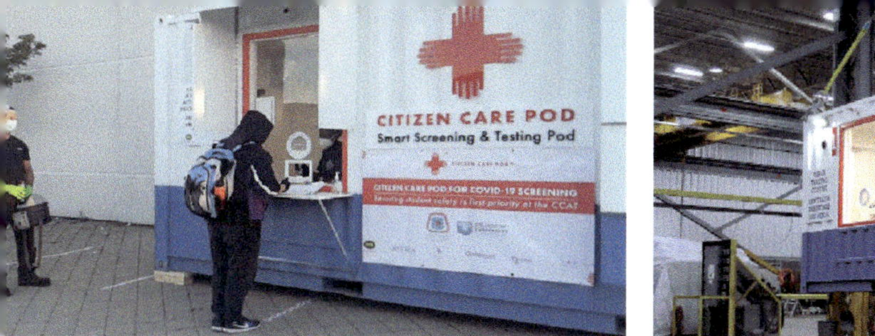
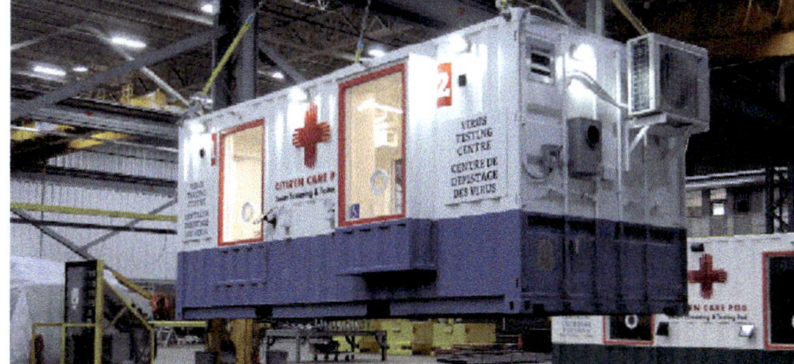
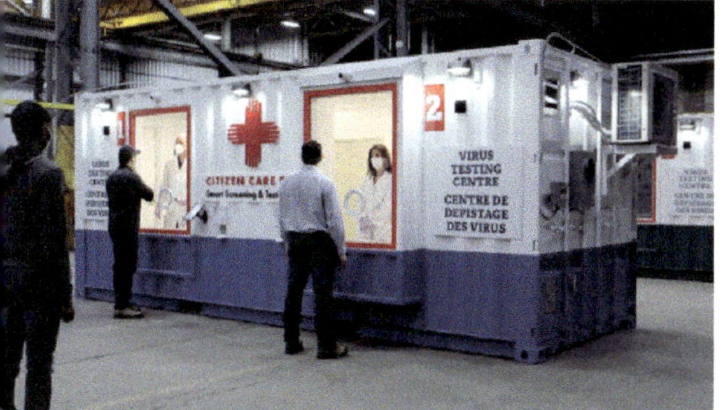
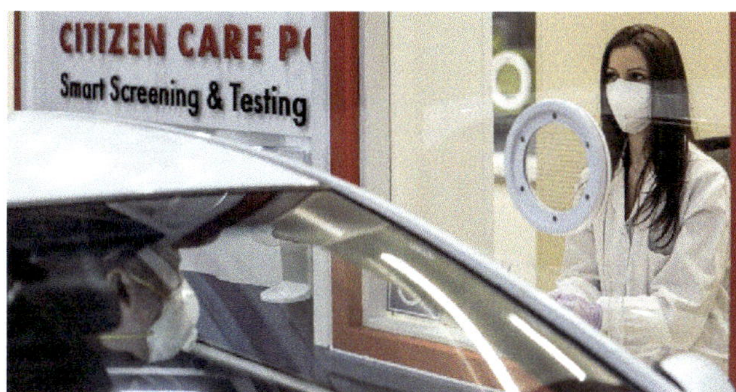

Figure 3.4. Citizen Care Pod, prototype, Canada, 2020. Courtesy of WZMH Architects, Parkin Architects, and PCL Construction, Toronto, Canada

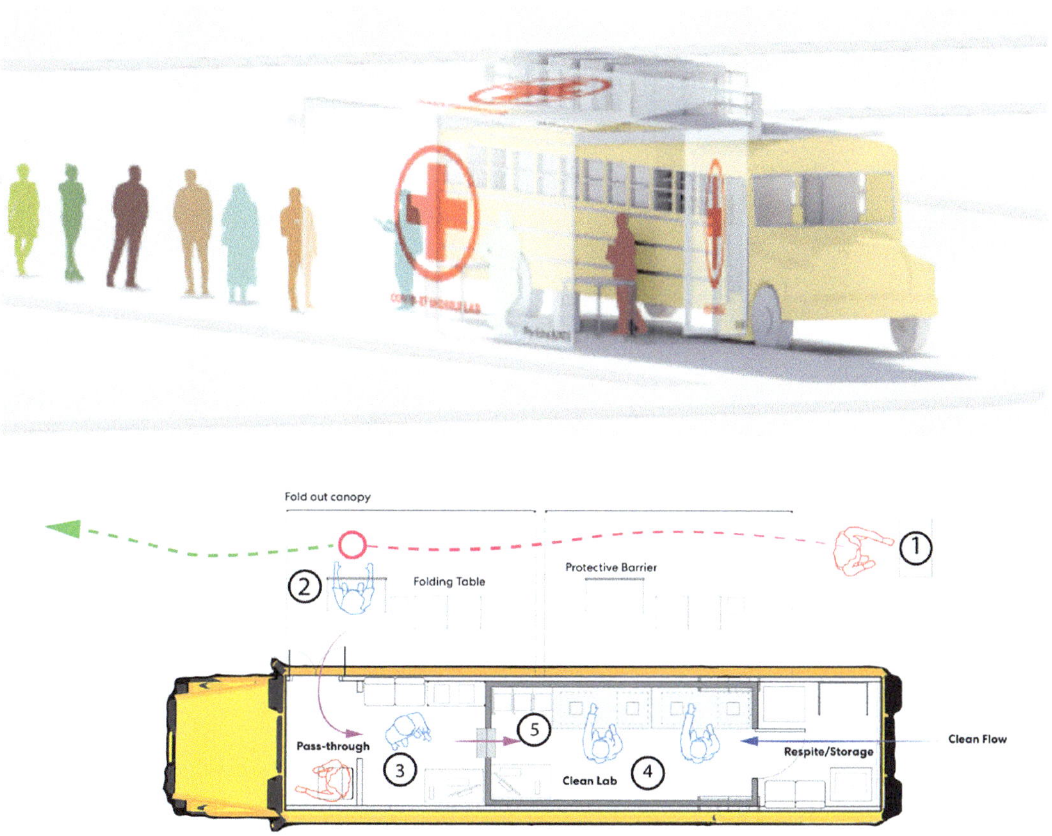

Figure 3.5. School Bus Mobile Unit, unbuilt proposal, United States, 2020. Courtesy of Perkins & Will, Los Angeles, California.

Pop-up Units in Repurposed Host Structures (Type 3)
COVID-19 Superhospital

This unbuilt prototype, designed by Opposite Office, Munich (Germany), is shown installed in the Brandenburg International Airport, recently opened in Berlin (figs 3.6 and 3.7). This pop-up is proposed for installation in one of the terminals close to where travelers board and deplane. With international air travel so drastically curtailed in the pandemic, many airports installed on-site testing units to control community contagion and distribute PPE. This proposal, rather minimalist in appearance, consists of dozens of close-packed semicircular modules, with each module fabricated of Plexiglas. The semicircular patient room modules are equipped with circular white fabric pull curtains and open ceilings, with the curved wall panels of the modules repetitively interweaving, creating an interlocked grid of potentially dozens of modules. The circular patient bedrooms and diagnosis and treatment modules are all housed in this interlocking grid. The airport terminal's HVAC system, electrical and plumbing systems, and restrooms are presumably repurposed in support of this pop-up COVID-19 superhospital. The honey-combed building-within-a-building's modules are visually open, to allow a view of the ceiling high above the patient's bed. The overall visual effect would likely be rather ethereal, if not a bit eerie.[15]

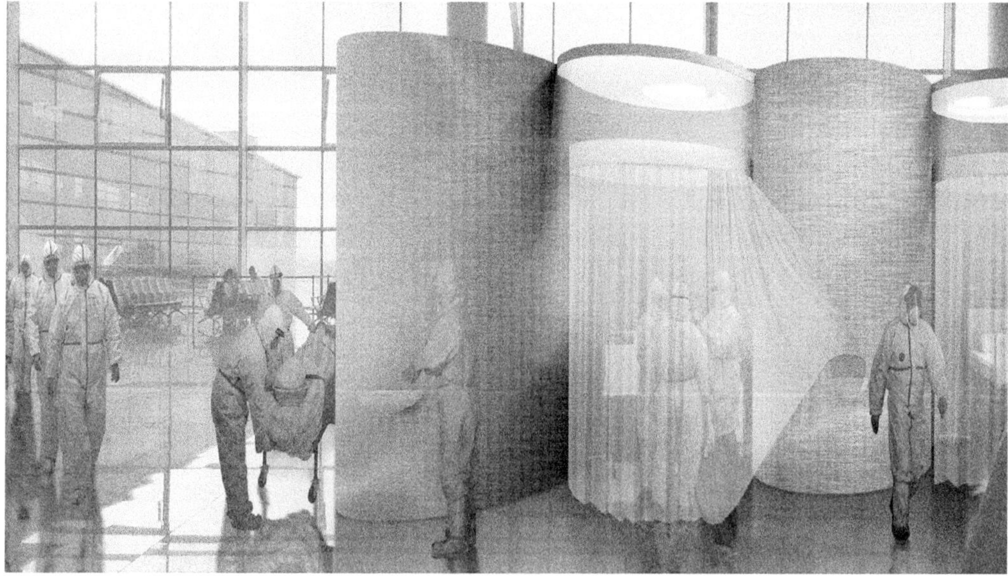

Figure 3.6. COVID-19 Superhospital, unbuilt proposal, Berlin Brandenburg International Airport, Germany, 2020. Courtesy of Opposite Office, Munich, Germany.

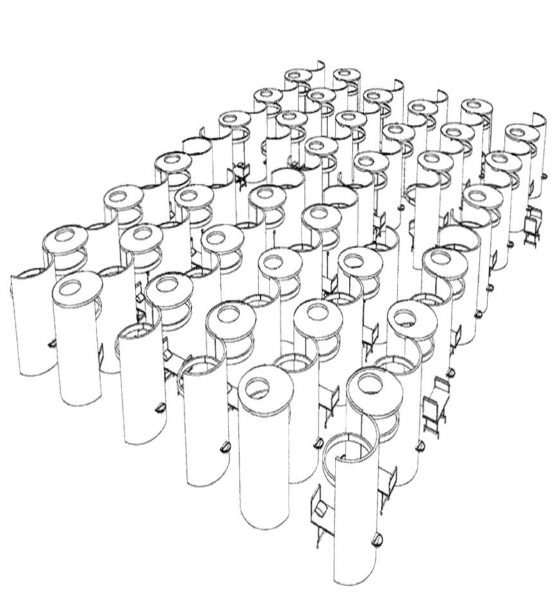
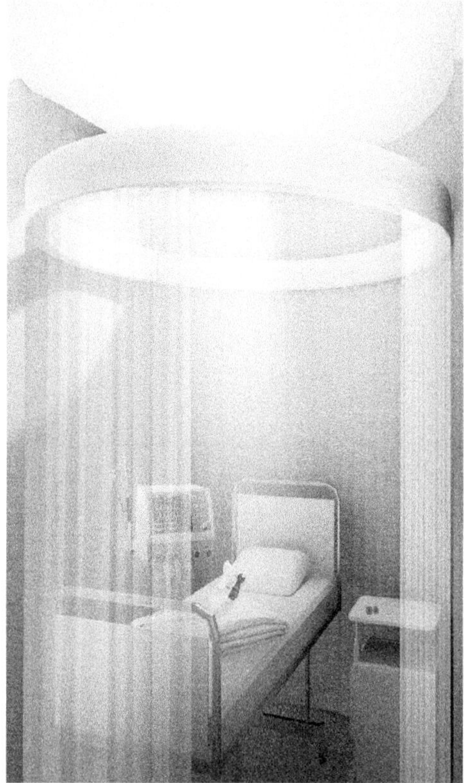

Figure 3.7. COVID-19 Superhospital, unbuilt proposal, Berlin Brandenburg International Airport, Germany, 2020. Courtesy of Opposite Office, Munich, Germany.

COVID-19 Testing Center/Laboratory

In January 2021, more than 22 million people were ordered to lock down in their homes in three cities in China—double the number of citizens the central government required to be locked down the January before in Wuhan (where the coronavirus was first reported in China in late 2019). When this second lockdown was imposed in Shijiazhuang, the local public health authorities mandated the collection of more than 10 million CNSTs over the next three days, totaling nearly one COVID-19 test per every resident in these quarantine zones. Test specimens were immediately sent to the Shijiazhuang pop-up lab (fig. 3.8) and others that had been quickly deployed and installed as pop-up facilities within a wide range of repurposed host structures.[16] As shown here, ten barrel-vaulted, pneumatically supported pop-up testing/lab units are configured in six rows, located in a large, repurposed gymnasium. Each module is structurally autonomous, with its own HVAC system to ensure negative air pressurization. Staff at a sign-in window receive test samples, and the units' vinyl sheathing is manufactured for indoor as well as outdoor installations.

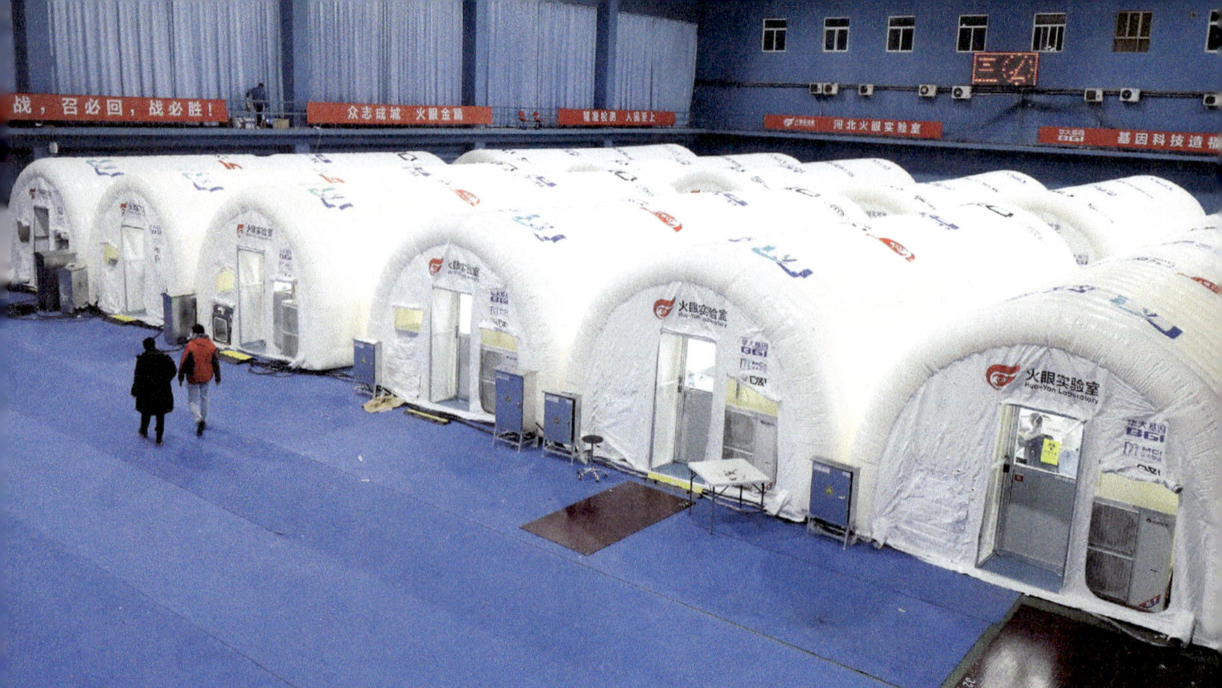

Figure 3.8. COVID-19 Testing Center/Laboratory, Shijiazhuang, China, 2020. Courtesy of Yang Shiyao/Xinhua News Agency and the Associated Press.

University of Toronto Prototypes

The work of architectural students also contributed to this public health/ architectural discourse during the pandemic. In fall 2020, the Architecture + Health graduate-level design studio at the University of Toronto produced a series of proposals for a prefab pop-up testing and immunization unit for (hypothetical) installation in a number of repurposed host structures located across the greater Toronto area (Canada).[17] Two of these prototypes are presented below.

The Circle Clinic: Many outpatient health clinics are needlessly institutional, with their windowless waiting areas, staff work zones, examination and treatment rooms, open-plan staff cubicles, and dreary corridors. Visual interconnectivity between a clinic's constituent rooms and zones is often minimal, at best. This pop-up installation rejects drab institutionalism in favor of color, transparency, and nonorthogonality. The system's components are premanufactured off-site, transported to the host building site in standard shipping containers, brought indoors, and then erected and commissioned. The host structure shown here (fig. 3.9) is a pneumatically supported recreational sports facility, built in 2012, in a large suburb of Toronto. This system's circular modules have interlocking curvilinear walls, fabricated in a mix of full-height translucent and opaque polycarbonate panels. The varied colors of the panels provide differing degrees of translucency while simultaneously affording privacy, as required, thus allowing

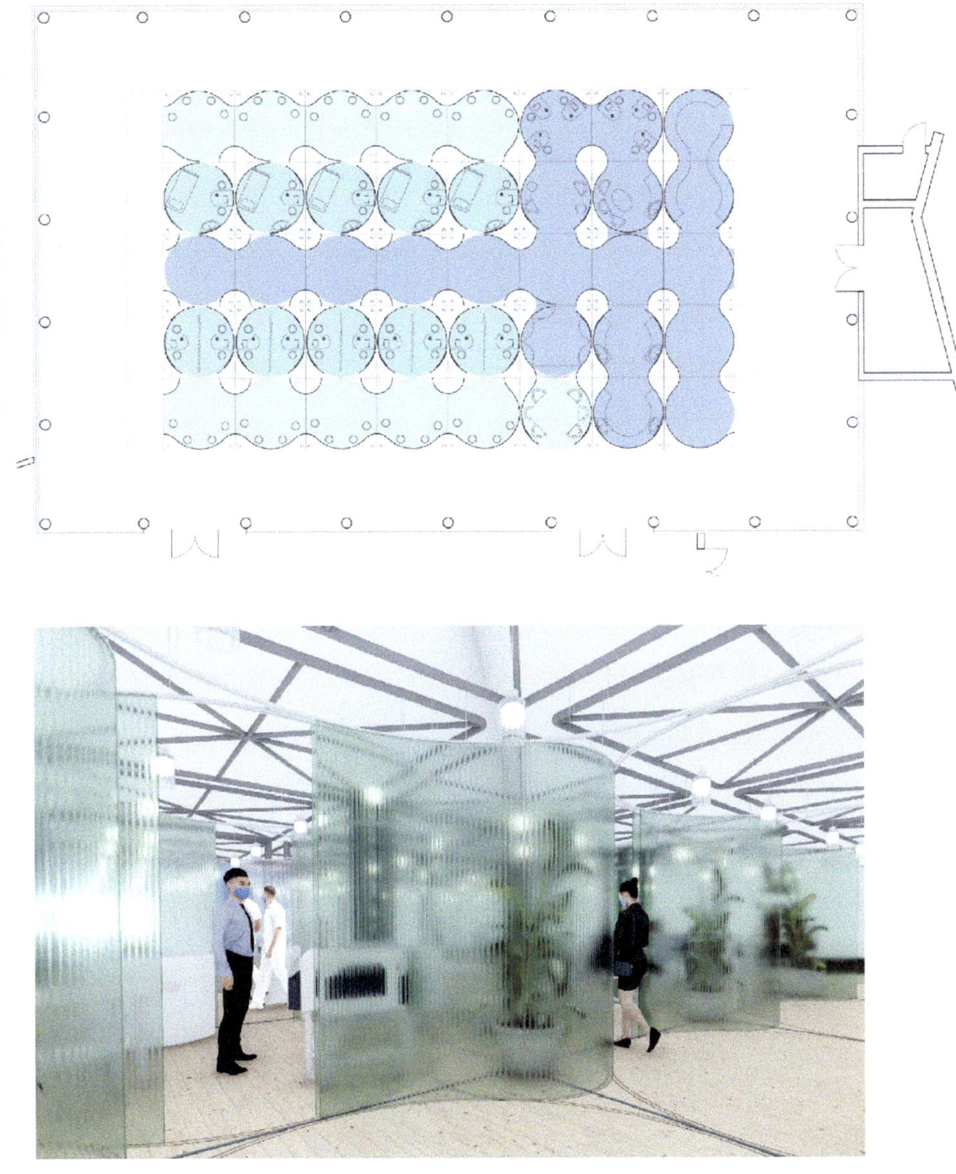

Figure 3.9. The Circle Clinic, unbuilt proposal, University of Toronto, 2020. Image and drawing by Zohar Hekouian Fathi, Yijie Dai, and Stephen Verderber.

daylight and artificial lighting to penetrate into the interiors. This system consists of closely packed modules that are all identical in size and shape, with open ceilings. Its three main internal areas are variously color coded: arrival/intake/waiting/administration zone; examination and testing zone; and treatment zone. Design team: Zohar Nekouian Fathi and Yijie Dai.

The Art Walk Clinic: Evidence-based design research for health care has identified the importance of artworks as a source of positive therapeutic distraction, providing a cognitive benefit to patients, caregivers, and patients' families. This type of positive sensory stimulation has been empirically linked with stress reduction in health care built environments (discussed in greater depth in chapter 4 and appendix B). In response, this proposal, also a lift-pack pop-up system (fig. 3.10), features the work of established as well as rising Toronto artists. Artworks are displayed on translucent polycarbonate panels installed along the clinic's circulation paths and in the main waiting room. In the installation configuration shown here, a suburban church serves as the clinic's host structure. The judicious placement of art on the various panels establishes a series of coordinated "event zones" and, for facility occupants, perhaps provides an unexpectedly positive distraction. Theatrical staging and illumination further accent the art via footlights installed in the modular floor's inset panels. The design's intent is to alleviate the mental fatigue and stress associated with COVID-19. Design team: Bronte-Morris Poolman and Damian Kercz.

Hybrid 24/7 Autonomous Infectious Disease Treatment Facilities (Type 4)

QurE

The Quarantine Unit for Recovery, Emergency and Ecology (QurE) prototype (not shown) is a prefab emergency quarantine and medical treatment shelter for COVID-19. It was proposed by the National Cheng Kung University (NCKU) and Bio-Architecture Formosana (BAF)—a joint venture between academia and private industry—in Taipei (Taiwan) and unveiled in April 2020 at the NCKU in Tainan City, Taiwan. QurE was jointly developed by NCKU and Taipei city–based BAF. Construction documents and specifications were subsequently made available online through open access. QurE can be constructed in three days and is adaptable to sites with irregular terrain. Airtight floor and wall panels, metal alloys, and thermal insulation panels ensure its continuous negative air pressurization. The goal of this system is to isolate an infected patient in an intensive medical care setting. Natural daylight is transmitted to the interior and perimeter, and double-loaded circulation is provided, as is a patient isolation area. The system is expandable at need, and this prototype was placed on public display on NCKU's campus in spring 2020.[18]

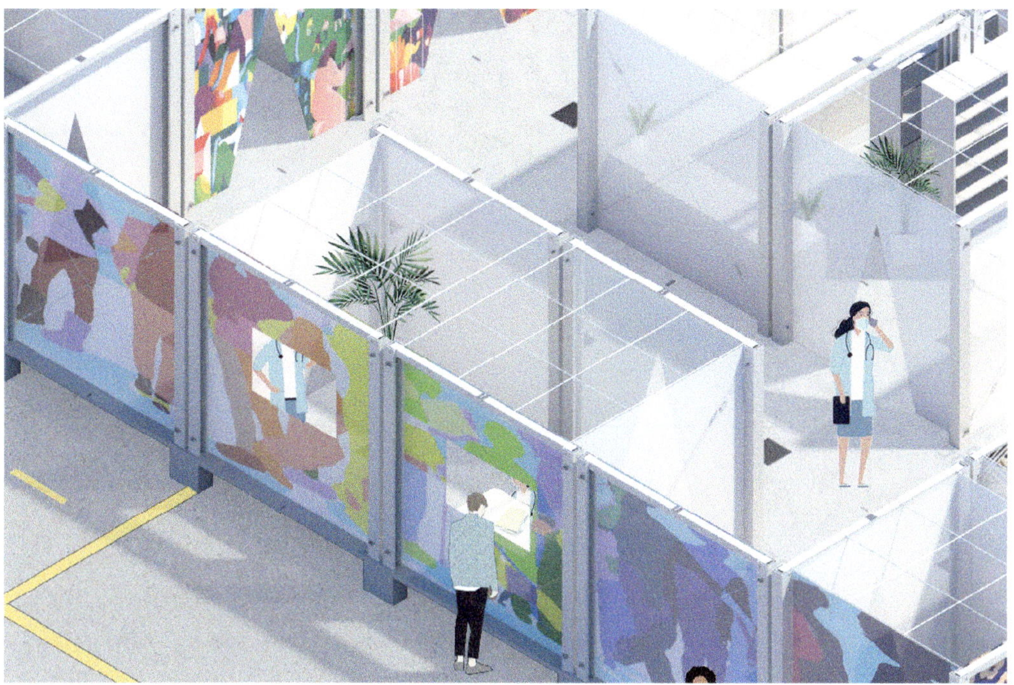

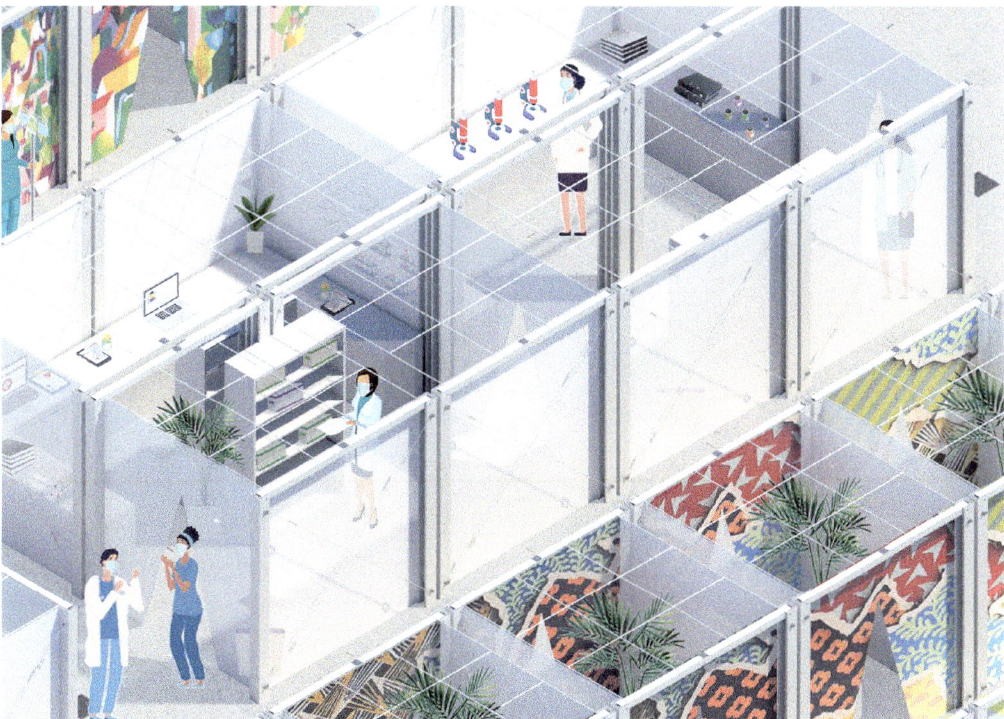

Figure 3.10. The Art Walk, unbuilt proposal, University of Toronto, 2020.
Images by Bronte Morris-Poolman, Damian Kercz, and Stephen Verderber.

Modular Mobile Hospital

VHL Architecture, based in Vietnam, teamed with Da Nang University's School of Architecture to design this unbuilt hybrid pop-up/containerized prefab surge hospital for COVID-19 (fig. 3.11). Based on a 6-meter^2 standard cube, subdivided into three internal zones, the module is 3 meters × 6 meters, and its raised platform consists of lightweight concrete panels. Medical supplies and staff workspaces are housed in cube modules designated with the iconic International Red Cross logo. The dozens of modules are positioned in long rows facing one another, either independently deployed or interconnected. Their interiors appear quite confining, however, and provide little in the way of views or daylight contact with the outside world—especially considering it was ostensibly designed for outdoor installation sites. The basic module can be manufactured as a monolithic unit or a lift-pack that is then fully assembled on-site. In either installation scenario, system components would be delivered by truck. The proposed installation, as shown, requires the ability to navigate a set of narrow exterior steps to reach the module, a condition that would allow scant room for easy egress and ingress. The module's HVAC system and its interlocking utility infrastructure presumably allow connectivity within the network of modules.[19]

Huoshenshan Hospital

The massive Huoshenshan Hospital was very quickly constructed in Wuhan (China) in early 2020 by the Chinese government. The 1,000-bed COVID-19 field hospital shown here (figs. 3.12 and 3.13) was built in fourteen days near Zhiyn Lake in Wuhan. A second field hospital in Wuhan, Leishenshan Hospital, was built just as rapidly, using a nearly identical prefabricated modular concept. This second installation opened in February 2020.[20] These two facilities were based on the Xiaotangshan Hospital, which the government had built in six days, years before, in a suburb of Beijing during the SARS pandemic in 2003. Both of the new prefab hospitals in Wuhan were fully modular, with two levels housing thirty ICUs, nursing and medical support, and dozens of multi-bed quarantine units. Each module was 10 meters × 10 meters and housed two patient beds. All rooms were negatively pressurized. Each of these surge capacity hospitals was staffed by 1,400 medical personnel. The Wuhan hospitals garnered extensive international media coverage for their extremely rapid construction and massive size.[21] In retrospect, it is fair to view them as the mother of all specialized COVID-19 facilities built worldwide during the COVID-19 pandemic. Nonetheless, the interior spaces were strikingly bare bones, with occupants lacking nearly any visual contact with the outside world.

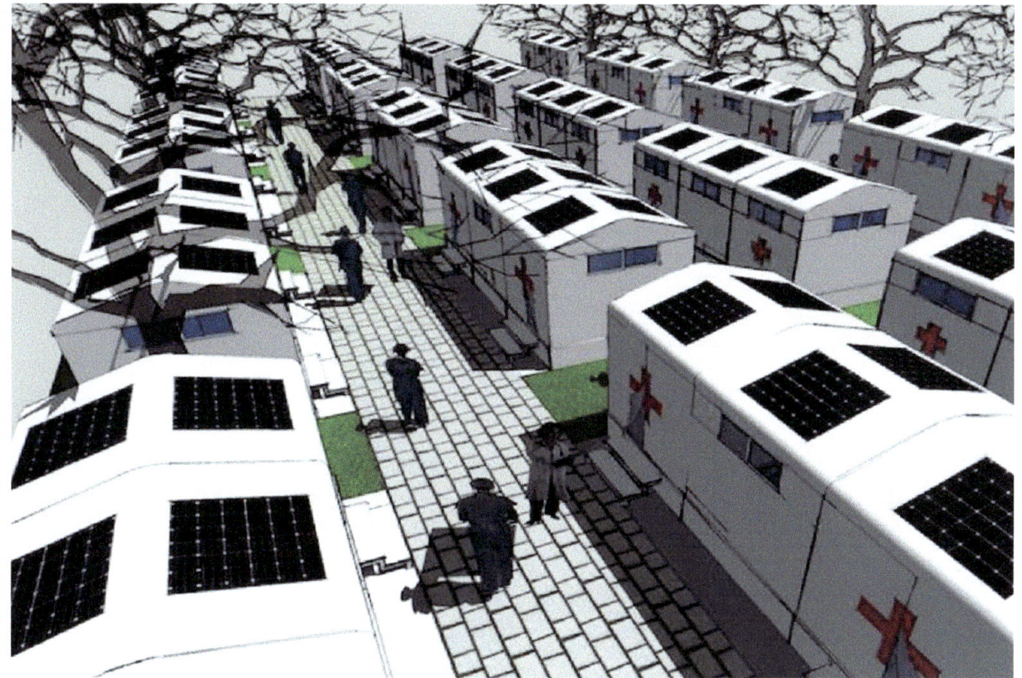

Figure 3.11. Modular Mobile Hospital, unbuilt proposal, Da Nang, Vietnam, 2020. Courtesy of VHL (Vo Huu Linn) Architects, Ho Chi Minh City, Vietnam.

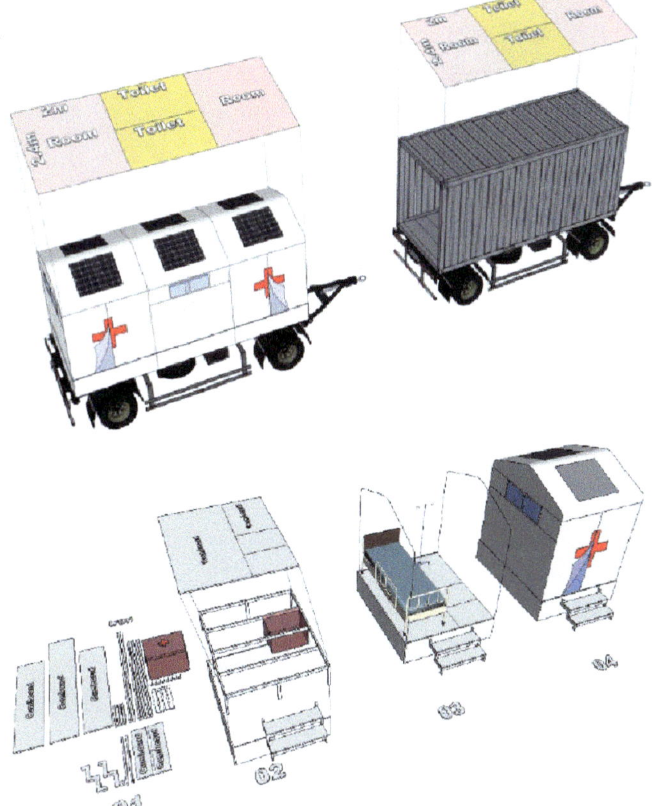

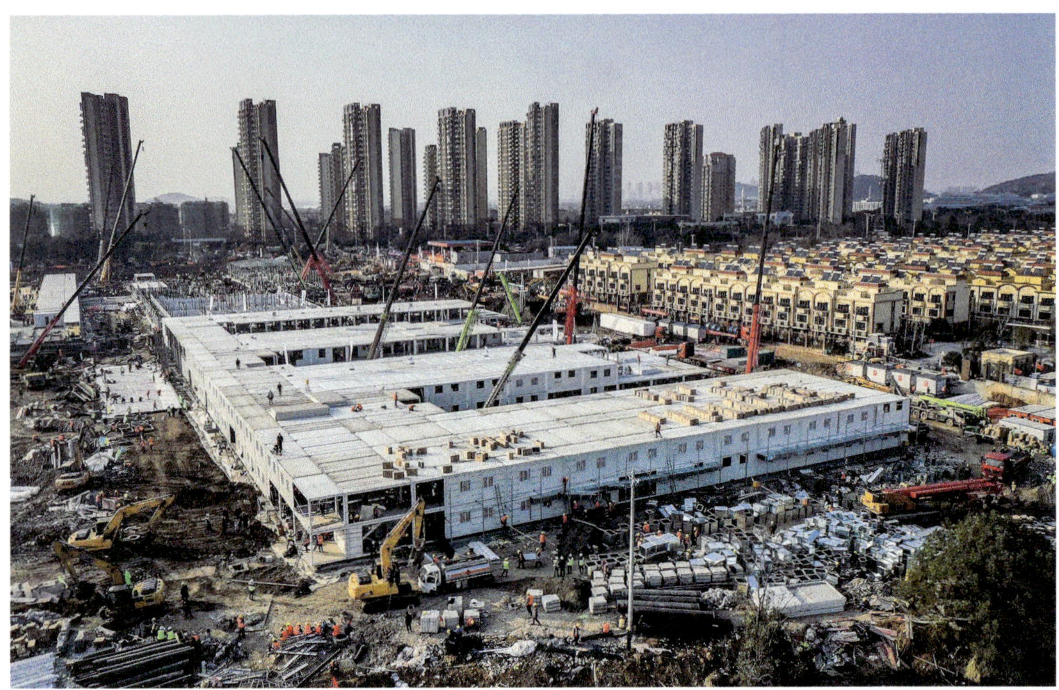

Figure 3.12. Huoshenshan Hospital, Wuhan, China, 2020. Courtesy of Stringer / Getty Images.

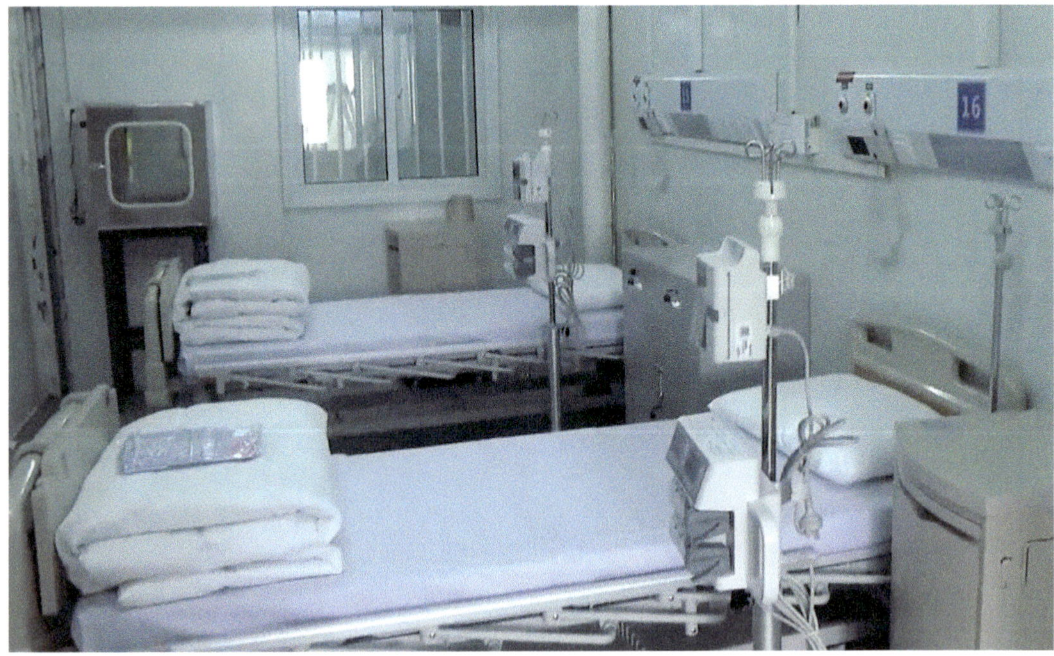

Figure 3.13. Interior view of inpatient isolation ward, Huoshenshan Hospital, Wuhan, China, 2020. Courtesy of Stringer / Getty Images.

Field Rescue Center

The Field Rescue Center (FRC) prototype—designed by HAHA Architects Group, Warsaw (Poland)—is a rather architecturally sophisticated clip-on/plug-in mobile diagnostic and treatment facility (fig. 3.14). It was expressly designed and built for emergency response uses—including pandemics, natural disasters, refugee crises, and humanitarian missions—where overflow emergency ICU surge capacity is required on short notice. This one-level facility consists of numerous interlocking 20-foot-equivalent FRC modules that are closely packed to create a grid. Its HVAC, plumbing, and electrical systems and IT equipment are housed in roof-mounted modules that service spaces directly below. Within this facility, circulation occurs via translucent perimeter clip-on modules that feature tinted polycarbonate wraparound panels. These simultaneously function as wall/roof elements, and their aqua-tinted paths are visually striking when viewed from the exterior. A modular inset-panel platform floor grid supports the entire installation, similar to virtually all the examples discussed in this chapter. This facility can house ICU beds, emergency diagnostic and treatment services, or a combination of them. The FRC installation, as shown, literally plugs into an existing acute care hospital mothership.[22]

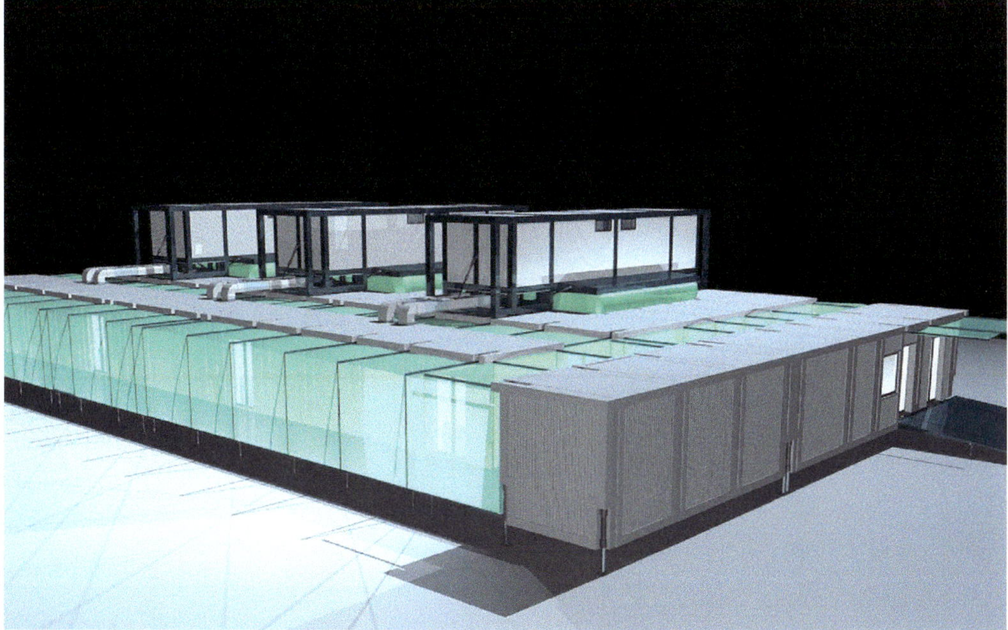

Figure 3.14. Plug-in Field Rescue Center, unbuilt proposal, Warsaw, Poland, 2020. Courtesy of HAHA Architects Group, Warsaw, Poland.

The CURA Pod

This container-based modular prototype, designed by Carlo Ratti Associates with Italo Rota, was built at a Turin (Italy) hospital in March 2020. Named the Connected Units for Respiratory Ailments (CURA), the first prototype was installed as part of a surge field hospital at the Officine Grandi Riparazioni complex in central Turin. Based on a generic 6.1 meter-long intermodal shipping container, each pod houses two beds and all required medical support equipment (figs. 3.15 and 3.16). The main design challenge was to ensure that "physicians would accept treating COVID-19 patients in a shipping container." Containerization offers quick assembly for ICU-level patient care, allows rapid transit, and ensures reliable negative air pressurization—all attributes the designers of fabric tents and pneumatically supported modular structures for rapid response cannot fully guarantee. Specially fitted ozone filters ensure negative pressurization. Each container

Figure 3.15 (right). CURA Pod, proposed installation adjacent to mothership acute care hospital, Italy, 2020. Courtesy of Max Tomasinelli and CRA-Carlo Ratti Associati, Turin, Italy.

Figure 3.16 (below). CURA Pod, prototype, showing custom-designed shipping container with attached pneumatic support space, Turin, Italy, 2020. Courtesy of Max Tomasinelli and CRA-Carlo Ratti Associati, Turin, Italy.

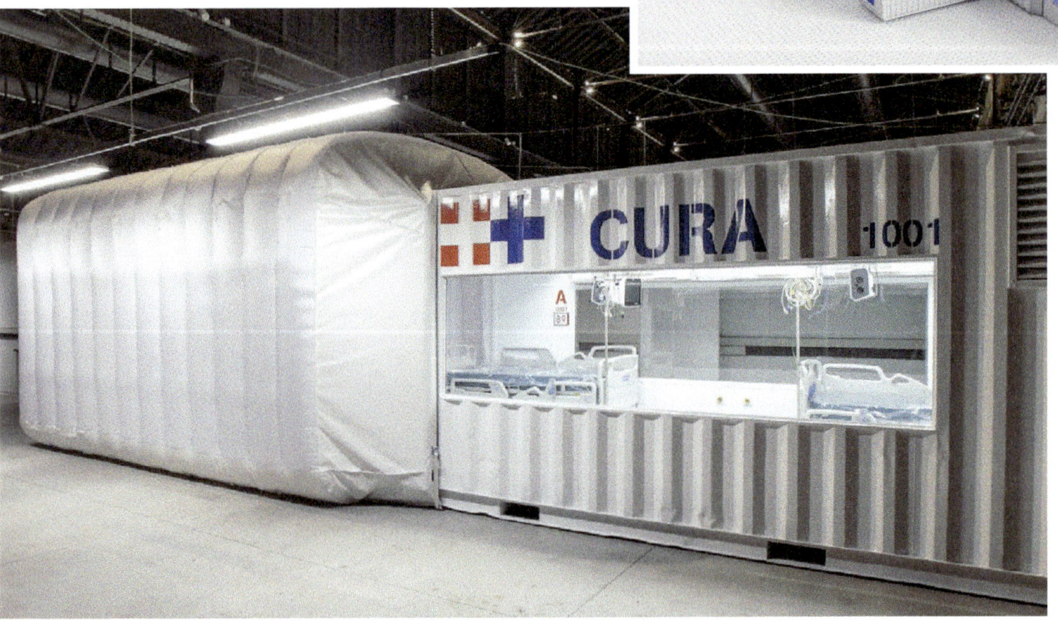

functions either autonomously or in tandem with a fabric-sheathed circulation spine, permitting larger-scale installations. Small glass windows are punched into the sides of the container, allowing patients to view out and staff and family to look in. At the time of this writing, technical drawings and specifications are available online as open-source documents, and the CURA Pod was adopted for fabrication and deployment in Italy and beyond.[23]

STAAT MOD

The Strategic, Temporary, Acuity-Adaptable Treatment Module (STAAT MOD™), a prefab modular system, was designed by HGA architects and constructed by the Boldt Company (US) for COVID-19 patient care. It is designed for installation either inside a large host structure or as a free-standing medical unit adjacent to an acute care mothership (figs. 3.17 and 3.18). Unit variations consist of a two-room module for interior installations; an eight-bed ICU module consisting of four two-bed modules plugged into an existing hospital; and a twelve-bed module with negatively pressurized open bays (four open bays with three beds each) linked by a central support spine. The system allows modules to be added or subtracted without compromising their individual functionality. Modules are 12.5 feet × 40 feet × 10 feet in height. This pilot system used stationary, virtual-reality-simulation walk-throughs with caregivers, including nurses, infection control

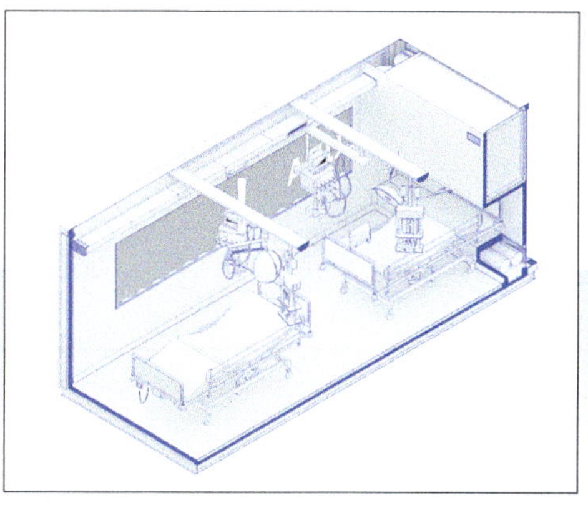

Figure 3.17 (left). Interior view, STAAT MOD™ COVID-19 Hospital, proposal, United States, 2020. Courtesy of HGA Architects, Boston, Massachusetts.

Figure 3.18 (below). STAAT MOD™ COVID-19 Hospital, proposal, United States, 2020. Courtesy of HGA Architects, Boston, Massachusetts.

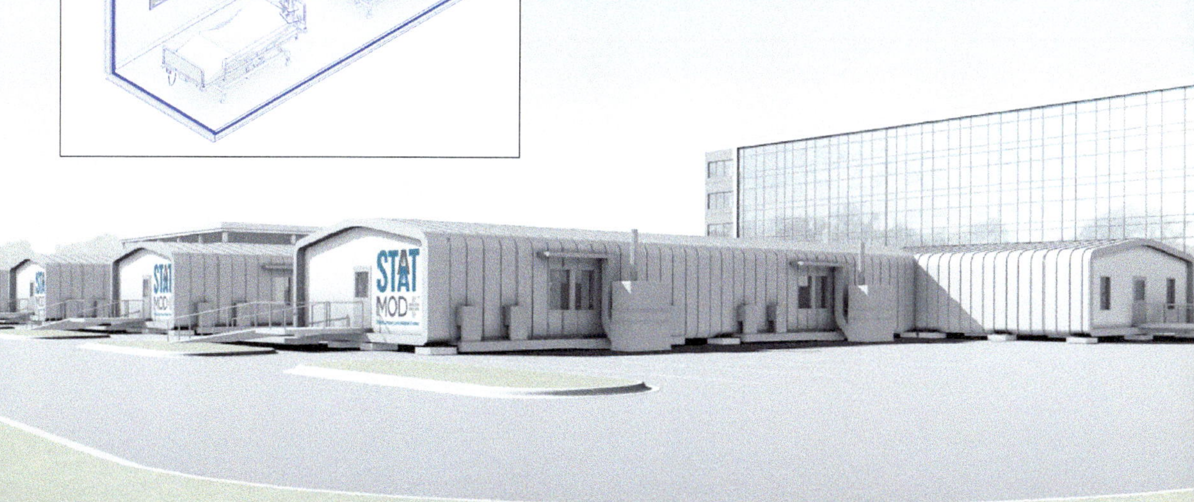

specialists, and lean-system engineers, who focus on efficiency through minimizing waste. The STAAT MOD system's full footprint is reminiscent of the spine-and-finger configurations typical of nineteenth- to early-twentieth-century Nightingale hospitals (see chapter 2). Somewhat ironically, these patient-housing modules feature small windows, versus the large windows and high ceilings so characteristic of classic Nightingale hospitals.[24]

Monash Health RESUS Facility

Australia's first COVID-19 RESUS ICU surge facility—developed by the architectural firm SPACECUBE—was designed and built in Melbourne (Australia). It was fabricated in three weeks' time. This off-site–built prefabricated hospital system was installed next to Monash Medical Centre's emergency department in fifteen hours. Erilyan Construction produced the internal fit-out for the system's medical support equipment. This portable field hospital (figs. 3.19 and 3.20) was commissioned to provide emergency surge capacity while the acute care hospital mothership's emergency department was undergoing renovation and expansion during the COVID-19 pandemic. The installation shown here consists of twenty-five lift-pack modules, totaling 360 square meters, configured on two levels, with each patient module housing six negative-pressure ICU beds, together with nurse's stations, medication rooms, and support spaces (including a staff breakroom). These isolation rooms feature sliding glass doors and windows, affording exterior views. Architecturally, the system is minimalist, with its interior and exterior not unlike a conventional hospital, to a certain degree. The iconic International Red Cross logo is contrasted here against these modules' bright white exteriors.[25]

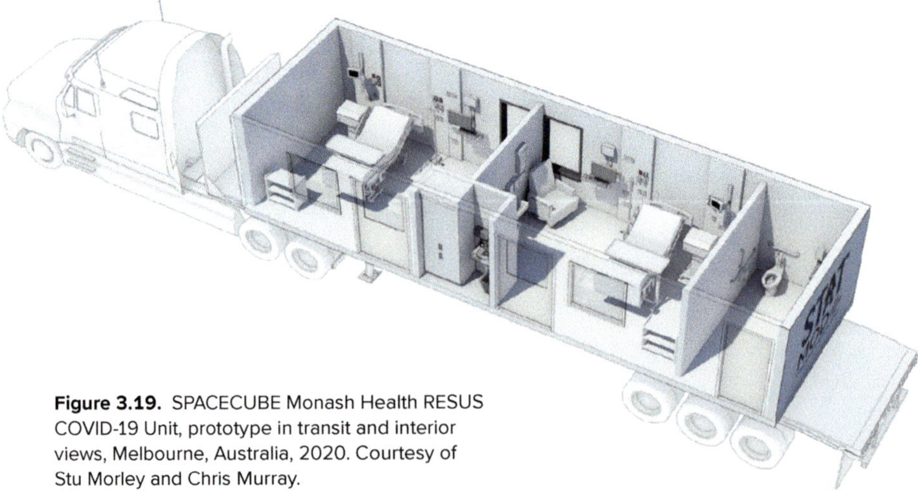

Figure 3.19. SPACECUBE Monash Health RESUS COVID-19 Unit, prototype in transit and interior views, Melbourne, Australia, 2020. Courtesy of Stu Morley and Chris Murray.

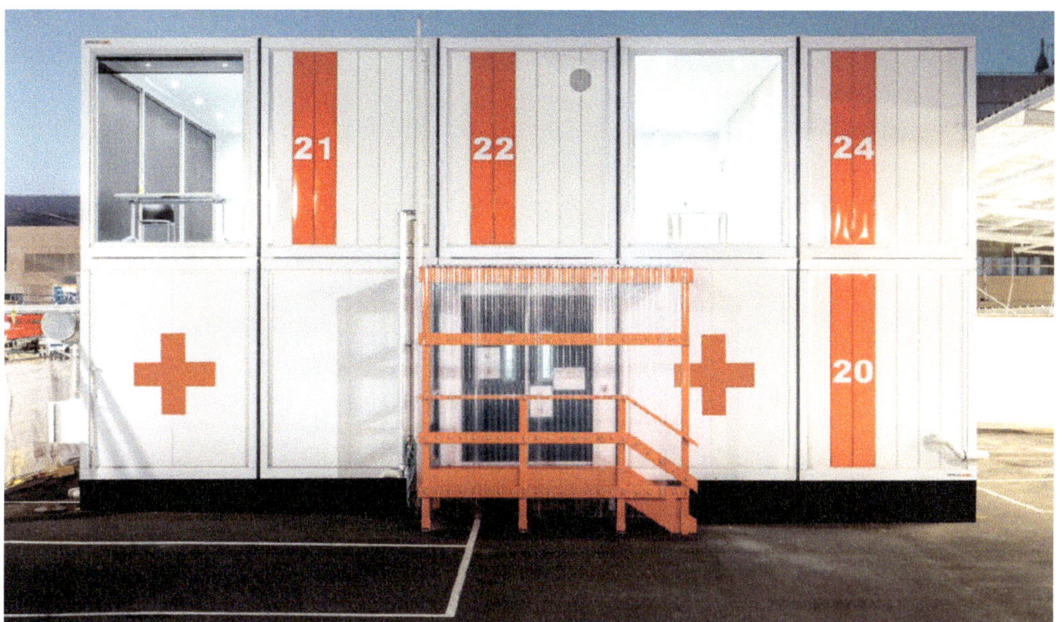

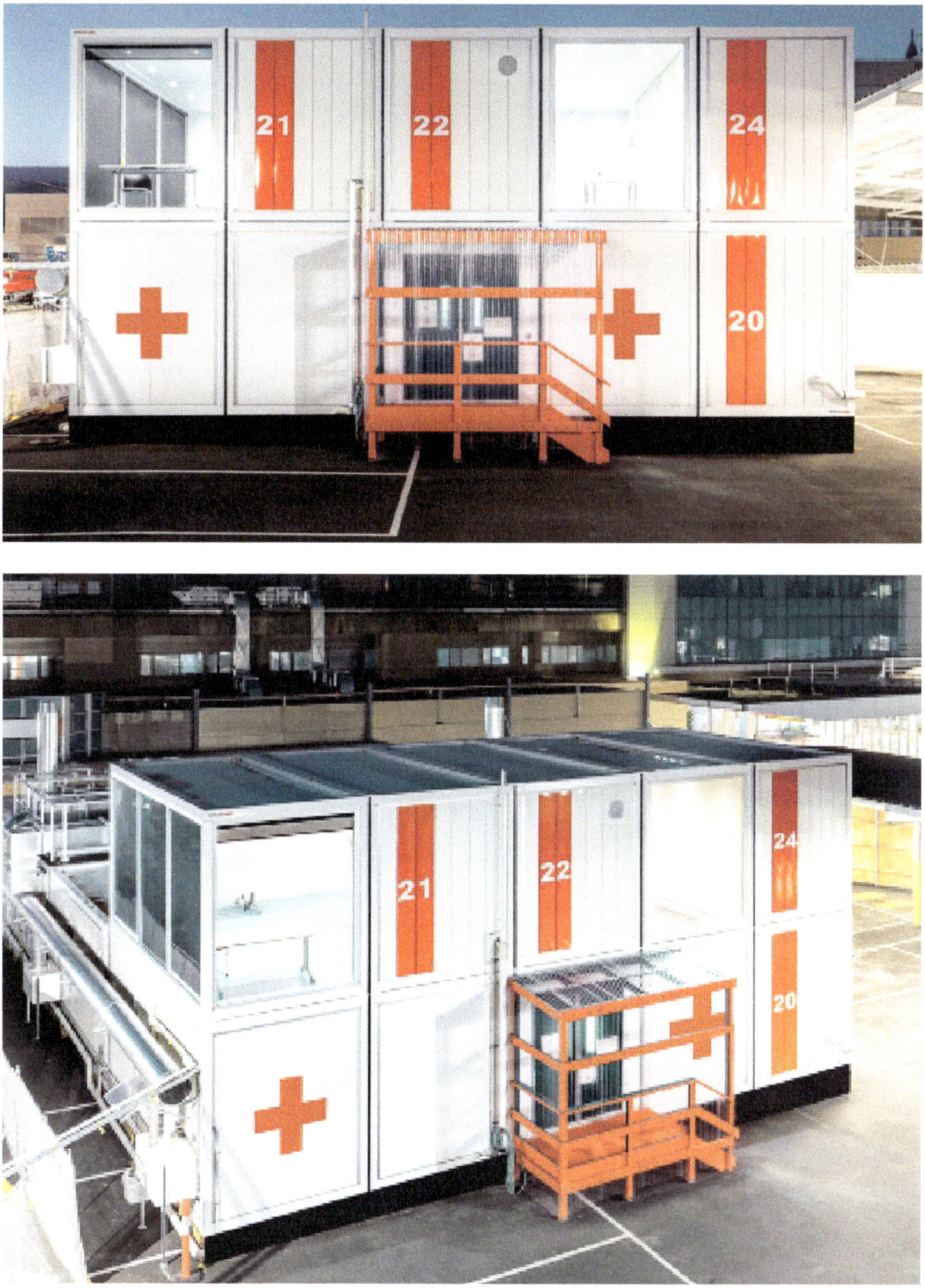

Figure 3.20. SPACECUBE Monash Health RESUS COVID-19 Unit, prototype, 10-module installation, Melbourne, Australia, 2020. Courtesy of Stu Morley and Chris Murray.

University of Toronto Prototypes

In fall 2020, the graduate-level Architecture + Health design studio at the University of Toronto also mobilized quickly—rapid response in practice—to (hypothetically) design a redeployable type 4, 24/7 infectious disease transportable treatment facility. The program brief called for an off-site–built modular prefab prototype in a fifty-bed (phase 1) configuration and a hundred-bed (phase 2) configuration on the same site, for redeployable installation adjacent to an acute care hospital mothership. Diagnostic and treatment support—MRI, surgery, nutritional services, counseling, administration, materials management, security, housekeeping, central laundry, and so on—is to be provided by the hospital mothership. The functional part of the brief called for incorporating salutogenic and biophilic design features (discussed further below). Two proposed designs, Crystal Hospital and Plug-in Hospital, are presented below.

Crystal Hospital: This proposal for a 24/7 redeployable infectious disease treatment facility is a biophilia-inspired architectural response to Arctic weather, accommodating challenges routinely encountered in Canada's circumpolar region and the deeply rooted vernacular building traditions in the country's Far North (fig. 3.21). This system is to be flown to the nearest airfield by cargo aircraft, and then trucked or airlifted (in stages) again via helicopter to the installation site. The architectural vocabulary is inspired by Indigenous building traditions of First Nations communities in Canada's Far North. Low-to-the-earth, circular, traditional healing lodges are known as *sweat lodges*. In the Crystal Hospital, every patient has a private window affording outdoor views, and, from the exterior, its vaulted forms and overall silhouette reflect Indigenous cultural traditions in Canada's Far North.[26] This architectural vocabulary is in opposition to the legacy of failure-prone colonialist hospitals and their associated medical protocols that, more frequently than not, proved to be insensitive to local cultural traditions. Beloit General Hospital in Wisconsin (US), built in the late 1960s and designed by Flad Architects, is a modern precedent. Its design plan, too, resembled a snowflake or snow crystal, presumably referencing its wintery locale in the Upper Midwest. Beloit General was a prominent example of American radial hospitals of the 1960s in the US, as was Bertrand Goldberg's now-demolished (in 2015) Prentiss Women's Hospital, built in 1974 on the campus of the Northwestern University Medical Center in Chicago. Design team: Emily Moore and Jiawen Lin.

Plug-in Hospital: This portable, two-level, prefabricated modular 24/7 treatment facility features interlocking, custom-designed, adapted inter-

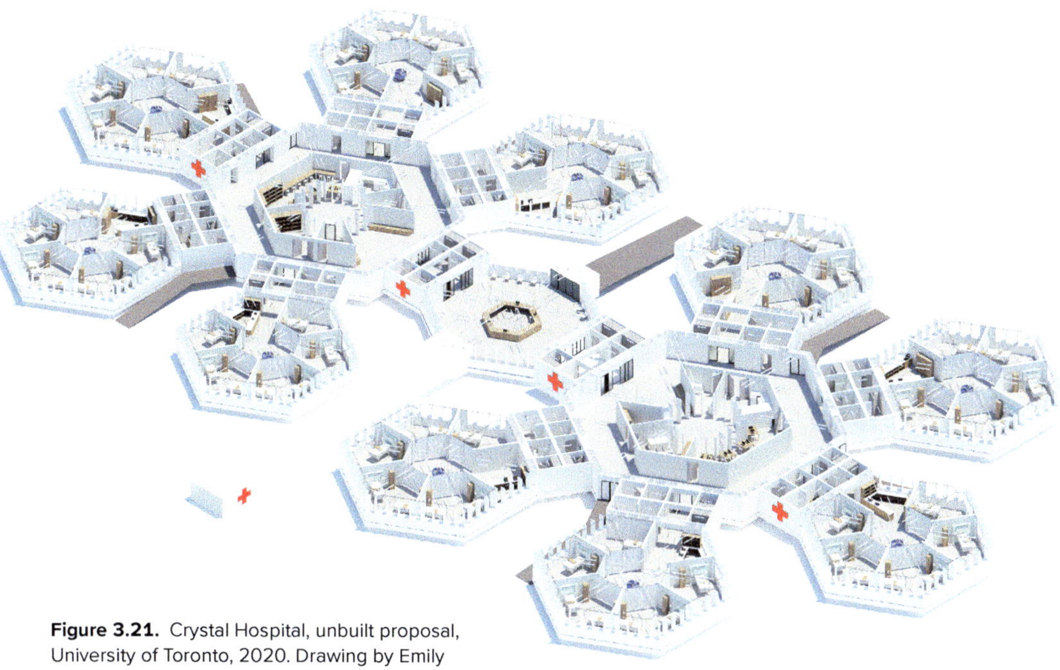

Figure 3.21. Crystal Hospital, unbuilt proposal, University of Toronto, 2020. Drawing by Emily Moore, Jaiwen Lin, and Stephen Verderber.

modal shipping containers with multiple pop-out elements, allowing the interior space to be doubled (figs. 3.22 and 3.23). In full deployment, this network of contiguous containers forms an A/B/A/B footprint, punctuated by exterior microcourtyards adjacent to the various patient units. In accord with the principles of biophilic design, these exterior spaces give occupants an opportunity to engage with nature while allowing natural daylight to be transmitted within. The containers are transported in close-pack mode, in specially designed "packaging." This system is deployable in fifty-, seventy-five-, or hundred-bed configurations. The upper-level containers feature solar panels and mechanical equipment that service the patient units immediately below. A high degree of visual transparency and openness is achieved—at least to a medically feasible extent—as opposed to the nearly windowless COVID-19 ICU surge hospitals built by the Chinese government in early 2020 (fig. 3.12). Instead, this off-site–built containerized system features full-height windows overlooking green AstroTurf in the patient housing zones, with the upper-level containers overlooking abstracted "green lawns" (the painted rooftops of the containers on level 1). The HVAC, electrical, and plumbing systems run beneath the floor and in overhead ducts suspended from ceilings. Design team: Francesca Lu and Feibi Pan.

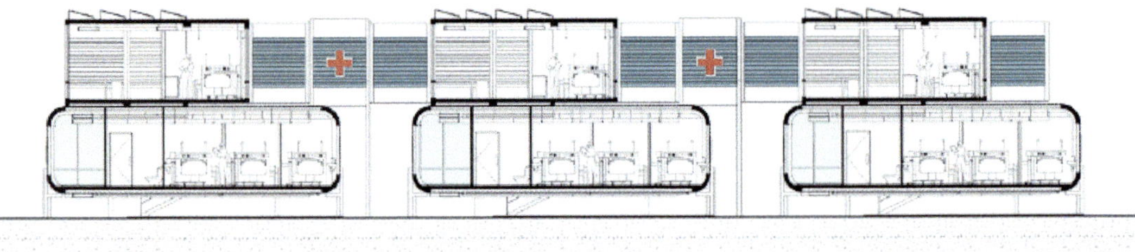

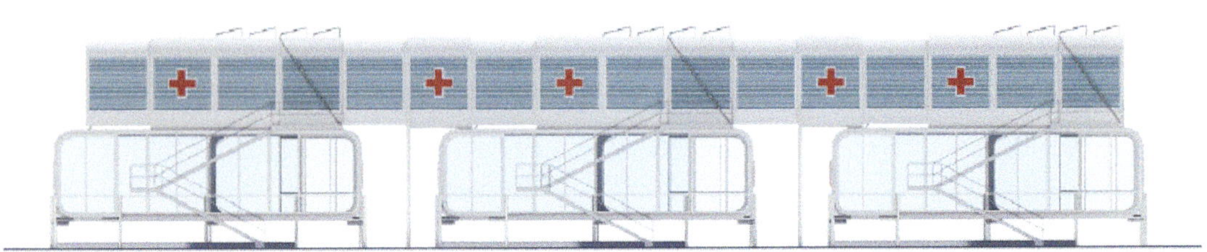

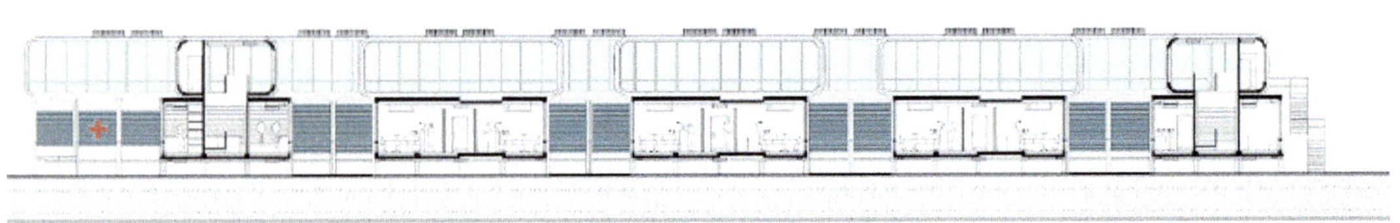

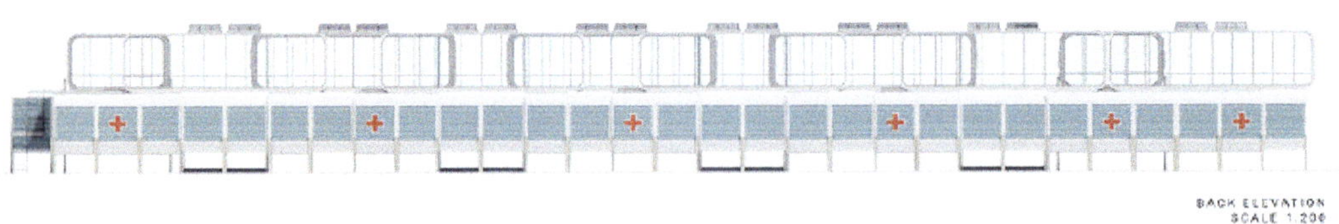

Figure 3.22. Plug-in Hospital, unbuilt proposal, University of Toronto, 2020.
Drawings by Francesca Lu, Feibi Pan, and Stephen Verderber.

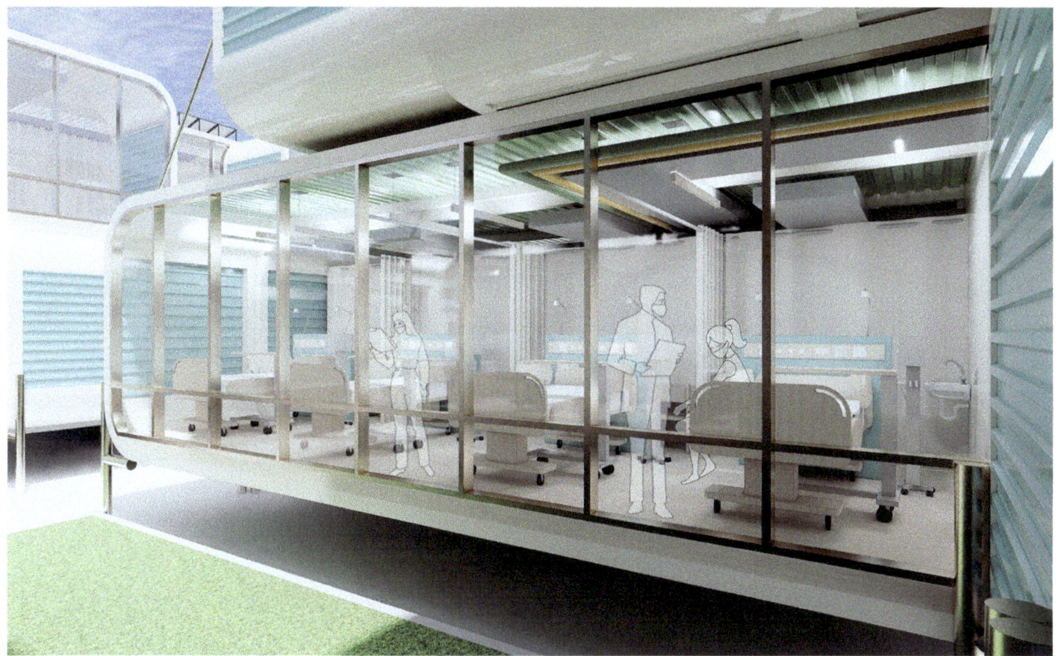

Figure 3.23. Plug-in Hospital, unbuilt proposal, University of Toronto, 2020. Image by Francesca Lu, Feibi Pan, and Stephen Verderber.

WHO INITIATE2 INFECTIOUS DISEASE TREATMENT UNIT

In the early days of the COVID-19 pandemic in 2020, the global health community was thrust into the spotlight like never before. Early on, many nations contacted the World Health Organization (WHO), based in Geneva, requesting technical guidance in the face of a rapidly escalating public health emergency. WHO responded by launching its own initiative for a transportable infectious disease treatment facility. The overarching aim was to integrate the best ideas from currently available civilian and military systems. Its INITIATE2 project was overseen by Techne (Technical Science for Health Network). Techne is an internal research and development arm of the World Health Organization—a consortium of global universities working in tandem with WHO—that was established in the early months of the pandemic. Its members collaborate with WHO on a range of activities dealing with infectious disease outbreaks and public health emergencies. Specifically, INITIATE2 focuses on medical facilities for the containment and eradication of infectious diseases. The *infectious disease treatment module* (IDTM) is its prefabricated, off-site–built, redeployable modular medical facility prototype.[27]

The programming and design processes for the IDTM were guided by ten provisos for dignified, humane care:

1. psychiatric care,
2. pediatric care,
3. care for older persons and maternity care,
4. an environmentally sustainable modular facility,
5. disaster resiliency,
6. socioeconomic and health equities,
7. cultural sensitivity in diverse geographic contexts,
8. rapid deployment and installation, based on modularity and constructability, efficient internal functions, sustainable maintenance, and repairability,
9. compatibility with local health care systems in diverse field deployment scenarios in medically underserved locales, and
10. ease of day-to-day operations.

In addition, this system must be easily transported to potentially highly diverse installation sites. At the outset, the team identified thirty-two commercially available pop-up tent and containerized systems and then studied a subset of these in detail: tents, containers, tent-container hybrids, pneumatics, and pop-up systems. In an on-site workshop held in Italy in August 2022, the project team articulated forty-nine schematic design precepts. A full-scale mock-up of the IDTM field hospital prototype (figs. 3.24, 3.25, 3.26, and 3.27) was field tested in Germany in October 2002 and in Italy in August 2023. It was evaluated each time by a team of emergency infectious disease medical specialists, engineers, and the WHO-led architectural team—of which this author has been a member since the start of the project.

Aaron Antonovsky, an Israeli American sociologist (1923–1994), first defined the health-promoting concept *salutogenics* as the confluence of factors in support of heightened human health and well-being.[28] This flew in the face of then-prevailing, negativity-based definitions of sickness and disease traditionally associated with pathogens, or *pathogenesis*. The term *salutogenesis* comes from the Latin *salus*, meaning "health," and the Greek *genesis*, meaning "origin." Antonovsky believed humans seek out socially, psychologically, and physically life-affirming experiences and places to cope with the stresses of everyday life—and avoid or minimize conditions that threaten to destroy our sense of well-being and place attachment.

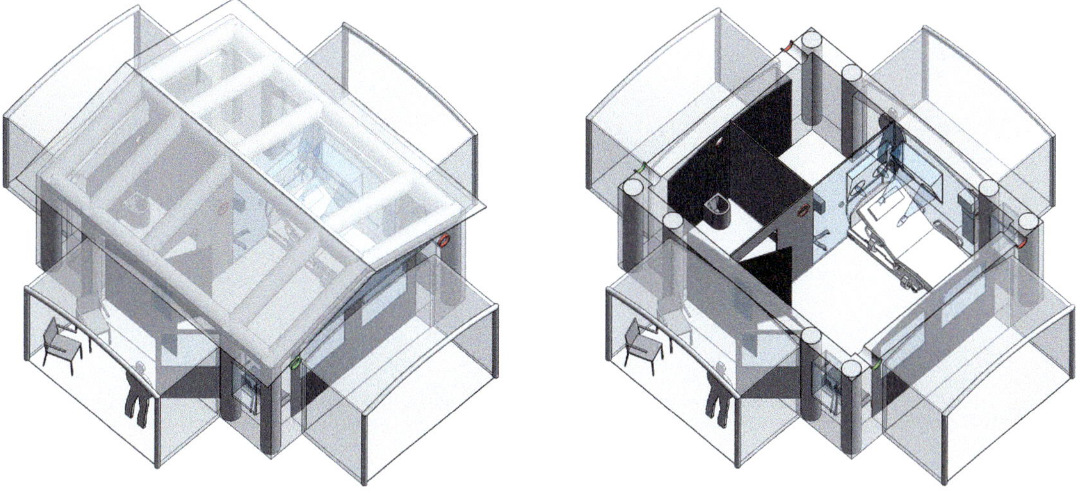

Figure 3.24. Infectious Disease Treatment Module (IDTM), prototype, 2024.
Courtesy of IDTM Team and Stephen Verderber, University of Toronto.

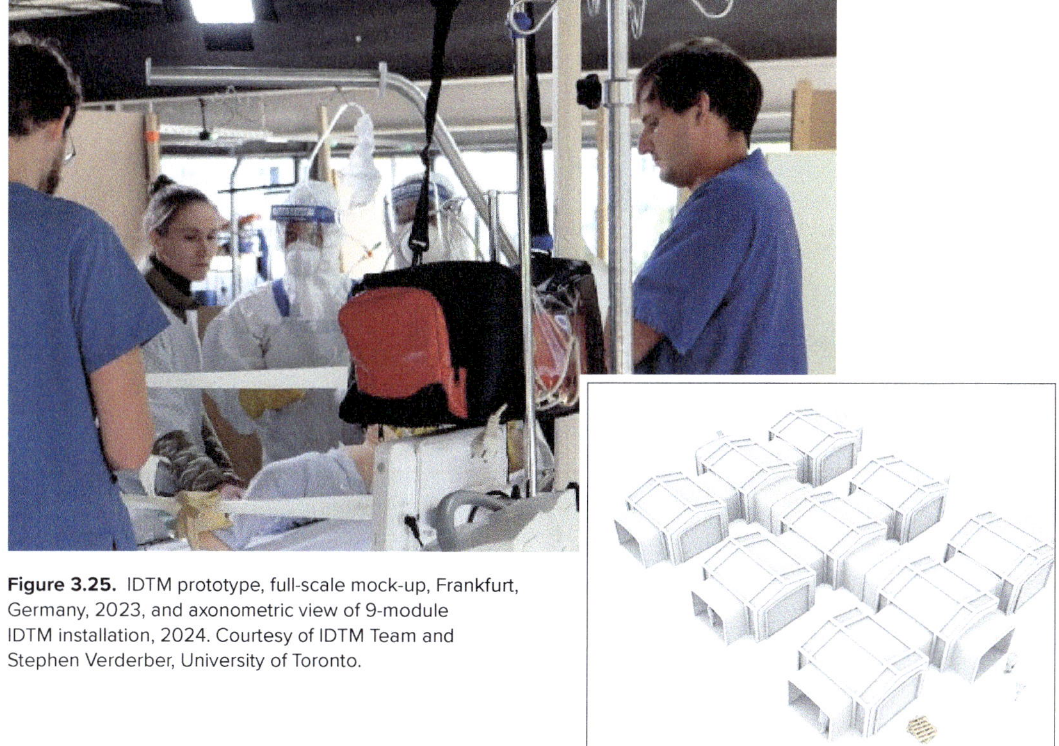

Figure 3.25. IDTM prototype, full-scale mock-up, Frankfurt,
Germany, 2023, and axonometric view of 9-module
IDTM installation, 2024. Courtesy of IDTM Team and
Stephen Verderber, University of Toronto.

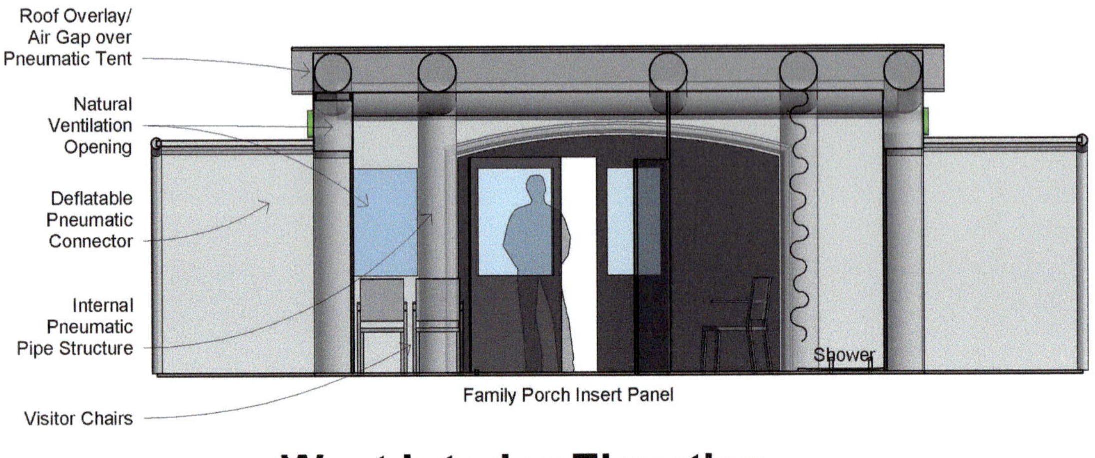

1 **West Interior Elevation**
1 : 50

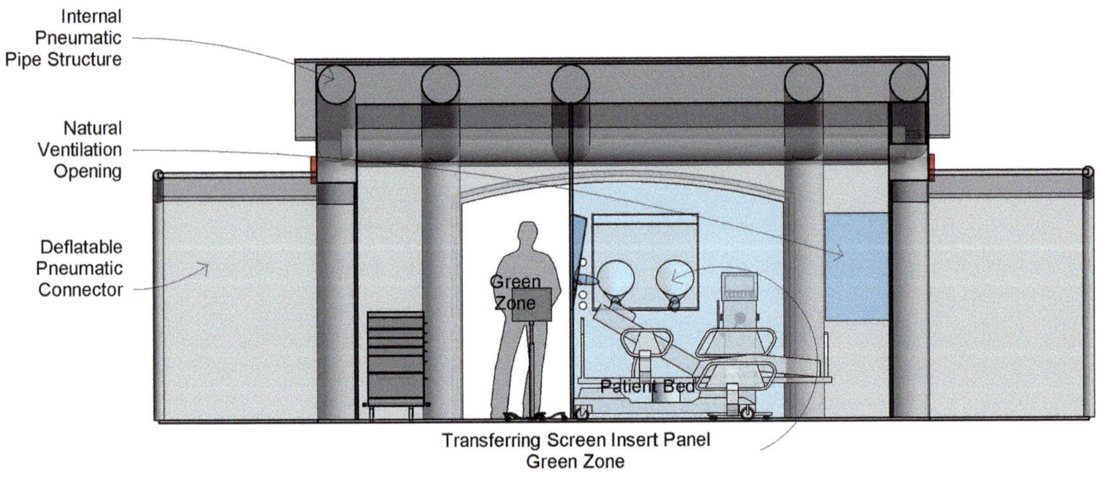

3 **East Interior Elevation**
1 : 50

Figure 3.26a. IDTM prototype. Courtesy of IDTM Team and Stephen Verderber, University of Toronto.

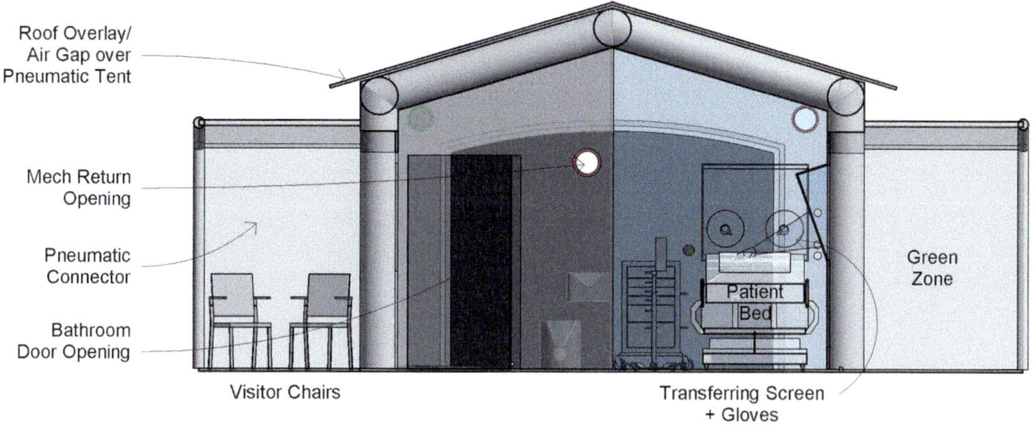

North Interior Elevation
2 1 : 50

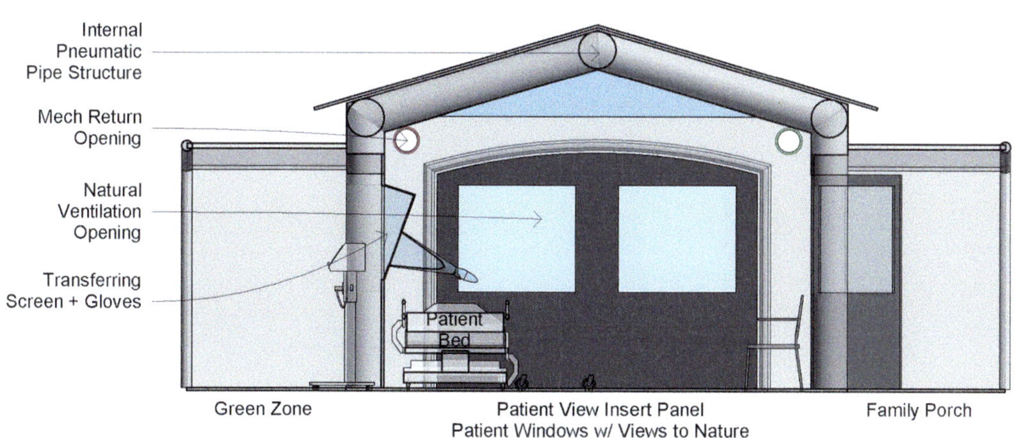

South Interior Elevation
4 1 : 50

Figure 3.26b. IDTM prototype. Courtesy of IDTM Team and Stephen Verderber, University of Toronto.

He defined *cognitive coherence* as a three-faceted phenomenon, consisting of (1) *comprehensibility*, or the belief that things occur in an orderly and relatively predictable manner, allowing humans to reasonably predict future events; (2) *manageability*, the belief that humans possess the capability to successfully solve problems, so a given situation is therefore potentially soluble and within one's grasp and range of control; and (3) *life meaning*, or the belief that life, which is intrinsically interesting and a source of fascination, is worth living, with each person possessing a unique purpose and mission in life.

The mental and physical challenges of being hospitalized for COVID-19 or another infectious disease are obviously intense. Jan A. Golembiewski and others have applied salutogenic concepts in the planning, design, and management of psychiatric facilities. The core argument is essentially that unsupportive or countertherapeutic physical environments challenge our coping abilities.[29] Meaning is derived from our capacity to recognize and find interest in normative elements in everyday life—whether one is confined to a community hospital two miles from where one lives or in a portable trauma center facility after a major disaster event far away—by having a window with a view outside, or at least a surrogate mural of intrinsic interest to relieve the monotony of the space. This human predilection for nature is recognized by architects, landscape architects, allied designers, and others as *biophilia theory*. Kellert has defined the fundamental tenets of biophilic design as consisting of two primary dimensions: the *organic* or *naturalistic*, and the *place-based* or *vernacular*.[30] Its theoretical tenets had previously been explored in the work of Edward Wilson.[31] This theoretical perspective has been applied to the analysis of other health care building types, including long-term care residential homes for older persons (see chapter 5 and appendix B).[32] Kellert defined six additional biophilic design elements: (1) environmental features; (2) natural shapes and forms; (3) natural patterns and processes; (4) light and space; (5) place-based relationships; and (6) evolved human-nature transactional relationships.[33] Subsequently, W. Browning, Catherine Ryan, and Joseph Clancy have further distilled a more directly applicable, design-based compendium of biophilia-related concepts for use in health care architectural design, as well as in the design of other building types.[34]

The architectural design team for the IDTM project sought to incorporate salutogenic and biophilic design features (fig. 3.27). This team included members from Parkin Architects' Vancouver office in British Columbia, Carleton University in Ottawa, and the University of Toronto (this author and assistants), all based in Canada, plus additional members based in Europe. Many organizations contributed expertise to the development of INITIATE2's IDTM under the direction of WHO, including the Alliance for International Medical Action (ALIMA), the International Medical Corps (IMC), Doctors with Africa (CUAMM), Médecins Sans Frontières (MSF), the Ministry of Health of Malawi, the Ministry of Health of Guinea, Samaritan's Purse, and the World Food Programme (WFP). The IDTM's prototype pilot pretest deployment was in 2024. Its specific architectural features include the following:

- Patient triage, an isolation zone, and compartmentalized toilet/ shower units physically separate from the medical staff's work zone, plus an adjacent, exterior patient viewing zone for family use. A residential-like silhouette establishes aesthetic compatibility in diverse installation settings.
- A pneumatic structural system that provides maximum stability without interior columns. The IDTM is either solar powered or mechanically powered, as local site conditions dictate. The system inflates with multiple interconnected modules, so if one or more modules fail, others can pick up the slack, ensuring uninterrupted caregiving.
- A modular-components kit, containing parts featuring a "clip on," pop-up, transparent patient module to facilitates staff's physical contact with patients via clear tubular arms, allowing the caregiver to reach inside to treat the patient.
- A modular system that can expand to up to twelve modules on a single site (twenty-four beds), featuring a raised, rigid, modular floor platform, elevated on tripod legs above ground level.
- Windows with transom screens, so patients and caregivers can look outside from within the treatment module and, conversely, families can see the patients within. A sunscreen attached above the module functions as a rain guard, and the pitched roof, color scheme, and aesthetic features are adaptable to Indigenous cultures and their local traditions, as encountered in the field.

Infection control is of top priority with respect to this prototype's design, layout, size, medicinal and nutritional supports, provision of staff safe zones and places for respite, adequate waste disposal zones, and vector and pest control amenities. There is no such thing as a routine deployment of a field hospital. Confronting a highly contagious pathogen places extraordinary demands on any facility. In the IDTM prototype, the patient is isolated in a single-bed lift-pack pop-up pod. Two domains are required—a high-risk zone and a lower-risk one—each with isolation. An internal corridor allows immediate transitioning from one realm to the other without blurring the line between the respective isolation zones. Since direct interactions among patients, personnel, supplies, and visitors would potentially be deadly, the physical spaces must be compartmentalized to preclude contamination, with separate showers/toileting and patient visitation zones—totally *unlike* the central "gray zone" corridors that proved so problematic in the Ebola treatment facilities deployed in West Africa in 2014–2016.[35] In the case of the Ebola outbreak, early projections of needed bed capacities in the region's hospitals were quickly exceeded, and some hospitals had to be entirely abandoned.[36]

The size and staffing of a deployable field hospital has direct ramifications for its architectural design, mechanical systems, and structure. The day-to-day staff should take the lead in determining what gets built and how it will function. From the early design stage forward, this requires the involvement of medical personnel highly trained in triage, infection control, preventive medicine, decontamination, epidemiology, behavioral health, and environmental engineering. The type and intensity of training and pre-

Figure 3.27. IDTM prototype model, 2024. Courtesy of IDTM Team and Stephen Verderber, University of Toronto.

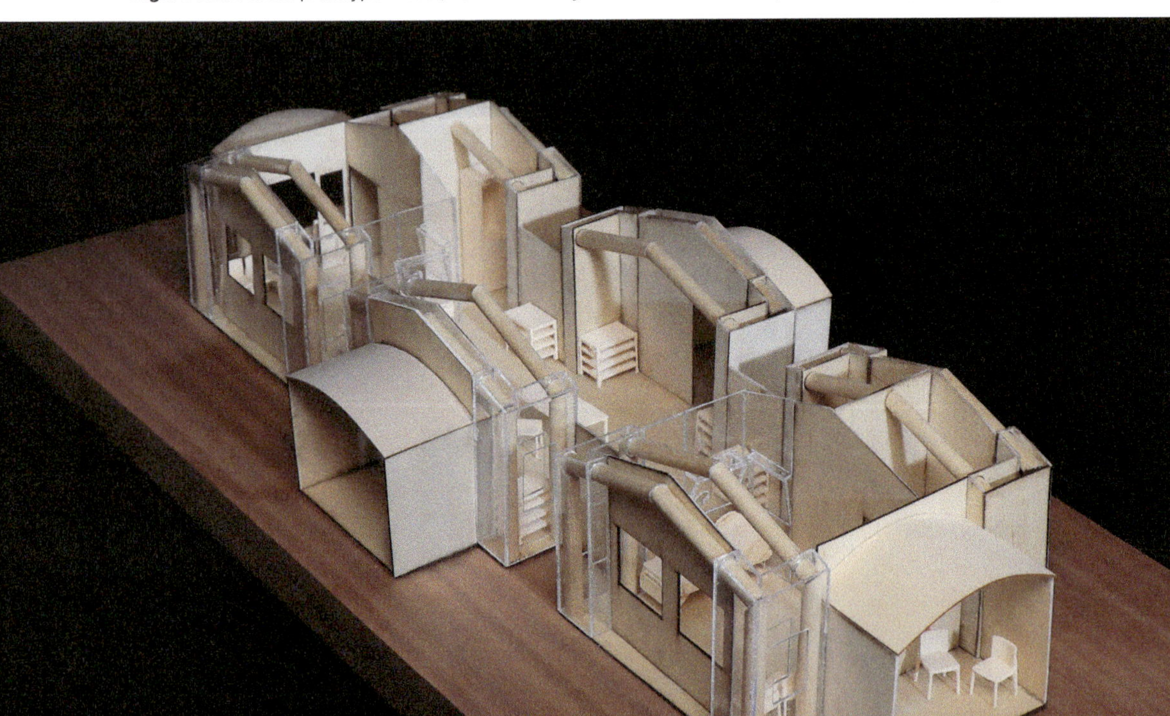

deployment preparation is dictated by the type of care to be provided in the field. Accordingly, the mental health stresses associated with working in a highly contagious field hospital setting are best addressed *a priori*, including training in how to store, retrieve, and don personal protection equipment. Contingency planning is essential at every step during predeployment. Otherwise, troublesome gaps in care delivery, medical record-keeping, and communications are likely to occur. Remaining adaptable is a prerequisite condition at all stages during facility deployment and the on-site commissioning period.

EQUITABLE REDEPLOYABLE ARCHITECTURE FOR HEALTH IS PROSTHETIC

A transportable building is similar to a human artificial limb. Both are built in a factory, fabricated from modular components and assembled by a repetitive manufacturing process. Both must be lightweight, malleable, and readily adaptable to sudden changes in the face of occasional blunt force impacts, reflecting the theoretical premise that architecture should ecologically tread as lightly as possible on the earth (see chapter 4).[37] A prosthetic device and a building must both be capable of returning *resiliently* to some approximation of their previous initial functional state, before the disruptive event. Both must somehow continue to function, should one portion cease to work or go offline, if only momentarily. Both must be made (to the extent possible) of biodegradable parts in a manufacturing process that minimizes the production of ecologically harmful waste products. Both must maintain fluidity to interdependently function while the larger system (human body / total installation) readjusts in response. The limb, and the facility, must be ambulatory—that is, capable of being positioned where most needed—in direct opposition to the inherent limitations of an immobile person or a permanent-site health care facility. Finally, both must remain relatively fully operational in diverse topographic, cultural, and climatic contexts.[38] From a project's inception—that is, in the programming and design phases—two questions must be answered, both in prosthetic and architectural designs. First, will this intervention provide the functional support needed to operate in diverse situations? For architecture this would include global public health emergencies. Second, will it express Vitruvian principals, which, in architecture, consist of providing *commodity*, *firmness*, and *delight*?[39]

In this regard, Attention Restoration Theory (ART) posits that humans seek out and crave opportunities to obtain respite from stressful and over-stimulating conditions (also see chapter 4).[40] Staff burnout is a major concern in humanitarian relief operations. A normal tour of duty may last for three months, and new personnel are rotated in according to a repetitive pattern. Thus staffing situations can become difficult, especially when one is so far from home. A person may just need to get away for a moment from a chaotic, unpredictable, discombobulated situation, particularly in tight, overcrowded work settings with few relief valves to depressurize the work atmosphere. Every bit of a portable structure must therefore be spatially designed for maximum efficiency and adaptability. Understandably, the pressure is great to overprogram—overpack—these tight quarters, given that X number of modules must support Y number of procedures each day, and even each hour.[41] With that disclaimer, to varying degrees, many of the walk-up/drive-up and 24/7 surge field hospitals reviewed above tended to suffer from the following:

1. inadequate space for patient confidentiality, privacy and personal distancing, and pediatric care,
2. inadequate space to allow proper isolation of the symptomatic patients from asymptomatic ones,
3. inadequate staff workspaces and insufficient storage areas for supplies (such as PPE equipment) and refrigerators,
4. inadequate protection from the elements,
5. inadequate natural daylight, outdoor views, and ventilation systems,
6. in many cases, the absence of real windows or "surrogate" views, such as attractive murals in windowless spaces,
7. aesthetically understimulating interiors, compounded by confusing spatial layouts and ineffective directional graphics, and
8. overcrowded diagnostic and treatment zones, as well as inadequate bedside amenities.

FIELD DEPLOYMENT

Historically, the type and quality of redeployable field hospitals (FHs) and infectious disease treatment units (IDTUs) vary greatly, although no empirical data on this have ever been collected and analyzed. Every nation that has been or is likely to be impacted by a disaster responds in its own way, for better or worse. Regardless, it is imperative to not repeat past mistakes, inefficiencies, or wasteful duplications of effort.[42] Experiences from the earthquakes in Pakistan (2005) and Haiti (2010) fueled the effort from WHO and its partner nongovernmental organizations (NGOs) to develop minimum standards for emergency medical teams (EMTs) that operate facilities in response to disasters. These standards function as a reference source for governments and humanitarian aid organizations in impacted recipient countries, as well as for use domestically in disaster strike zones.[43] Correspondingly, FH and IDTU facilities operating in disaster zones are now classified according to the services they provide, rather than the types of physical structures themselves. Three types of foreign medical teams (FMTs), or types 1–3, were defined in 2013, and in 2015 the term "foreign" was replaced with "emergency," to allow a classification system that includes both national (N-EMT) and international (I-EMT) categories.[44]

Preassessment Protocol

Deployment of an FH or IDTU follows a protocol, where need is demonstrated and the host country has already been vetted for its ability to accept the facility and provide at least a modicum of operational support (fig. 3.28). This preassessment protocol includes the following:

- a documented request for assistance by the host country,
- a detailed description of the adverse event,
- its impact on human lives and property,
- the predisaster functional capacity of the local health care system in normal times and an assessment of the complex,
- associated logistical challenges involved in deploying an FH or IDTU to a given poststrike zone,
- the availability and suitability of one or more installation sites for the facility, once it has arrived in the host country,
- the nature of the local and national political climates in the host country, especially at the local level,
- the record of recorded disaster events in the host country,
- the record of past disaster response performances,
- a scoping review of the competition that nearly always arises between international disaster aid agencies vying to be the first on the ground and the first to set up a portable medical facility in the field within the strike zone, and

- perhaps most importantly, the ability to obtain the funding needed to launch and sustain the given field deployment as needed over the long haul.[45]

Verification Process

To register and become a WHO-certified EMT, a health care provider organization is required to complete a verification process. WHO periodically updates these criteria, classifying the three types of emergency medical teams.

Type 1 EMTs are limited to daytime outpatient services only, with a minimum capacity of 100 patients per day. The facility is physically designed for the staff to provide triage screening and certain types of trauma care. Special services include assessment, minor trauma care, stabilization, and

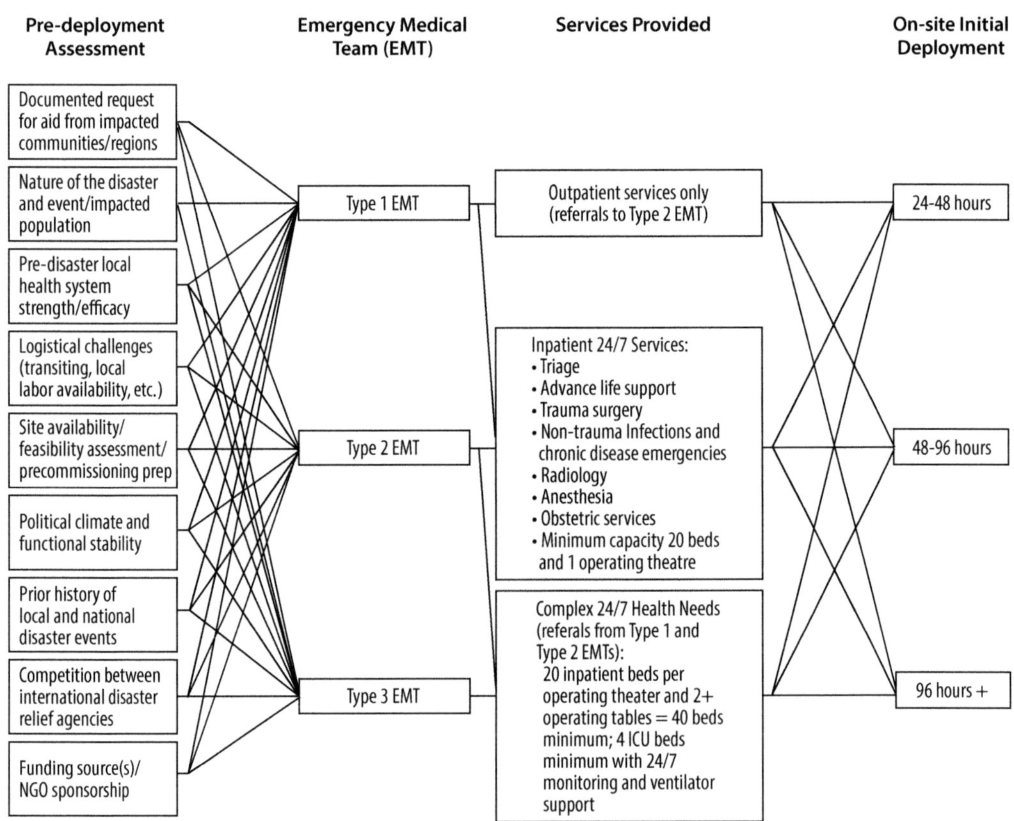

Figure 3.28. Redeployable field hospital needs assessment. Diagram by Stephen Verderber.

referral. Typically these facilities are modular, tent-based, or pop-up units, or mobile vehicular clinics. These units are quickly deployable after a disaster event, preferably within forty-eight hours. They can also be set up and commissioned within existing permanent structures. These facilities typically are on-site for two to three weeks after a disaster event, as was the case for Hurricane Katrina in New Orleans in 2005.

Type 2 EMTs receive referrals from type 1 EMTs and also admit new patients. Required 24/7 services include triage, advanced life support and trauma surgery, and inpatient care for nontrauma emergences, such as infectious and chronic diseases. Radiology and obstetric services are available autonomously or in partnership with a local fixed-site provider. These facilities have a minimum capacity of twenty inpatient beds and one operating theatre, with at least one operating table and a minimum operative capacity of seven major or fifteen minor operations per day. Type 2 EMTs take longer to deploy than type 1 facilities, as they are generally larger and more complex, due to their greater logistical transportation requirements, longer erection process, and multiple commissioning factors on-site. An exception to this occurred during the 2014–2015 Ebola outbreak in West Africa, during which type 2 EMTs were assigned more specialized services than would have been typical.

Type 3 EMTs for field deployment represent the highest level of disaster-related medical care and therefore receive patients referred from both type 1 and type 2 EMTs. The minimum capacity on-site is one operating theatre and at least two operating tables. A minimum of four ICU beds must be available, with continuous monitoring and ventilator support. For each operating area, at least twenty inpatient beds must be provided on-site. The minimum surgical capacity is fifteen major operations or thirty minor procedures per day. These facilities may take up to a week to deploy, erect, and commission. They typically remain on-site for a minimum of two months.

The three EMT types all provide surge capacity to support the local health care system and its preexisting network of facilities that may be within and near the strike zone. Unfortunately, during the 2010 Haiti earthquake, multiple international field hospitals were deployed and operated without any coordinating oversight from any central public health entity.[46] This led to significantly suboptimal care, a scenario that must assiduously be avoided. All EMT disaster events must be directed by an emergency medical team coordination cell (EMTCC) affiliated with WHO and its various partner NGOs, as well as the local ministry of health or an equivalent coordinating governmental agency.[47]

SUMMARY

In the first hours after a disaster event, remote assessments of its magnitude and scope are essential. The vulnerability of the impacted population(s) must be assessed, plus any potential newly arising threats. Beforehand, permission to enter the host country must be obtained. This typically occurs vis-à-vis WHO's assigned EMTCC communication channels on the ground. An essential prerequisite is a relatively sophisticated understanding of the epidemiological challenges, opportunities, and anticipated risks encountered in the days, weeks, and months ahead. Without question, unforeseen disruptions and knotty problems will likely arise, involving transportation snafus, political roadblocks, funding issues, staff shortages, and so on. Disrupted infrastructure deployment will exacerbate unmet health care needs and likely result in increased causalities. For example, a delayed facility deployment timeline can lead to a rise in malnutrition or dysentery cases. During the Ebola outbreak, the countries mainly impacted by it—Guinea, Sierra Leone, and Liberia—already had fragile public health systems, resulting in widespread unmet health needs during that public health emergency.[48]

Disasters and catastrophes can result in disease outbreaks becoming secondary, or collateral, adverse events—that is, ones caused by the deleterious impacts of the initial disaster.[49] Redeployable facilities are increasingly being designed to be tailored to a specific type of disaster event (such as WHO's IDTM prototype). Within the scope of a response, morbidity and mortality rates can surge, with over half all mortalities in refugee camps caused by measles, diarrheal diseases, acute respiratory infections, malaria, cholera, and meningitis.[50] Conditions associated with acute and chronic disease outbreaks often also include compromised water supplies and sanitation; nutritional vulnerability; and limited medicinal supplies to combat *Staphylococci*, *Streptococci*, and waterborne organisms, such as *Aeromonas*, *Vibrio*, and *Pseudomonas* species. Related illnesses requiring rapid treatment include hepatitis A, hepatitis B, parasitic diseases (e.g., amebiasis, cryptosporidiosis, and giardiasis), rotavirus, shigellosis, and acute typhoid fever.[51] Additionally, animal bites can lead to secondary infections, such as rabies, West Nile virus, encephalitis, dengue, and zika—all dangerous conditions requiring immediate treatment.[52]

Without question, the COVID-19 pandemic placed intense pressures on health care facilities and their caregiving staffs worldwide. In this discussion, four types of pandemic-inspired testing and treatment facilities were reviewed: (1) pop-up portable outdoor units; (2) pop-up vehicular nomad units; (3) pop-up units installed in repurposed host structures; and (4) 24/7 ICU-based surge capacity field hospitals / quarantine units (pop-up structures within host structures or freestanding side-by-side autonomous installations). Recent case studies of pandemical architecture for health care were then reviewed for their architectural, biophilic, and salutogenic content. This was followed by the presentation of an evidence-based case study initiated by the World Health Organization—its prototype Infectious Disease Treatment Module transportable field hospital. In *The Scope of Social Architecture*, C. Richard Hatch defined architectural education and practice as possessing the potential to serve a prominent advocacy role with respect to the marginalized in society.[53]

Professional architects are well positioned to assist in filling the unmet need for health-equitable built environments in a spirit of *rational transparency*—being predisposed and trained to critically respond.[54] A reflective public health and architectural practitioner offers the promise of achieving transformative outcomes, working alongside—and collaboratively—with frontline health sector clients and associated sponsoring agencies in times of crisis.[55] But too often, it is easy to dismiss innovative collaboration.

> *"We didn't have the time to plan for anything like this."*
>
> *"We didn't have the funds available on such short notice to consider windows, views, natural daylight, or matters of personal privacy for patients or their loved ones."*
>
> *"My medical center's board of directors is unwilling to pay for an expensive portable infirmary that will probably just sit in some warehouse gathering dust for years."*

Architects are empowered by their clients to act responsibly and ethically, yet innovation does not happen in a vacuum. The question for public health professionals, direct-care health care leaders and their chief financial officers is, *After the COVID-19 pandemic is over, will you just go back to the old ways of thinking when it comes to your health care facilities, or will you seriously consider the risk/reward benefits of portability as a compliment to old-school brick and mortar facilities*? The following is a cautionary tale from Canada about what can happen when a federal government's health agency mismanages its inventory of redeployable medical facilities:

> Ottawa allocated $300 million at the beginning of the pandemic for the construction of fifteen mobile hospitals, but only four have been completed and they are sitting in storage. The federal government gave a sole-sourced contract of up to $150 million to a joint venture between SNC-Lavalin and Pacific Architects and Engineers (SNC-PAE) in April 2020 to build five mobile respiratory care hospitals that can be set up in existing structures such as conference centres and indoor skating arenas. A similar no-bid multimillion-dollar contract went to Weatherhaven Global Resources Ltd. for ten stand-alone field hospitals that can be deployed either in urban or remote areas, each housing 100 beds. So far, Weatherhaven has delivered three units with none in use. . . . Two of the units were deployed early last year [2021] for several months at Toronto's Sunnybrook Health Sciences Centre, and at Hamilton Health Sciences. In October [2021] an oxygen concentrator from one of Weatherhaven's units was shipped to the Northwest Territories to handle an influx of COVID-19 patients in the local hospital's ICU. Since those contracts were awarded, SNC-PAE has received $71 million from the federal government and delivered just one mobile hospital unit, also sitting in a warehouse [in Ottawa], never deployed . . . although the SNC-PAE mobile respiratory unit can treat 100 patients in five wards including 20 ICU beds with oxygen respirators.[56]

As for the stated reason why these units remained unused at the height of the pandemic in Canada:

> The health ministries [in the provinces] have not requested the mobile pandemic hospitals because they don't have enough nurses or doctors to staff them. Katherine Smart, president of the Canadian Medical Association, said she can understand why the provinces haven't asked for the federal units, given staff burnout, attrition and COVID-19 infections among nurses, doctors and other staff: "Of course it would be nice to have more physical space but that doesn't help when you don't have the caregiver resources to staff it. . . . The crisis in front of us is we need people in order to properly staff more space. . . . What we learned from this pandemic is we have to understand that there is not healthcare without healthcare professionals."[57]

A CALL TO ACTION

Le Corbusier (1887–1965) wrote of the architectural significance of the earliest transportable building type: the primitive temple. He considered this to be a modest, demountable, nomadic structure, consisting of simple poles covered in animal skins that could be disassembled and then transported across deserts, grasslands, and forests. To Le Corbusier, its temporality embodied the essence of architecture.[58] The ancient yurt was a somewhat more sophisticated portable dwelling, also capable of being transported by mule or horse-drawn wagon from one place to the next and adaptable to diverse locations and climates. Seasonal and climatic factors weighed in, as did the necessity to suddenly relocate the structure due to war, conflict, famine, and other adverse events. Yet this building type endures to this day.[59] The recent work of noted Japanese architect Shigeru Ban exhibits gravity-defying lightness. Ban was the recipient of the 2014 Pritzker Prize in Architecture, the architectural profession's equivalent to the Nobel Peace Prize. After the Tōhoku earthquake and tsunami in Japan in 2011, his firm pioneered paper tubing as a structural design element in post-disaster housing. He installed restorative projects in the heart of the strike zone, traversing the line demarcating elitist from nonelitist public interest architecture and simultaneously demonstrating compassionate concern to ameliorate health inequities in that emergency.

In addition, transportable architecture must be resilient in the face of an unexpected adverse blow to its operational or structural integrity, with technology now making it possible to monitor a facility's "health status" and provide minute-by-minute information both on-site and remotely, assisting in enabling the facility to bounce back to some semblance of its prior state.[60] It is no longer a question of *whether* more catastrophes will strike, but *when*, *where*, and *how frequently*—with their compounding impacts placing unprecedented burdens on the planet's public health and medical infrastructures.[61] The need is growing for more *and better* public interest rapid-response architecture—including pandemical architecture for health.

Part II

Equitable Built Environments for Health in the Anthropocene

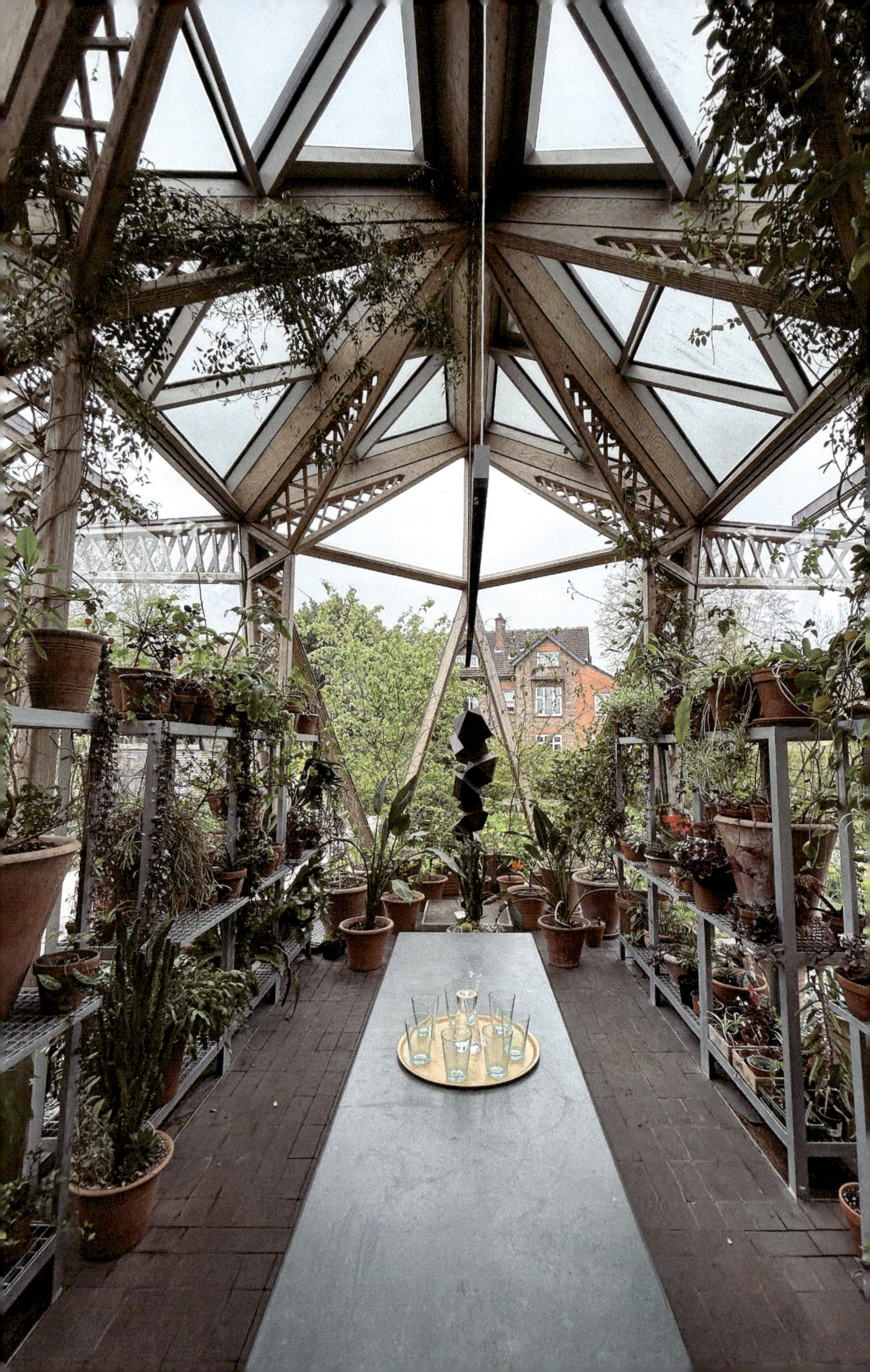

Theraserialization and Health Equity

The coyote only knows nature, for it is everywhere. It is not as if he looks at one thing and says, "That's nature," and something else and says, "That isn't nature." At one time our species was exactly the same, but no more.[1]

INTRODUCTION

Shortly after I was born, my parents moved to the suburbs from the near west side of Chicago. Right away my father planted ten trees across our treeless wide backyard. As a child I remember him saying, "I want you to love trees as much as I love them." Only two of the ten trees had survived when my sister and I sold the family home in 2019. On that last day, I gazed into the backyard, reflecting on my many positive memories of those trees. I was experiencing a case of ecological grief. The degradation and loss of valued animal species, environmental ecosystems, and nature is a source of growing feelings of grief and suffering. This grief is a legitimate response to ecological and habitat loss, and it is predicted to heighten as the climate crisis deepens.[2] But our understanding of this form of grief, anxiety, and, in the extreme, hopelessness remains largely unknown. Recent

Figure 4.1. Maggie's Centre, Manchester, United Kingdom, greenhouse, looking toward garden, 2023. Photo by Stephen Verderber.

empirical studies suggest that adverse mental health consequences are associated with specific types of ecological loss, and this occurs across diverse geographic regions and populations.[3] The adverse impacts of rising temperatures, extreme heat waves, floods, tornadoes, hurricanes, droughts, wildfires, deforestation, general habitat loss, disappearing rivers, and desertification are being felt.[4] Those most vulnerable to these adversities include the poor and the medically underserved, racial and ethnic minorities (including Indigenous populations), older persons, the unsheltered, and children. Restorative buildings and places are highly likely to be valued to counter these accelerated ecological losses (fig. 4.1).[5]

The World Health Organization defines health as "a state of complete physical, mental, and social well-being and not merely the absence of disease or infirmity."[6] This definition is interesting heuristically when applied to the architectural environment, as it calls attention to the multidimensionality of an individual's health status. The implication is that one can enjoy relatively good health or, conversely, poor health in different ways at the same time, as well as when in different places. A physically and mentally fit person can still experience poorer health, due to inequitable access to health care. While our personal abilities can carry us a long way, even in difficult circumstances, the human affinity for meaningful nature and landscape experiences is timeless and deep-rooted. For instance, Neolithic cave dwellers sought shelter and refuge to cope with a highly uncertain, threatening external world. Humans strive to perceive, evaluate, and assign meaning to phenomena encountered in the immediate world. Experiences with nature and landscapes have been broadly described and defined over the past century in fields as diverse as quantum physics and fine art. It is a multidimensional, iteratively interpretative relationship, scalable from a single object, building, or open space to the entirety of the earth's physical realm. In the Anthropocene, this relationship is under intense pressure, due to the rapid *denaturization* of the planet as the degradation and destruction of nature and natural ecosystems accelerates. The destruction of the Amazon rainforest is but one example, since the earth suffocates as the carbon dioxide provided by this once-vast resource evaporates. The melting glaciers in the mountainous regions of the world and the loss of massive ice sheets in the Arctic and Antarctic are harbingers of enormous changes to come. If ecological and habitat loss mitigation efforts prove ineffective, an enormous species extinction looms on the horizon—a period now referred to by climatologists and social scientists as a possible sixth mass extinction.[7]

In 2022 alone, 3 million Americans were internally displaced, due to wildfires that burned hundreds of thousands of acres of forests and grasslands; hurricanes that destroyed tens of thousands of mature trees, while permanently disrupting natural wetlands and river systems; and sudden floods caused by intense rainstorms. Many of these disasters lack precedents in recorded history.[8] Yet this is only part of the story, since the climate crisis also causes population displacement and new migration patterns. The risk is that these migratory patterns will exacerbate the ecosystem's mass extinction domino effects. Take the case of extreme drought and desertification. The impact of prolonged drought alone can be devastating, resulting in tree and plant die-offs as poor and wealthy countries alike experience ever hotter extreme temperatures.[9] The loss of one species can cause others within the same ecosystem to decline and eventually disappear—a process known as *co-extinction*, with the power to drag down entire ecosystems, collapsing them in a species regime shift.[10] This will have direct and unintended consequences for all living species. One study examined the psychological condition of ecological grief experienced by mountain dwellers bereft by the changes now underway in their lifelong relationship with their immediate natural environment, due to deforestation caused by warming temperatures.[11] It concluded that further quantifiable metrics are urgently needed to assess shifting person/environment codependencies that, for millennia, defined where humans live and how we experience our immediate natural habitats. In addition, population displacement is caused by the impacts of war and constant political conflict, most recently the Ukrainian War (2022–present), tsunamis, and earthquakes, such as the Turkey-Syria earthquake in 2023, which killed 45,000. Worldwide, in 2022 nearly 100 million persons were displaced, meaning that 1.2 percent of the *entire* global population was forced to leave their homes either temporally or permanently.[12] Among them were 32.5 million refugees, with 76 percent of these displaced persons coming from just *six countries*. Even worse, wrecked landscapes of damaged and destroyed natural ecosystems, cities, and buildings are left behind.

Unspoiled green space is vanishing at ever-increasing rates globally, due to excessive urban development and industrial land uses, which pave it over at a rapid rate. In the US alone, for each day in 2022, an estimated 6,000 acres of formerly green open space was devoured by the unrestrained march of urbanization.[13] Canada's biggest cities have lost open green space at staggering rates over the past two decades, as reported by Statistics Canada.[14] Urban "greenness," as they define it, declined in every province, averaging 8 percentage points across the country. This decrease was greatest in large urban population centers where, on average, 10.5 percent of urban greenness disappeared.

Worldwide, humans are traveling farther and farther to reach once-remote places—such as islands, mountain regions, seashore resorts, and other ecotourist settings—to obtain psychological respite from hyperurbanization and *denaturization*. This explains why 100,000 tourists visited Antarctica in 2022, whereas only four decades ago, that continent saw only a few hundred visitors each summer. Despite the increased cost of accessing these natural settings and resort locales, fewer and fewer such places remain unaffected by the imprint of human destruction.[15] While the wealthy have always been able to access the psychological and physical health benefits of nature, regardless of its financial expense, *what about everyone else*? Since the seventeenth century, during times of plague and pestilence, the wealthy and privileged could afford to vacate cities and towns and be immersed in the health-promoting benefits of natural landscapes, including rural spas and natural-spring resorts.

In our contemporary, information-obsessed world of competing demands on our attention every day, the therapeutic, or *restorative*, functions of nature and landscapes are gradually being eroded—relegated to a lower priority if not entirely dismissed—due to a quixotic form of learned helplessness:[16] "Why bother with species and habitat destruction, because I can't do anything about it anyway." A century ago it was different. The public health fervor that led President Woodrow Wilson to establish the National Park System in the US in 1916 simply does not exist today. Paradoxically, that nation's national parks are now being overrun by thoughtless over-tourism, without due consideration of its ecological consequences. At the same time, hypercapitalistic forces consistently fight the establishment of new urban parks or designations of wilderness conservation areas for rivers, forests, and oceanside seascapes. This is a harbinger of trouble ahead, a classic case of "out of sight, out of mind." This *ecological apathy* symbolizes a cultural desensitization to nature and landscapes and is part of a larger denaturization syndrome. This syndrome has been attributed to a lack of effective environmental education, beginning in elementary and secondary schools. Environmental apathy is the direct outcome of a broken educational system, with nearly everyone seemingly online nearly all the time. We are no longer engaging in real time experiences with each other or with the outdoors as much as we did even a decade ago. This ecological apathy is attributed to an obsession, especially among youth, with settling for indirect abstractions—digital mediation, or AI-generated digital replicas of nature and landscapes—versus experiencing the real thing. Other oft-cited reasons for this apathy (e.g., crime and increasing daytime heat) are based on parents' fear for the safety of their child to justify disallowing outdoor playtime for their children.[17]

NATURE AND LANDSCAPE

Synopsis: Nature and landscape (N-L) ecosystems encompass features and related built forms that humans see and experience. This consists of the multisensory experience of trees, forests, prairies, and other vegetated habitats, bodies of water, and organic life forms and their ecological habitats, as well as the weather, sunlight, clouds, and seasonal changes. With respect to architecture, "nature" denotes its active incorporation within a building, and "landscape" denotes the immediate outdoor environs safely viewable from within a building.

Our evolutionary past is rooted in our species' interdependency with nature and landscapes (hereafter abbreviated as N-L) and successfully coping with uncertain, complex, and often highly contradictory N-L experiences. In the open spaces of the savanna, tribal hunter-gatherer communities had to become adroit at coping with dangerous conditions. Sensory modalities—specifically, our eyesight, hearing, sense of smell, and sense of touch—were paramount in being safe and secure in life-or-death situations. Being able to perceive and construct cognitive maps of the physical world was critical to this process.[18] Therefore, the aim of this chapter is to examine how architecture for health can help humans experience the therapeutic benefits of N-L. A second, closely related aim is how architecture for health can equitably improve the psychological and physical health of medically underserved individuals and populations. The underlying assumption is that this is becoming imperative, due to the ongoing denaturization of formerly naturalistic landscapes worldwide.

The terms natural environment, natural landscape, landscape, and nature are used interchangeably in the social sciences and, to some extent, in architecture: *natural environment* and *natural landscape* typically signify a place or landscape not altered by direct human intervention, whereas *landscape* in architecture typically refers to a direct or indirect view from a building over or into a parcel of land. *Nature* is often applied to denote elements of this, but it generally refers to nonhuman biological habitats, animal species, natural vegetative species, and natural ecosystems. To further complicate matters, in the case of architecture, divergent cultural interpretations come into play, such as the terms *romantic* or *pastoral* to define and analyze the experience of nature and landscapes.[19] The *biophilia hypothesis*, *prospect-refuge theory*, and *attention restoration theory*, can, to varying degrees, help in understanding person/nature/landscape transactions that, at one extreme, can be highly health promoting (positive) and, at the other, highly health threatening (negative). Some midpoint condition, combining positive and negative assessments, or synchronicity, occurs in each building or place. The emerging psychological condition known as *nature deficit disorder* consciously draws on elements of all three of these pertinent theories.

Biophilia Theory

Expanding on the discussion of biophilia in chapter 3, this term was introduced by Erich Fromm in 1964 to describe humans' attraction to the various spheres of life, life processes, and all that lives and is vital in the physical world.[20] This term was subsequently popularized by Edward O. Wilson, who defined biophilia as the connection that humans subconsciously seek with the rest of life in the physical world.[21] The core idea, or hypothesis, is that all humans share an innate affinity with every other life form. It assumes that for the millions of years during which our species evolved, humans existed codependently with the natural environment. Most adaptations in the human organism, including those of the brain and related behavioral systems, developed as an evolutionary response to external N-L demands imposed on our species.[22] More recently, fourteen composite biophilia-based design patterns for application in the built environment were identified.[23] These patterns, together with Kellert's dimensions (see chapter 3), are hypotheses suitable for application in specific N-L environments with respect to behavioral and social cost benefits, the climate crisis, and the medically underserved. Biophilia tends to manifest in two dimensions in the architectural environment—the *organic* and the *naturalistic*, incorporating vernacular aesthetic features, methods of construction, and building materials (e.g., natural wood structural beams, walls, floors, and finishes), as well as the use of natural, organic shapes, forms, and spaces.[24]

Prospect-Refuge Theory:

The psychological advantage of seeing without being seen drove Jay Appleton's 1970s definition of landscape prospects, refuges, and hazards.[25] He defined *prospects*, or views outward, as belonging to two general types. *Direct prospects* are views available from a stationary or primary vantage point. Examples include panoramas and vistas. *Indirect prospects* are views attainable if one can see or physically reach points farther off in the landscape (i.e., secondary vantage points). A *refuge* is a shelter or hiding place. Nonetheless, a shelter may provide refuge from a storm yet not from the eyes of a predator. A perceived or actual *hazard* (e.g., a hazardous situation), impedes free, unrestricted spatial movement within a given landscape encounter.[26] In 1991, the architectural historian Grant Hildebrand was the first to directly apply this theory to architecture, in the Prairie School residences designed by Frank Lloyd Wright (1867–1959). Hildebrand added several new spatial dimensions to the concept of *prospect*, including an involuntary interest in complexity, exploration, and affordances.[27] He concluded that these design concepts exist intuitively in the work of insightful architects to control precisely how and where bright spaces are framed, along with ceiling heights, the degree of spatial complexity, and carefully choreographed person/N-L interactions. The discussion here hypothesizes that *orchestrated balances between prospect-refuges in the architectural environment can be of positive psychological and physical benefit*. The basic elements of prospect-refuge in architecture consist of

- a building's immediate site context and setting,
- the building in its contextual context or frame of reference,
- spatial refuge attributes relative to spatial prospect attributes,
- the ability of occupants to strike attain a preferred balance between their frame of reference and attainable views outward from a favored vantage point or fixed station,
- the degree of perceived/actual safety from this vantage point,
- the ability to mitigate external hazards or threats, and
- its intrinsic richness, complexity, and multisensory attributes.[28]

Attention Restoration Theory:

The third theory of direct relevance to the phenomena of experiencing N-L content in architecture is attention restoration theory (ART). It is based on an extrapolation of psychologist William James's 1892 definition of involuntary attention, described by him as experiences of a fascinating, intrinsically interesting quality, including the perception of "strange things, moving things, bright things, pretty things, metallic things."[29] In his taxonomy of involuntarily interesting phenomena, he included the sight of blood and views of animals, especially when they are in motion. In buildings and places perceived to be uncertain and threatening, directed attentional fatigue is likely to set in. It is a neurological phenomenon resulting from an overtaxing of the brain's inhibitory attention mechanisms, which can have difficulty accommodating incoming informational distractions while concurrently allowing one to maintain a focus on a specific task, place, or object. It is natural for an individual to alternate between periods of intense attention and periods of avoidance or distraction. This latter condition is due to having to cope with (suppress) excessive incoming environmental stimuli difficult or impossible to comprehend (make sense of). A symptom of mental fatigue is humans' inattention to events in the physical world.

Two types of attentional behaviors identified as prerequisites in this process are *involuntary attention*, which refers to an aspect requiring little or virtually no effort at all—such as when something in a building or landscape is seen as intrinsically fascinating—and, on the other hand, *voluntary attention*, or highly directed attention. This latter condition often requires considerable effort, such as when something is perceived as being monotonous, undifferentiated, tedious, or simply boring.[30] In the architectural environment, ART hypothesizes that buildings and their attributes that humans find aesthetically pleasing, inherently compelling, and even fascinating, attract interest for their promise of a safe or positive informational experience. This assessment will have a direct impact on psychological and physical satisfaction and recovery, particularly in situations where an individual suffers from excessive attentional (mental) fatigue. Natural environments, such as forests, mountain landscapes, and beaches, are particularly effective in this respect. They offer a positive, attention-restoration perspective, as these places provide tangible *affordances* perceived as intrinsically interesting, if not outright compelling, and are therefore worth pursuing further.[31]

The Influence of Nature-Deficit Disorder

While not (yet) officially listed in the *Statistical Manual of Mental Disorders* (DSM-5), nature-deficit disorder (NDD) has been broadly defined as the psychological, physical, and cognitive costs of humans' alienation from nature, particularly for children in their developmental years. The term NDD was first introduced by Richard Louv in his bestselling *Last Child in the Woods*.[32] He hypothesized that humans are increasingly disconnected from nature. This separation fosters myriad social disfunctionalities and dramatic, some-what paradoxical decreases in awareness of or concern for the well-being of N-L (and, by extension, the well-being of the planet).[33] Here, a proper exposure to (dosage of) nature immersion is hypothesized to be of thera-peutic benefit in our everyday lives.[34]

The Nature Conservancy, the world's largest environmental NGO, con-tends humans are "increasingly disconnected from nature and as a result are less likely to value nature."[35] This doom-loop dynamic, it warns, may well be the world's greatest environmental threat right now. Restorative N-L immersion experiences hold tremendous promise in therapeutically treating individuals and populations especially vulnerable to experiencing the adverse effects of NDD and related sensory deprivation disorders.[36] Recent research on this issue has reaffirmed the currency of NDD, including its affordances, as viewed through the lens of political ecological theory and practice.[37] Political challenges lie ahead, however, in developing sustain-able, geographically transferrable public health policies in order to foster greater environmental awareness of N-L engagement across all segments of society, including the medically underserved and those who experience chronic health inequities. Shared, as well as divergent, underlying assump-tions and associated behavioral outcomes are diagrammed in figure 4.2.

PRECURSORS IN HEALTH-PROMOTING ARCHITECTURE

Perhaps the earliest landmark contribution regarding environmental (and indirect) architectural precursors in habitat was *On Airs, Waters, Places*, a treatise traditionally attributed to the Greek physician Hippocrates of Cos (460–370 BC). This seminal work, forebearer to the field of public health epidemiology, explained the predictive causes of diseases that afflict the population of a city and how these adverse events can be better under-stood by taking cognizance of that city's specific environmental circum-stances, such as its proximity to stagnant bodies of water and exposure to harsh seasonal winds. He called attention to the particulars of physical locale, which, to Hippocrates, warranted full consideration in the planning of any new town or city, in order for the living conditions of current and future residents to be "salubrious," rather than inadvertently harmful or

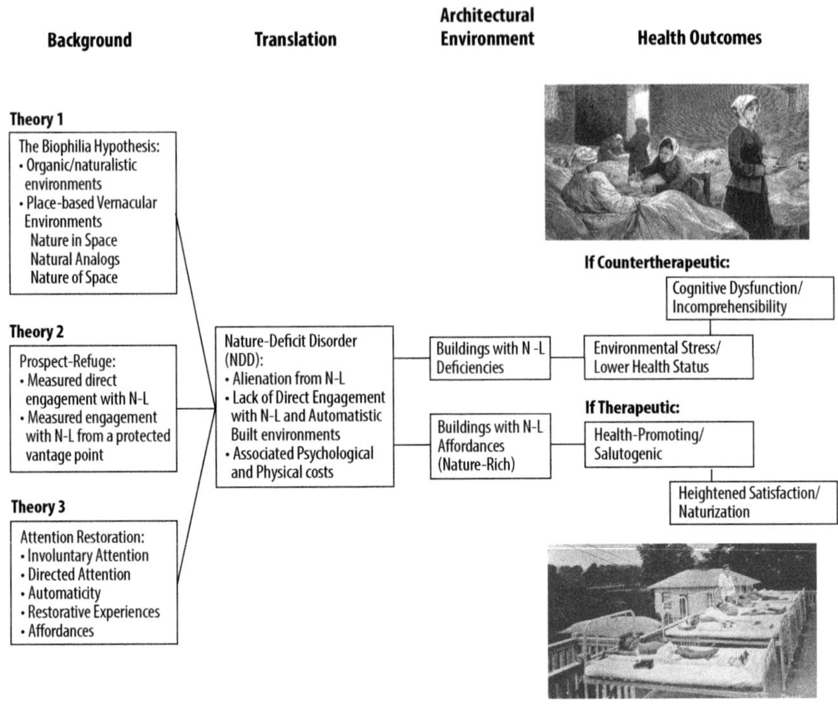

Figure 4.2. Salutogenic determinants of theraserialization. Diagram by Stephen Verderber.

otherwise deleterious from a public health standpoint. At the time, humans' physical and mental health were held to be an expression of percipient, seasonally manifesting imbalances among what Hippocrates termed the four humors (blood, black bile, phlegm, and yellow bile)—a fundamental health-promoting concept that may have predated Hippocrates but one that remained a legitimate theoretical perspective, with continued widespread usage well into the nineteenth century.[38]

The ancient Greeks developed a sophisticated approach to the treatment of human aliments. The Asklepieon at Pergamon, completed in the fifth century BC, was not a hospital per se. It was more akin to a civic institution whose function was to serve the general populace, conceived of as a combination temple and wellness retreat (as defined by contemporary standards). It was a place to obtain respite through the worship of Asclepios, the god of healing. The patient (referred to as such, since one had to wait patiently for a time when the god would turn his attention to the human subject at hand) would be instructed, through dreams and meditation exercises, to undertake an individually prescribed therapeutic treatment regimen. Nature was the most essential component of this regimen, perhaps involving a thermal bath, supplemented with physical exercise, periods of quiet contemplation, time spent outdoors and in a garden, heliotherapy sessions, proper nutrition, and rest. The Asklepieon complex featured a large open-air central courtyard, flanked on two sides by open-air wings housing patients. The patients—whose beds were arranged in long rows within these porticoed, adapted commercial stoas—could view the healing temple from the location of one's bed. The beds were positioned along the hall's length, a 24 foot × 108 foot space, open on the south-facing side. In the winter months, taut animal hides hung from pulleys above would be lowered to screen out any inclement weather.[39]

A succession of Roman emperors believed that populations who lived in the conquered lands throughout the empire should be able to benefit from an array of civic buildings and complexes. If such egalitarian amenities were provided, it was reasoned, there would be significantly less probability of a local uprising against their far-off occupiers, based in Rome. This was the period when health-inspired Roman public baths were conceived of and constructed. The most extravagant of these many dozens of public complexes were built in Rome, notably the Baths of Caracalla (212–217 AD) and the Great Baths of Diocletian, constructed between 298 and 306 AD. Less expansive but functionally similar natural spring baths were built in town centers and cities, including the unearthed, reconstructed complex at Bath in the UK (completed in the second century AD). At Bath, an intricately constructed warren of preparatory rooms typically opened directly onto a large open-air bathing pool at the center of the structure and its larger, surrounding complex. Notably, massive load-bearing partition walls and other types of room-to-room partitions were minimized in these elaborate public bath complexes.

Many centuries later, the wellness spa / retreats of the nineteenth and early twentieth centuries in North America would, in part, be inspired by Thomas Jefferson's University of Virginia campus (1819–1830) and, to some extent, by the Roman bath complexes as architectural precedents. The typical American spa/retreat featured a hotel-like manor house, surrounded by numerous freestanding pavilions situated in expansive, attractive grounds, far from the contagious diseases and miasmas that frequently plagued cities and towns during this period. The Age of Enlightenment in the fifteenth century brought not only advancements in the application of reason and scientific method, but also a profound shift toward an appreciation of naturalistic environments and wildlife. This was fueled by a newfound belief in the thoughts and intent of God being more ideally revealed, and hence received, through an individual's immersion in the pastoral wilderness.[40] Beginning in the 1600s, wealthy individuals and families would travel to a nearby or not-too-distant spa/retreat to partake in its calming, restorative waters, physical exercise, and ancillary social activities. Later, in the Romantic Movement, cities and towns would be harshly critiqued as the main causes of nearly all deleterious effects on individual humans and on the public's health. This included the mental, social, and moral threats that cities and towns inflicted on the rhythms of everyday life, an anti-urban bias that remains to this day. This persistent, unfavorable critique manifests in the current century with respect to the dichotomous relationship between urban centers versus mor-spacious, greener suburbs and remote rural cottages, especially idyllic retreats directly located on bodies of fresh, uncontaminated water, far from the impurities of potentially contaminated cities and towns.

By the late nineteenth century, the tuberculosis sanitorium had emerged as a distinct architectural building type for human health promotion (see chapter 2). Their broad, expansive open-air terraces demonstrated how modern architecture could aptly accommodate both the ancient Greek practices and the then-recently rediscovered treatment regimen known as heliotherapy.[41] Many TB hospitals were constructed in rural settings, far from the putrid, contaminated city. All were based on the nearly identical rationale that had governed the location of spa/retreats a generation or two earlier. A contemporary example is a hospital's therapeutic garden, which began to appear in the 1980s as a reaction against the nature-devoid modern megahospital.[42] Florence Nightingale, 120 years earlier, in her pioneering book *Notes on Hospitals* (1859), had extolled the therapeutic benefits of nature to patients in a hospital environment. In what would become internationally known (in time rather generically) as Nightingale Ward Hospitals, these buildings featured rectangular open wards, with green courtyards situated between them. These one- or two-level hospitals were an updated version of the open, rectangular hospital wards at the Hôpital Lariboisière in Paris (1846–1854), which Nightingale had toured before the Crimean War (1854–1856) and was most impressed. Not coincidentally, *miasma theory* became predominant at this time, postulating that the filthy, foul air of Industrial Age cities was the primary agent for nearly all contagious disease transmissions. To Nightingale, a patient's exposure to natural ventilation, sunlight, and sanitary conditions would be antithetical to this new reality: "There shall be no enclosed courts with high walls, for they stagnate the air. All enclosed courts, narrow cul-de-sac, high adjacent walls, closed angles, overshadowing trees, and other obstructions to outer ventilation should be sedulously avoided at whatever cost."[43]

Regarding public health advancements at this time, the Garden City Movement, promulgated by Ebenezer Howard and his contemporaries in the late nineteenth century, represented an attempt to ameliorate the downsides of toxicity and the overcrowded living conditions in Industrial Age cities. Howard—in his influential treatise *To-morrow: A Peaceful Path to Real Reform* (1898), which he expanded a few years later into *Garden Cities of To-morrow* (1902)—presented a well-received alternate paradigm to the status quo.[44] During this same period, *germ theory* had gained widespread popularity. By the end of the nineteenth century, it had supplanted miasma theory. The advancement of germ theory would prove effective in combating infectious illnesses previously requiring hospitalization, although it could not fully account for the continued prevalence of chronic conditions, such as cardiovascular disease and diabetes. Meanwhile, the celebrated landscape architect Frederick Law Olmsted (1822–1903)—who, in time, would receive praise as the father of the urban park movement—advanced the same prevailing medical and scientific theories, extolling the public health virtues of naturalistic open spaces in urban centers, with the intent of helping to mitigate mental illnesses, urban malaises, and the general unhealthfulness of urban populations.[45]

Early-twentieth-century architects, including Austrian-born Rudolph Schindler (1887–1953), expressed a high regard for a significant presence of naturalistic content in architecture. After studying with Adolf Loos for a year, Schindler had left Vienna in 1914 for the US, working in the office of Frank Lloyd Wright in Chicago from 1917 to 1920. He relocated to California in 1920, where he established his own architectural office. Schindler was influential in what he referred to as *organicism* in his buildings. These early commissions were mostly single-family residences, allowing him to exhibit his keen interest in maximizing numerous salutogenic interdependencies: views, fresh air, natural daylight, and layered, visually interconnected (theraserialized) transparency between the indoors and outdoors. He was unequivocal in a belief that buildings needed to be designed in reverse—from inward to outward, and vice versa—making extensive use of stepped sections on their irregularly sloping sites, thereby creating a more naturalistic condition for gardens, terraces, and courtyards, all elements incorporated in Wright's best residential work. Schindler had been influenced by Wright's introduction to the 1908 Wasmuth Exhibition and Wright's accompanying masterful drawings, in which he advocated for extensive horizontal sectional stepping and for situating buildings into naturalistic "prairie horizons."[46] This version of transparent two-way fluidity characterized Schindler's best residential work in California. His buildings opened unrestrained to the horizon, as if to actively reach outward, touching the immediacy of nature and beyond, thus inversely pulling nature back within.

Architect Richard Neutra (1892–1970) was another modernist highly influenced by the International Style. His work also broke down barriers previously isolating a building's occupants from their fuller expose to nature and its myriad psychological affordances. Neutra was a mid-twentieth-century modernist whose private residences, most of which were also built in California, established an international reputation. His Lovell "Health House" (1929) in Los Angeles is now recognized as an International Style masterpiece. Its formal composition was open in plan. This residence featured full-height windows, sliding glass doors, abundant natural daylight, and dramatic views of the city and its surrounding canyons. Neutra's Von Sternberg residence, completed in 1935 (demolished in 1972) and once owned by author Ayn Rand, continues to serve as an architectural exemplar for the dematerialization of static, opaque wall planes. Its generously proportioned interior living spaces and delicate steel-frame structure visually transition into an outdoor pool area, establishing an unbroken continuum of health-promoting, transactive connectedness. His Kaufman Desert House (1947) in Palm Springs and the Tremaine House in Santa Monica (1948) are similarly strong examples of health-promoting design as applied to private residential commissions.[47]

Wright, Schindler, and Neutra all championed the rejection of Victorian era stuffy, rigid, unyielding architectural aesthetics and the obsession with rigid formal symmetry (something especially afflicting hospitals). It was a time when a building's perimeter wall functioned primarily, in retrospect, as a visual guillotine, with its exterior wall plane slamming to the ground, disconnecting occupants from landscape and nature.[48]

THERASERIALIZATION

Synopsis: Theraserialization is the two-way fluidity between a building and its nature and landscape (N-L) environs in a manner that contributes to the restorative health of a building's inhabitants. Its theoretical imperatives are drawn from environmental psychology and nature-deficit disorder. The term—a conjunction of the terms "therapeutic" (effects) and "serialize" (buildings)—is of potential significant benefit in clinical treatments by restoring a patient's transactive relationship with the timeless affordances of N-L and countering the human-inflicted denaturization of the planet.

Theraserialization is an architectural design strategy premised on drawing nature into health care architecture and, in turn, opening up these specialized buildings to proactively project outward, thereby revealing the building's passive/active symbiosis with nature and landscapes. In a broader historical context, theraserialization dates from the ancient Greeks, as well as from the nineteenth and early twentieth centuries, in precursors cited earlier in this chapter and in chapter 2. It seeks to architecturally recreate the experience of walking through an untouched forest, as well as that of someone viewing this forest from within. The phenomenal experience of theraserialization in architecture draws inspiration from a variety of naturalistic narratives, both real and abstracted. Passive design strategies are fused with active strategies, including incorporating technology in an appropriate, humane manner. This facilitates surrogation by means of sampling nature (i.e., geographically remote landscapes, including deserts, polar regions, dense tropical jungles, or any other landscape) and representing it within an architectural setting. Extemporaneous experiences, reproduced through simulation and replication—either naturally in place of actual content or via AI-based surrogate representations of the real thing—are incorporated in a supplemental manner as passive or active design strategies, or in hybrid combinations. This concept is grounded in humans' timeless predilection for a balanced level of multisensory informational contact with the exterior world, as experienced from within a building.[49]

Theraserialized architecture is premised in spatial collage, superimposition, and the layering of spaces, stepped setbacks, and visual transparency as a two-way transactive continuum, revealing the building's ability to breathe. It is a strategy potentially redefining aesthetic and functional relationships between the four principal realms inherent in architecture for health: public, semipublic, semiprivate, and private realms. It by no means is an entirely new concept in architecture (I first introduced this term in my 2010 book, *Innovations in Hospital Architecture*).

MAGGIE'S CENTRES

In 1995, Maggie Keswick Jencks, the founder of the first Maggie's Centre, wrote about her difficult personal experiences while coping with breast cancer for a protracted period. Over the course of her final seven years, she dealt with a cancer diagnosis, treatment, remission, and recurrence. During this time, she diarized her insights from repeated dehumanizing hospital experiences into an innovative, nonmedical alternative to conventional cancer treatments. She envisioned a wholly alternative place where architecture, nature, and landscapes are symbiotic. Her philosophy would soon manifest in a network of, to date, twenty-six Maggie's Centres, with the first having opened in Edinburgh, Scotland, in 1996. It was designed by Frank Gehry.

These outpatient, health-promoting counseling centers are typically built on land donated by a nearby or next-door collaborating mothership medical center. Charles Jencks, a noted architectural historian (and Maggie's husband), worked tirelessly up to his death in 2019 to promote the mission of the Maggie Keswick Foundation. Architects' fees are covered by private fundraising activities, as is the cost of the building's construction, landscape design, and daily operating expenses. The formal program brief, which is provided to every architect involved in designing a Maggie's Centre, states, in part:

> The building, the landscape, the design of the interior . . . are to provide
> significant emotional impact. . . . If they [the Centres] raise your spirits,
> if even for a moment, they will have done a good job. Our buildings
> must look friendly. . . . The [architectural] footprint will be minute in
> relation to the [nearby] hospital and a Maggie's must shine like a beacon
> of hope. . . . Our buildings and our garden landscapes invite you in.
> The path must beckon and guide you clearly to the front door. The
> plantings help one shed the stress of a hospital atmosphere. . . . The
> immediate landscape [should] provide breathing space between the
> two worlds of hospital and everyday life. . . . All too often the person
> who turns to a Maggie's does so because cancer has turned their world
> upside down. . . . Our Centres must look and feel joyous, while calming.
> . . . The impression they must give is "I can imagine feeling different
> here". . . allowing each individual to take charge of how they want to
> use the outside and inside space, the built and the natural environment
> while reminded of the seasonally changing scene outside. . . . We want
> our buildings to encourage people to talk to each other, while offering

corners to tuck up in with a book, where one can sit and watch but not necessarily join in. Furnishings and artworks are very important. . . . What we are looking for in our architects and designers is imagination and thoughtfulness beyond the normal boundaries of mere function. Hospitals seem hopelessly large and confusing and their sites enormous, compounded by the proliferation of signage, endless corridors, and long treks between departments. The patients who must negotiate them feel like very small cogs in a very large machine. . . . The scale of a Maggie's is deliberately domestic, the antithesis of a hospital.[50]

In other words, theraserialization is a primary design intent. *A theraserialized building for health care salutogenically reconnects its occupants with the timeless, restorative properties of N-L through the provision of involuntarily interesting spaces and experiences. It provides a range of indoor and outdoor immersive N-L experiences, in contrast to the human desecration of the earth's natural ecologies in the climate crisis and the dehumanizing qualities of most hospitals today.*

Maggie's Oxford

Maggie's Oxford (figs. 4.3, 4.4, and 4.5), built in 2014 on the suburban campus of Churchill Hospital in Oxford, UK, was designed by Wilkinson Eyre Architects. It is surrounded by a dense grove of trees. An inviting atmosphere of warmth emanates from within. As one approaches, the colors of tree trunks and canopies coordinate with the exterior materials and colors of this inventively designed, informal, rather humble building. A small stream passes beneath it. Large windows with treelike diagonal frames afford views of a natural, undisturbed site, conveying a calming atmosphere throughout the building. A staircase is provided to invite direct use of this natural habitat. Natural light is abundant throughout the interior, further establishing its theraserialization. The structure resembles a treehouse, appearing to hover among the trees. It breathes outward from all sides, encompassing open space above and below. The Centre's occupants interact virtually everywhere within with the natural environment, through the sights and sounds of birds and animals inhabiting the immediate site directly below and surrounding landscape. The leaves of the trees rustle overhead, and indigenous plant species thrive, bathed in the sunlight nourishing all living things sharing this site. The undisturbed exterior environs below aptly reinforce multisensory connectivity between architecture, living species, and nature-landscape.

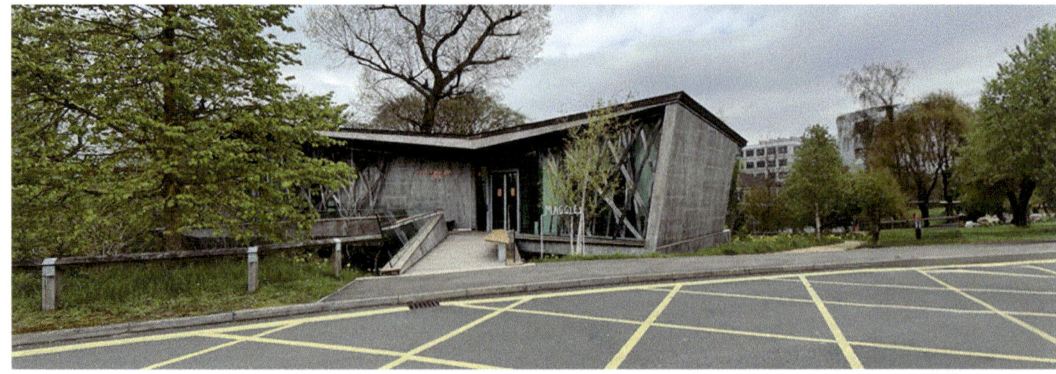
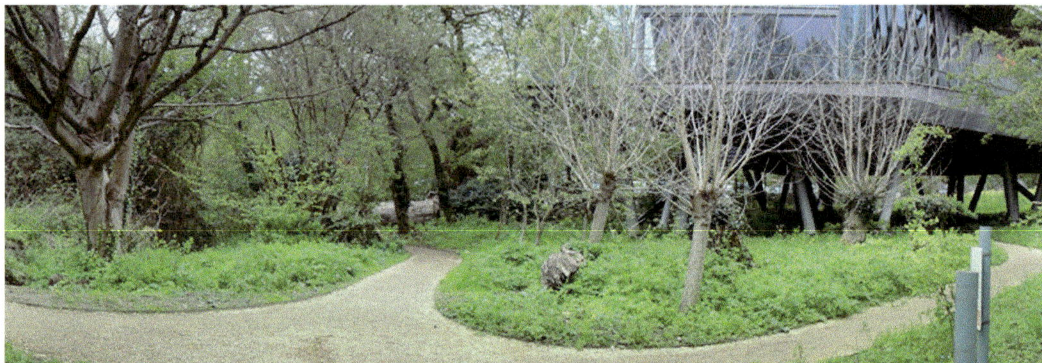
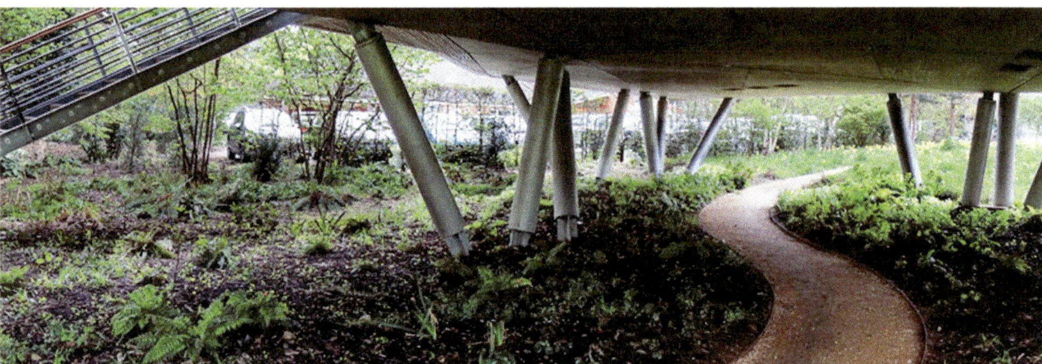
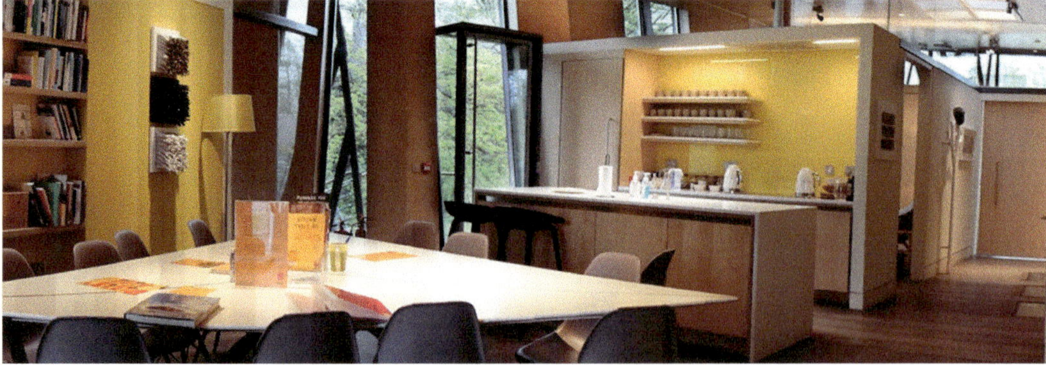

Figure 4.3. Maggie's Centre, Oxford, United Kingdom, theraserialization, 2023. Photos by Stephen Verderber.

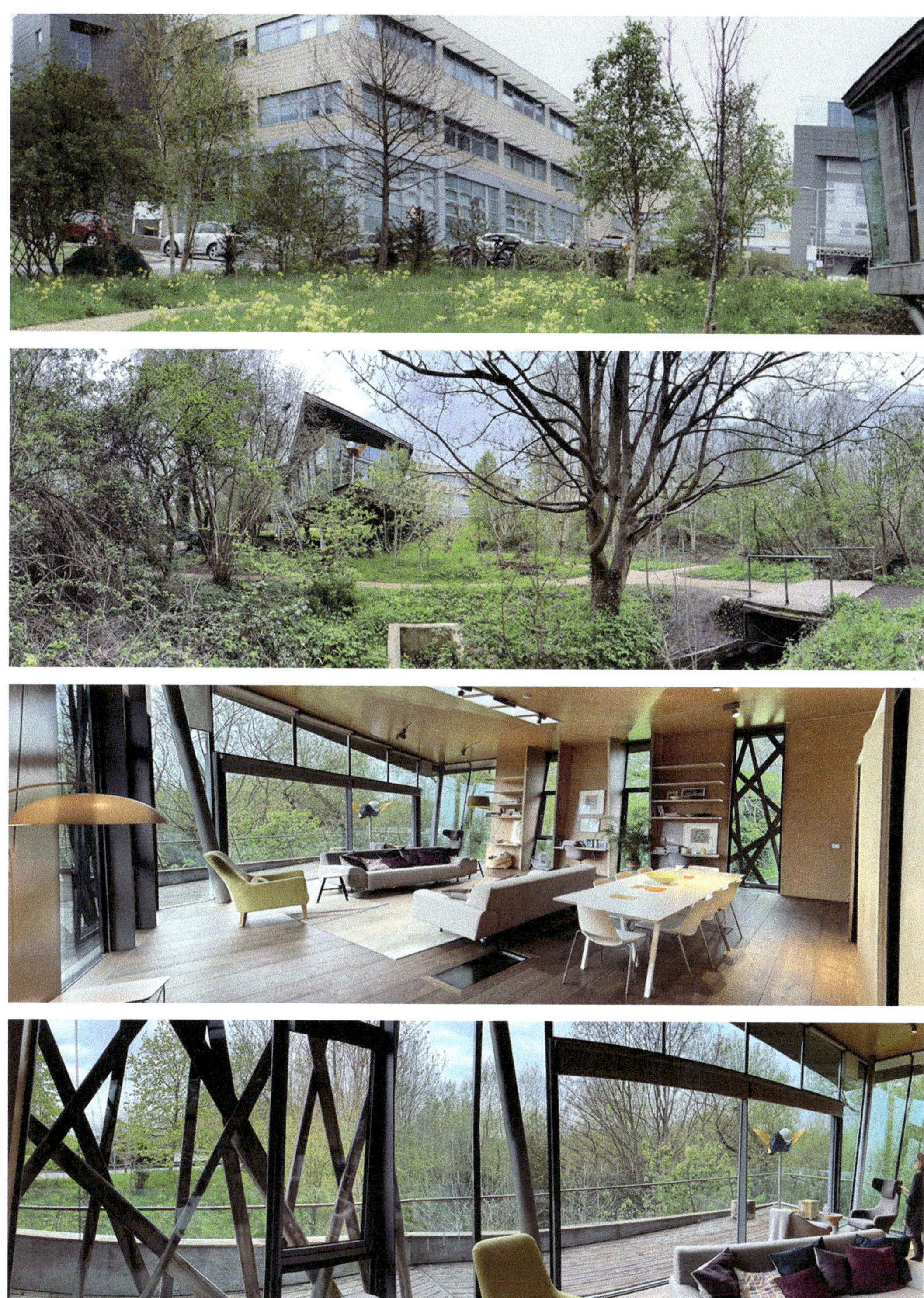

Figure 4.4. Maggie's Centre, Oxford, United Kingdom, theraserialization, 2023. Photos by Stephen Verderber.

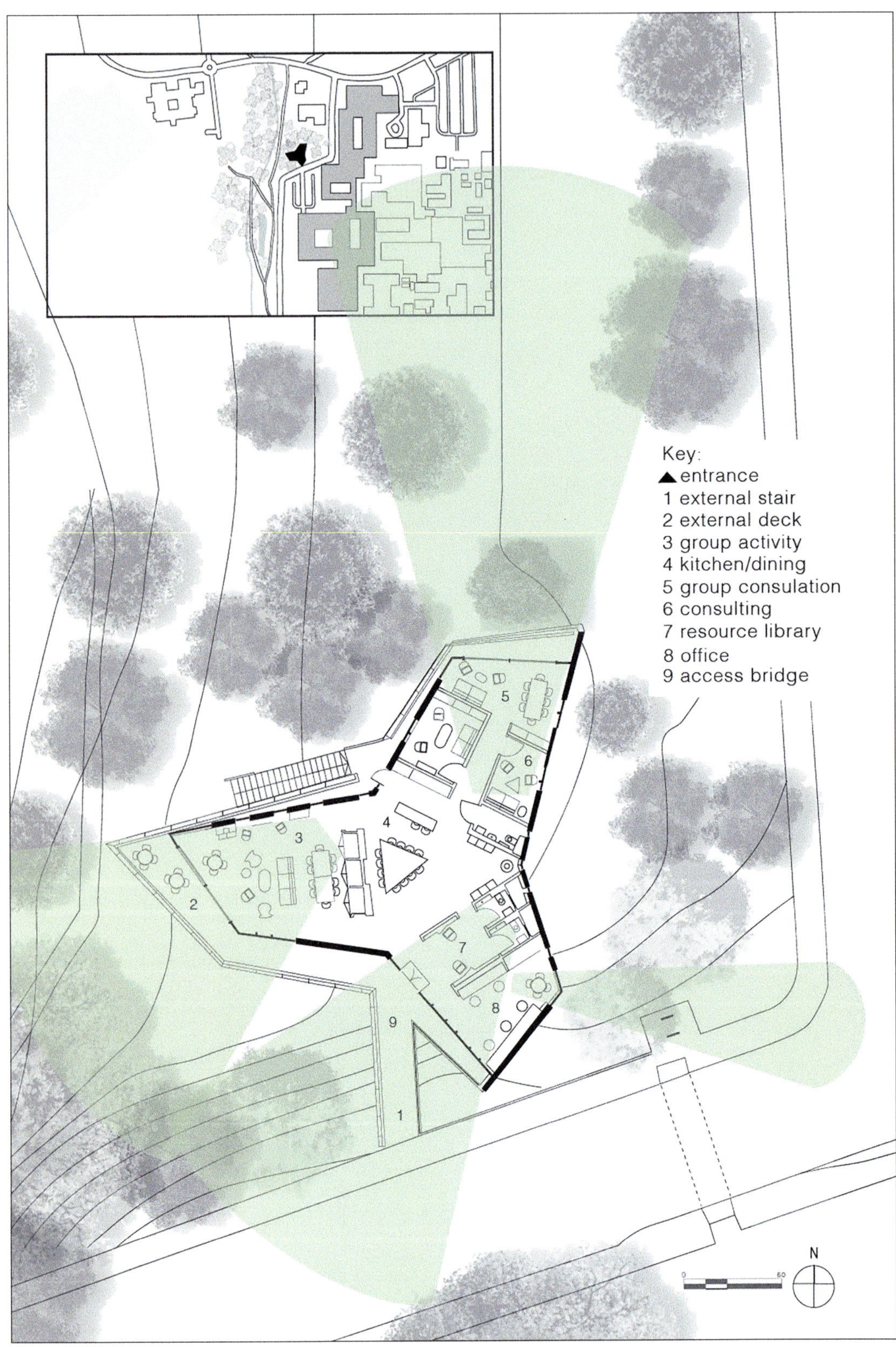

Figure 4.5. Maggie's Centre, Oxford, United Kingdom, site plan and floor plan, 2023. Drawing by Stephen Verderber and Gal Volovsky Fridman.

Maggie's Manchester

Maggie's vision has been to establish strong spatial and sensory connectivity with nature-landscape. In this regard, Maggie's Manchester, UK (figs. 4.6, 4.7, and 4.8)—which opened in 2016 and was designed by Foster + Partners, with Dan Pearson Studio as landscape architects—faced a somewhat unique set of challenges. Its parti is narrow, and the building gradually dematerializes into its surrounding exterior environs—actually a reclaimed site, formerly an asphalt parking lot. Interior spaces feature strong view connectivity with this recaptured urban site. Interior spaces flow into one another, on to the exterior greenhouse and its adjacent gardens. A repetitive, exposed timber structural framing system further establishes its theraserialized connectivity with site and nature-landscape. Exterior columns are covered with climbing vines, giving the structure the look of attempting to further dematerialize into the landscape. The adjoining greenhouse, with its semienclosed patios and long workbench, is a central feature, extending outward on an axis from the interior circulation spine. The surrounding garden invites its year-round use. Its abundant plantings evoke the process of spiritual renewal while concurrently functioning as a setting for various social activities and horticultural therapy. Several raised-platform gardening beds in the greenhouse invite use by those with limited physical mobility. An upper-level loft space spans the length of the building housing the Centre's administrative and volunteer staff. Numerous skylights transmit natural light into its various workspaces and the spaces on the main level below. The mothership-affiliated medical institution in this case is the nearby Christie Foundation Trust National Health Service (NHS) Hospital, one block away.

Maggie's Oldham

Maggie's Oldham, built in Oldham, UK, in 2017, was designed by dRMM Architects and is an integral part of the Royal Oldham NHS Hospital's medical campus. This Maggie's Centre is located right across the street from the main hospital's front door. Like the Centre at Oxford, this structure is also a virtual treehouse, rising above its downward-sloping natural landscape—once the site of a hospital maintenance shop. Theraserialization is utilized to lift the building off the ground, with a cut-out undulating circular volume at the building's center revealing views of an undisturbed site immediately below. Undulating full-height glass panels wrap around the courtyard. A single large tree occupies the courtyard below and activates the entire

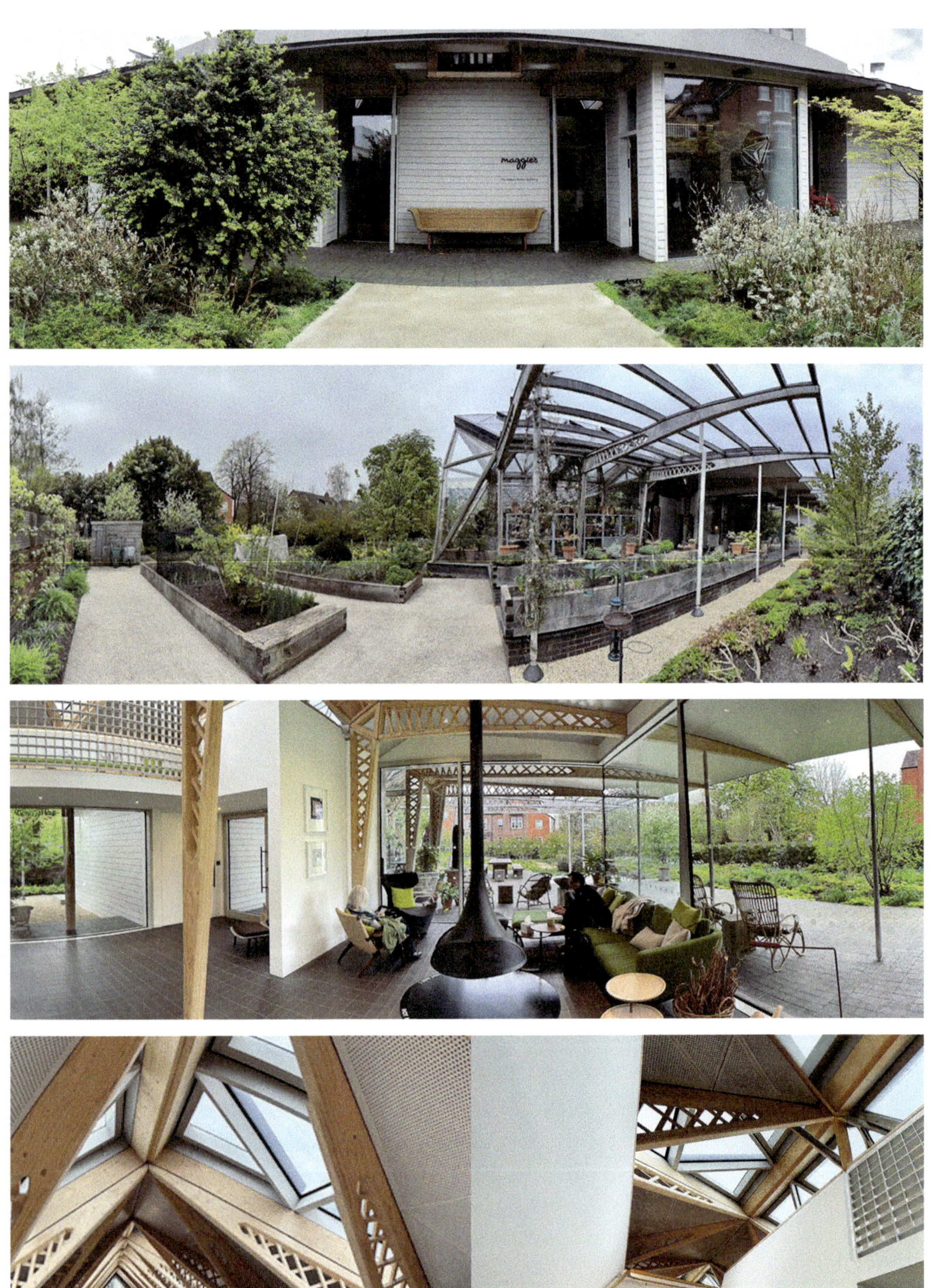

Figure 4.6. Maggie's Centre, Manchester, United Kingdom, theraserialization, 2023. Photos by Stephen Verderber.

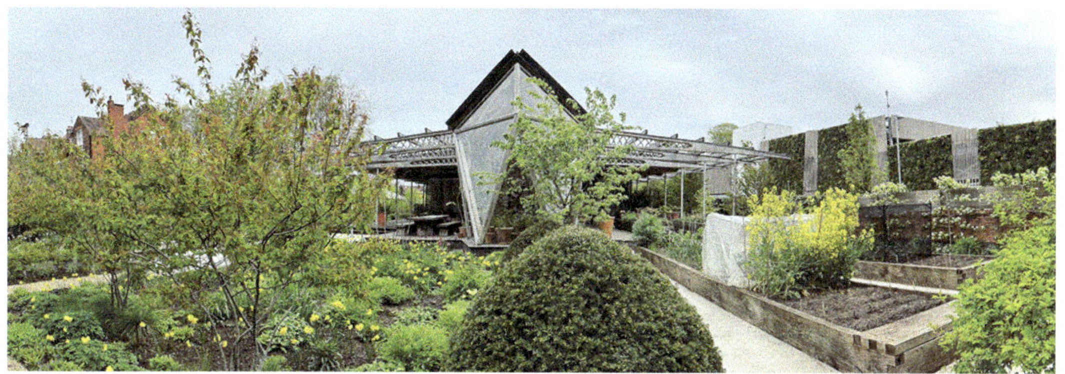
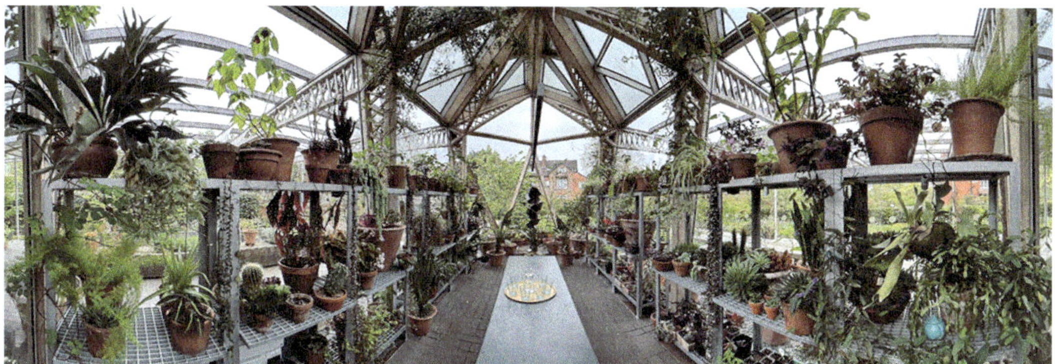
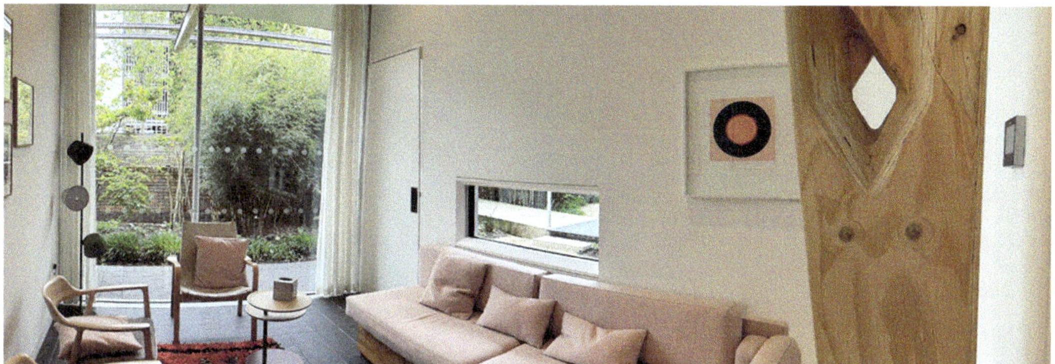
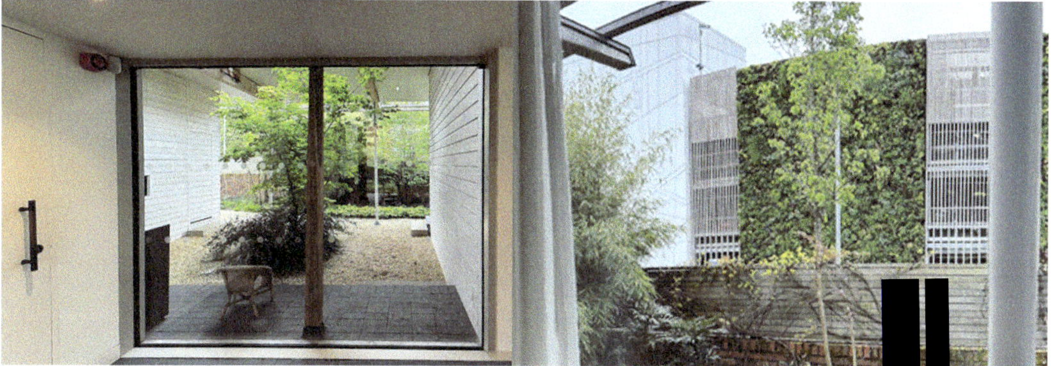

Figure 4.7. Maggie's Centre, Manchester, United Kingdom, theraserialization, 2023. Photos by Stephen Verderber.

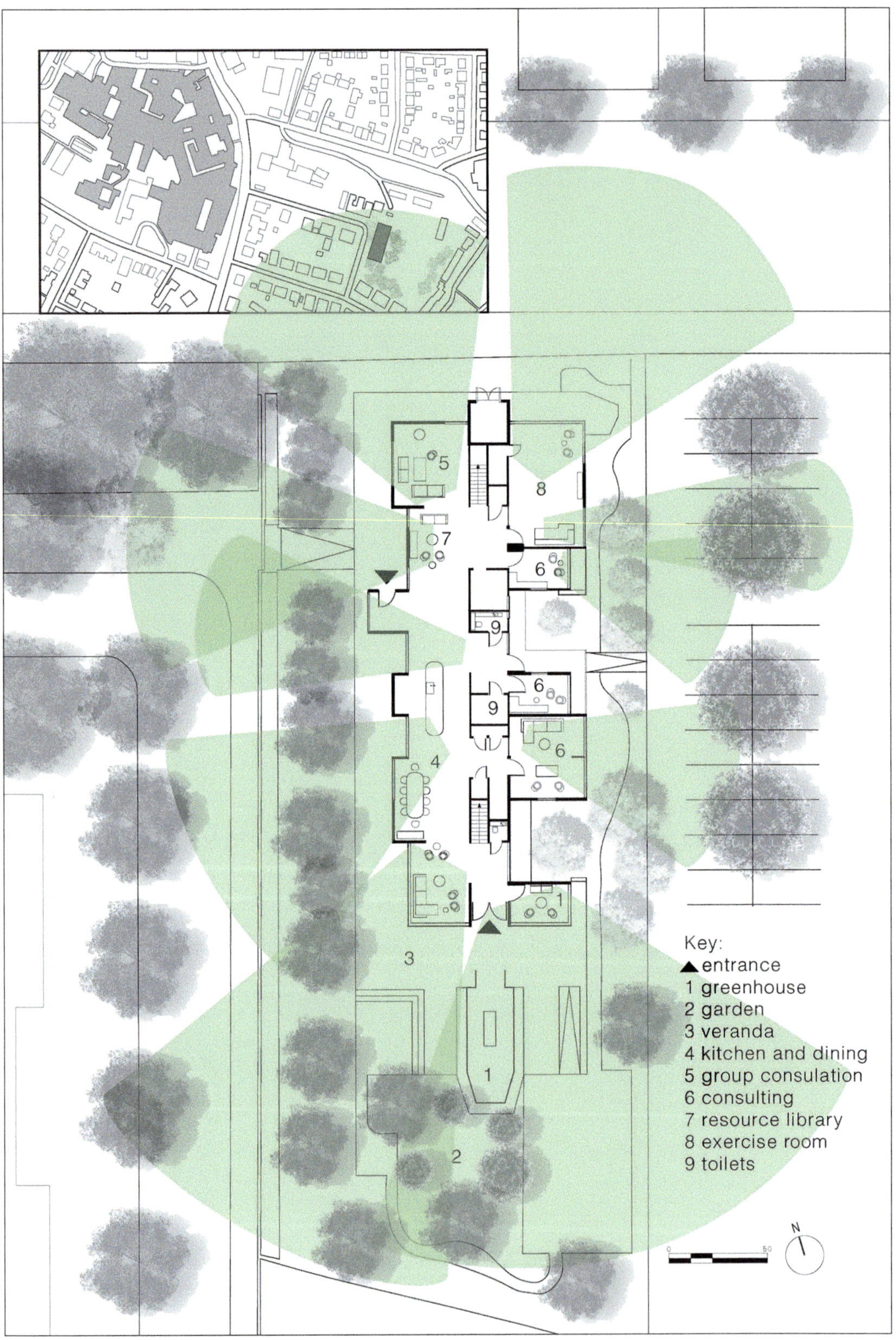

Figure 4.8. Maggie's Centre, Manchester, United Kingdom, site plan and floor plan, 2023. Drawing by Stephen Verderber and Gal Volovsky Fridman.

building. Interior spaces are essentially open plan throughout. A footbridge establishes a strong connection with the naturalistic green space beneath, continuing to either side. The undulating glass-paneled courtyard creates the sensation of standing inside a large aquarium. A small greenhouse for gardening and social activities is at the southern edge of the site. This amenity and the adjacent natural landscape are accessed by an exterior staircase. The treehouse structure contains open-plan administrative spaces, a small resources room / library, a large kitchen and dining area, a meeting table, and a multipurpose counseling room, featuring a single draw curtain. The latter space is subdividable into two smaller areas for counseling or more active uses, including yoga classes and music therapy. The curtain can be fully or partially closed or entirely opened, revealing expansive views of the surrounding neighborhood and hillsides beyond the city.

THE NATURE IMMERSION CENTER

These three Maggie's Centres express many fundamental aspects of posthumanism—and provide a promising way forward to inform and shape health care architecture in the twenty-first century. It is both an old and a new perspective, reprising certain essential qualities found in nineteenth-century wellness spa / retreats and the TB hospitals of the early twentieth century (see chapter 2). A proposed new building type, described below— the *nature immersion center* (NIC)—draws inspiration from Maggie's Centres and historical precursors, including ancient Roman bath complexes, the nineteenth- and early twentieth-century spa/retreat movement in Europe and North America, and the heliothropic architectural features of the hundreds of TB sanitoriums constructed in the past 125 years worldwide. This proposed building type for health is designed and operated to promote human health in the Anthropocene through restorative therapeutic treatments for individuals suffering from the symptoms of nature-deficit disorder, seasonal affective disorder, and related sensory deprivation conditions associated with physical, psychological, and spiritual disconnection from nature and landscape. The intent is to immerse a patient in restorative N-L experiences to help reduce and ameliorate stress, anxiety, and depression. Its basic premise, or mission, is to address psycho-emotional and spiritual health, with no overt medical or pharmacological intervention provided on site.[51] These places would be staffed by an interdisciplinary team of professional

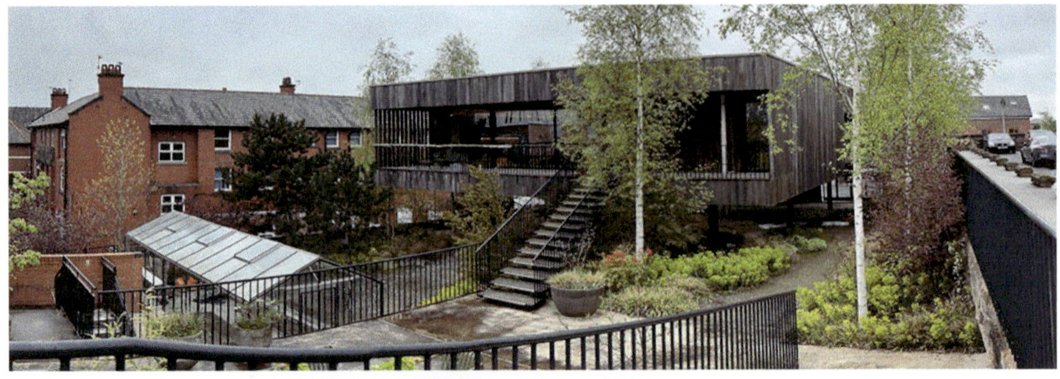

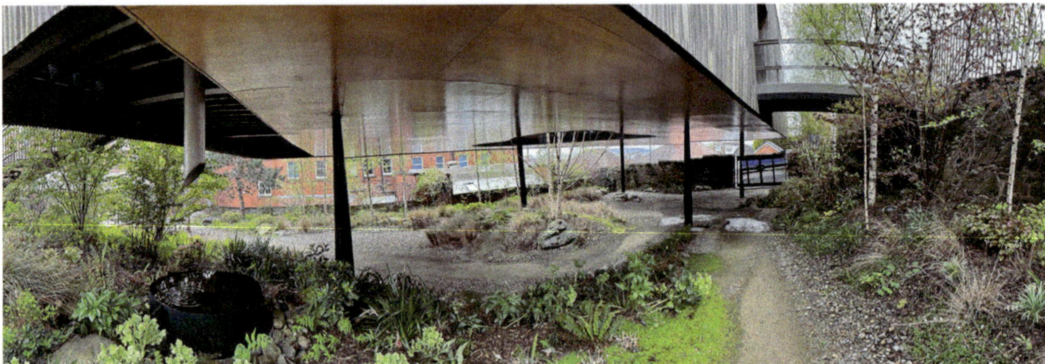

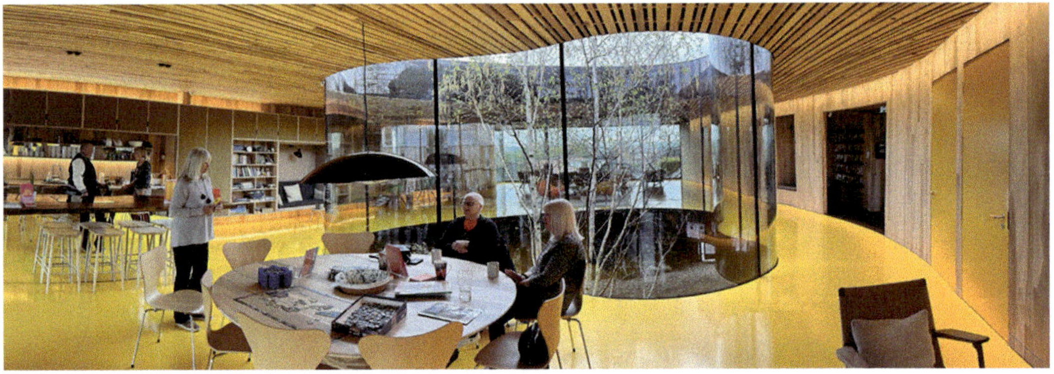

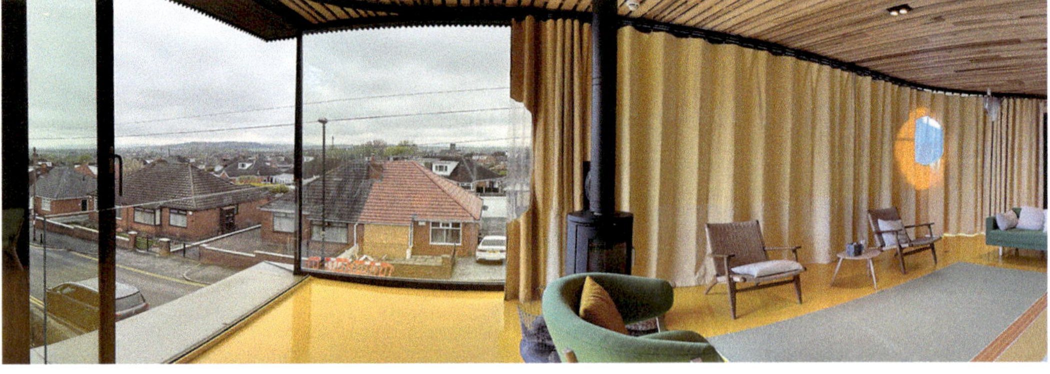

Figure 4.9. Maggie's Centre, Oldham, United Kingdom, theraserialization, 2023. Photos by Stephen Verderber.

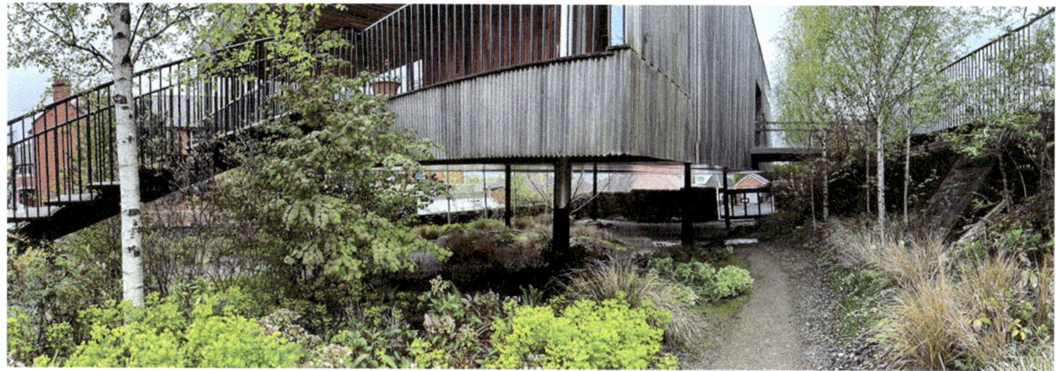

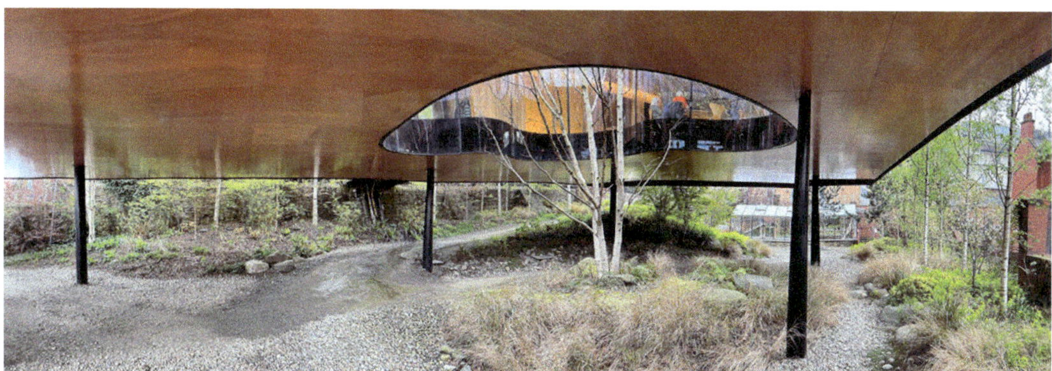

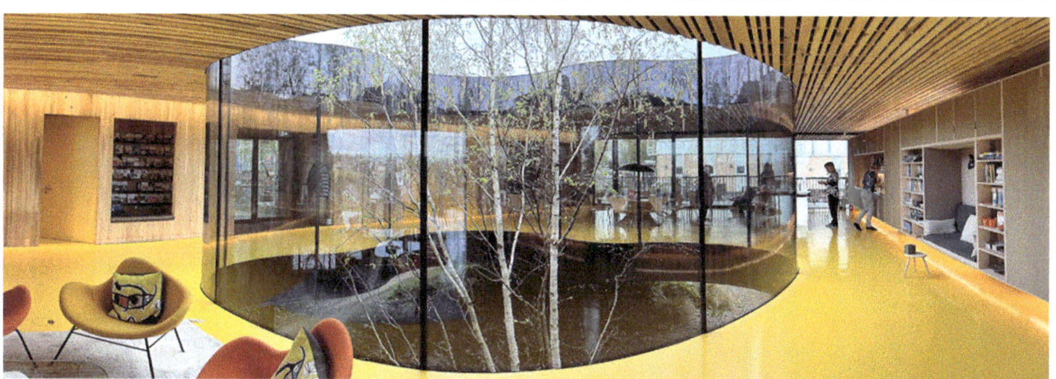

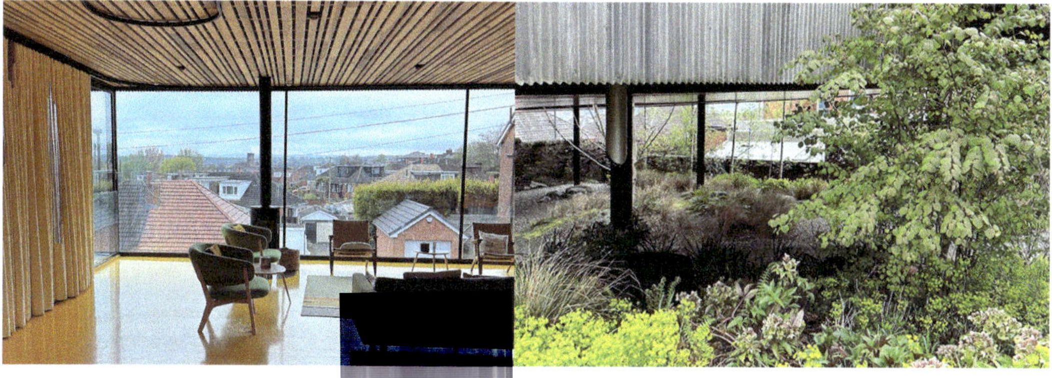

Figure 4.10. Maggie's Centre, Oldham, United Kingdom, theraserialization, 2023. Photos by Stephen Verderber.

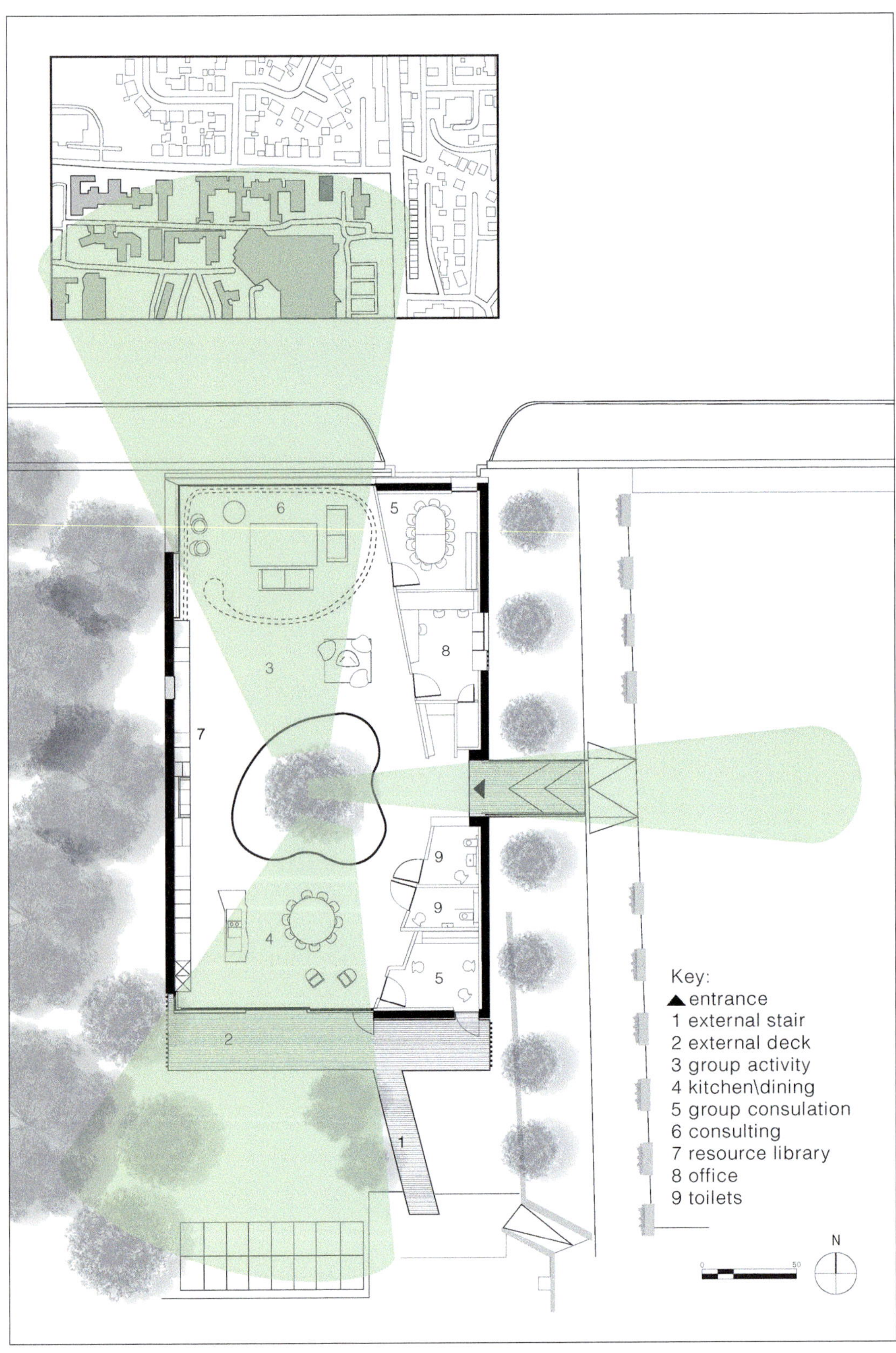

Figure 4.11. Maggie's Centre, Oldham, United Kingdom, site plan and floor plan, 2023. Drawing by Stephen Verderber and Gal Volovsky Fridman.

therapists and counselors, plus administrative and support staff, complimented by assistance from local volunteers. No physicians or nurses would work on site or be contracted from external organizations or agencies. Ideally, these places would be built near a mothership health care institution and, preferably, in proximity to a mainstream behavioral health treatment facility providing inpatient and outpatient services, not unlike Maggie's Centres. More broadly, these places can support the amelioration of adverse human health outcomes with regard to planetary ecological degradation. Architecturally, a nature immersion center would embody the following core functions:

- an inviting, landscaped exterior arrival sequence,
- a welcoming front door and arrival intake area,
- a living room overlooking landscaped exterior environs,
- clinical treatment areas affording abundant contact with nature,
- corresponding exterior and interior restorative treatment areas,
- opportunities for prospect-refuge behaviors, and
- theraserialized spaces throughout.

The nature immersion center and its immediate environs provide a reminder of the rhythms of seasonal change, related environmentally based dimensions of temporality, and one's reaffirmed relationship to the physical natural world. The NIC would provide multiple vantage points where people can look out into N-L from multiple viewing stations. These areas are to function as respites—semisequestered nooks to get away from a nature-degraded everyday routine—while supporting socialization when so desired. Diverse opportunities for prospect-refuge immersion in real and simulated N-L settings—that is, the ability to quietly, experience a green space or wooded area while reading, listening to music, or experiencing art or the sounds of nature. These places are not art galleries. Nor are they to be misconstrued as day spa/retreats, such as the wave of spas that have proliferated in North America and elsewhere in the past decade. They do borrow elements from the day spa as a building type. What would differ in the NIC is how every room and space is carefully programmed to therapeutically support N-L attention restoration practices. From a small consultation room to a reapportionable multipurpose room, each is furnished with treatment-appropriate accouterments. Bear in mind functional adjacencies and how everything blends together with the whole, greater than sum of the parts. Areas overlooking courtyards and other green spaces, as well as greenhouses, help foster N-L person/environment relationships. The size and ambiance of an NIC is deliberately *domestic* and assiduously *antihospital* in its aesthetic vocabulary and day-to-day functionality. A preliminary, foundational set of site-planning and architectural design considerations for this proposed new building type is provided in appendix A.

There will be skeptics, of course, those who see no need whatsoever for any such new building type for health care. As is being reported in the mainstream media nearly every day, the general public's trust in science, medicine, and public health as a profession is currently on the wane. Critics of this building type will argue against the very existence of nature deficit disorder and related environmentally based sensory deficit disorders, especially if linked with the continued degradation of the everyday physical world we live in. Unfortunately, the evidence of this declining public trust is real. The rates of childhood vaccination against dangerous diseases like diphtheria, tetanus, and measles have fallen in recent years, and nonmedical exemptions to kindergarten-age routine vaccinations in young children are on the rise. Increasingly, public health specialists view climate change skepticism as a global "infodemic." A recent survey published by the Pew Research Center substantiates this. Between 2016 and 2023, a decline in the public's trust in scientists and a corresponding decrease in the belief that science has a positive impact on society have become more pronounced.[52] What will happen if (and when) there is another global pandemic such as the avian bird flu, or a widespread climate catastrophe, or a biosecurity public health emergency such as anthrax? Further, this proposal for the NIC is as a nonclinical alternative, similar in this way to the Maggie's Centres. The sheer physical size, complexity, and organizational bureaucracies of conventional hospitals and medical centers—including mainstream mental health and substance abuse treatment facilities—warrant new antihospitalist architectural alternatives.

DENATURIZATION AND HEALTH INEQUITIES

Jill Suttie writes:

> Trees are important to our lives in many ways. Most obvious is their
> role in producing the oxygen we breathe and in sequestering carbon
> dioxide . . . but science suggests trees provide other important benefits.

> . . . Nature exposure helps to decrease our stress and anxiety. Much research has been conducted in forests . . . and the psychological benefits of walking through forested environments will have a more important role in promoting mental health in the future . . . through the practice of "forest bathing." Studies have shown that spending time in forests benefits our immune systems.[53]

One need not be a tree-hugging environmentalist to appreciate trees as essential sources of oxygen. Yet they provide both us and the planet with far more. Their root systems help stem soil erosion and provide essential shade, safety, and protection. When Hurricane Katrina struck metropolitan New Orleans in 2005, more than 400,000 trees were destroyed. It uprooted thousands of massive oaks that had survived for generations, and toxic floodwater brine poisoned their root systems. Eighteen years later, the city still struggled to restore the health of its urban treescape. In response, a nonprofit organization, Sustaining Our Urban Landscape (SOUL), was founded to combat the nearly 30 percent loss of the city's urban tree canopy over the past two decades. Approximately 4,000 acres of tree cover have been lost, confirmed by satellite imagery. SOUL established a relationship between the degree of urban tree cover, socioeconomic income levels, rising mean temperatures, and increased flood risks.

Research revealed the lowest-lying flood-prone neighborhoods and the hottest (not coincidentally), poorest neighborhoods tended to have the least amount of tree cover. These parts of the city are also health care facility deserts. SOUL strongly advocates for the preservation of existing urban treescapes, especially in the poorest parts of the city; more landscaped public parks and promenades that are accessible to these neighborhoods; a citywide tree replanting program; and the establishment of protective heritage tree covenants.[54] Without these shields, living in N-L disadvantaged neighborhoods in New Orleans and other cities will become more perilous for the poor and the medically underserved in the coming years, as these urban populations become ever more disproportionally vulnerable to the adverse impacts of local, regional, and global N-L denaturization.[55]

Important additional lessons can be gleaned from studying Indigenous communities' symbiotic relationship with their traditional nature and landscape attributes. The period of widespread Western colonialization of Indigenous lands and populations sought to forcibly reshape, and often destroy, tribal homelands. European settlers—driven by the perception that these tribal landscapes were empty, devoid, untamed, and uncivilized—saw them as justifiably ripe for the exploitation of and capital gains derived from their natural resources and their native animal species.[56] In stark contrast, Indigenous groups' self-conceptualization of their tribal homelands saw human/landscape transactions as an ecological continuum, characterized by a deep symbiosis where the survival of one always depended on the survival of the other. We walk *in* the forest, *among* the trees, *through* the brush, and *on* the grasslands. Tall forests, impassible scrublands, open meadows, and the vegetation along a shoreline constantly and collectively shape and reshape our physical, psychological, and spiritual transactions with natural ecosystems, with other living species, and with all inanimate objects.[57]

A major stumbling block in accepting the magnitude of the growing climate crisis is our archaic perception of nature itself.[58] Ecological grief—caused by the loss of valued animal species, environmental ecosystems, and naturalistic settings—is becoming a source of growing disillusionment. This grief is a legitimate response to ecological and habitat losses. Ecological posthumanists are relatively united in their call to equally embrace all living and inanimate things in the built and natural worlds. Yet this philosophical universality has set them on a collision course with ecological preservationists who, through narrowly constructed theories, policies and resultant actions, continually strive to conserve the natural world as if it were some sort of museum attraction to be viewed from afar but not to be experienced by means of direct, firsthand immersion. Nonetheless, these curiously divergent ideologies thankfully share one basic commonality: the conclusion that human overconsumption is rapidly destroying the planet. An emerging philosophical perspective, ecological posthumanism, offers a promising alternative to the status quo in the Anthropocene. This alternative is discussed further in the following chapters.

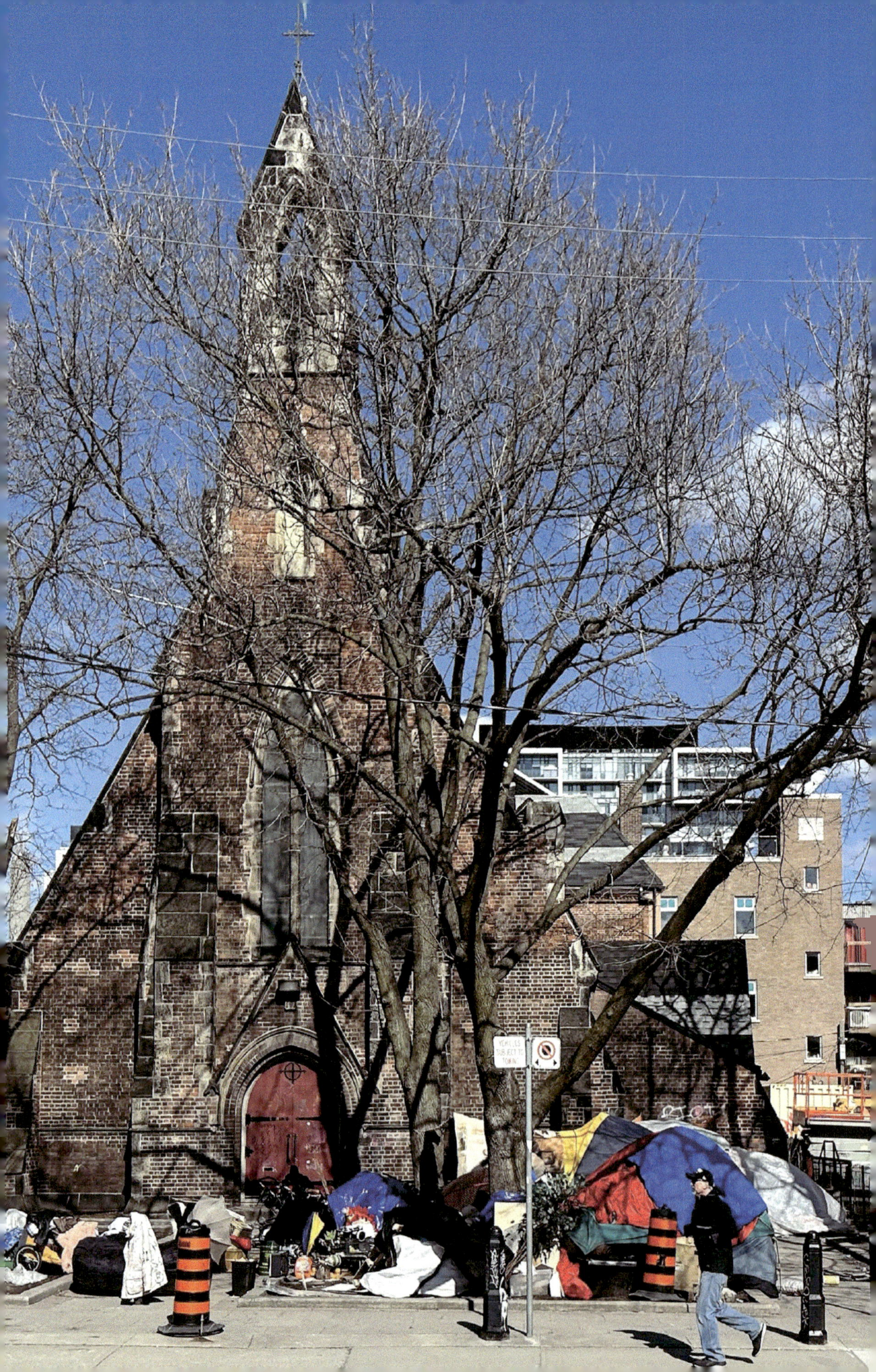

Equitable Places for Older Persons to Live

INTRODUCTION

The world is graying. By 2050 the global population aged 60 and older is projected to nearly double—from 12 to 22 percent—and while most older persons continue to experience relatively good health, many contributing importantly to society as family members, volunteering, and remaining active in the workforce, others are at heightened risk.[1] They are vulnerable to becoming unhoused, experiencing mental health and neurological/cognitive disorders, and being plagued by alcohol and substance abuse problems often combined with comorbidities, including diabetes, hearing loss, and osteoarthritis. As we age, our exposure to *comorbidities*, defined as multiple concurrent adverse health conditions, increases significantly.[2] Many colliding factors contribute to older persons' vulnerability and their experiencing chronic health inequalities. Another problem, ageism—that is, discrimination—takes on multiple uncomplimentary expressions. Unfortunately, this can translate into built environment–based ageism, of which housing discrimination is but one example with direct implications for architecture (fig. 5.1).

Figure 5.1. Homeless encampment, Church of St. Stephen-in-the-Fields, Toronto, 2023. Photo by Stephen Verderber.

AGEISM

Unhoused Older Persons

The number of unhoused older persons is on the rise in the US and elsewhere. The income level of the poorest older adults is becoming outstripped by soaring rents and real estate prices, leaving a growing number of older adult renters at risk of losing their apartment or home in the struggle to cover personal and family daily living expenses:

> On a recent rainy afternoon in Columbia Falls, Montana, just outside Glacier National Park, Lisa Beaty and Kim Hilton were prepared to sell most of their belongings before moving out of their three-bedroom, two-bath rental home. Hilton, recovering from a broken leg, watched as friends and family sorted through old hunting gear, jewelry, furniture, and clothes. . . . Hilton, 68, has type 2 diabetes, heart disease, and other health issues that have left him disabled and unable to work for years. He is covered by Medicare, but his only income is federal disability benefits. Because of a shoulder injury and fibromyalgia, 64-year-old Beaty—Hilton's partner of seven years—also relies on government disability benefits. Combined, their income is only roughly $1,500 a month. This is no longer enough. Investors bought their house this year and raised the rent from $1,000 (including utilities) to $1,800 (not including utilities). . . . "On a fixed income, I can't do it," Beaty said as she sorted through her belongings. They had nowhere else to go. The stress of this ordeal caused them to end their relationship. Despite his poor health, Hilton planned to live out of his truck while waiting for a bed in one of the few long-term care homes in Flathead County. Her wait could last days if not months.[3]

In the US, the number of renter households headed by someone aged 50 and older is expected to grow from 16 million in 2018 (35 percent of all renters) to 21.2 million by 2038 (a 40 percent rise).[4] These older adults enter retirement in worse financial shape than did same-age households in 2001. While many older adult homeowners have built up wealth and savings, renters aged 50–64 had a median net worth of only $4,990 (USD) in 2016, down in real terms from $8,860 in 2001. The drop was less pronounced for renters aged 65 and older, decreasing from $8,810 in 2001 to $6,710 in 2016, but still significant. The relative wealth of older renters is falling fast, while the percentage of cost-burdened older renters spending at least 30 percent of their total income on shelter in the US is increasing dramatically. This accounts for nearly 45 percent of all older adult renters. By 2017, this represented a new high of 8 million Americans, and it continues to rise.

Moreover, the overall poverty rate for people 65 and older had risen from 8.9 percent in 2020 to 10.3 percent by 2021, according to the National Council on Aging.[5] Greater numbers of older adults are showing up at shelters across the US as inflation and rising rents remain uncontrolled. In the US and Canada, thousands of older unhoused persons are being deprived of more-permanent housing options. Moreover, many nonprofit and for-profit residential long-term care (RLTC) 24/7 custodial facilities are fiscally strained, due inadequate governmental reimbursement rates.[6] It is impossible to know exactly how many older persons are unsheltered in the US on any given night, because national statistics do not break down the number of unsheltered people aged 25 and older into smaller age strata. Because these data are insufficiently granular, it is also impossible to ascertain how many older persons lose their home for the first time each year versus how many older persons are chronically unhoused on an annual basis. *Regardless, this crisis is expected to only worsen.*

Older Persons with Mental Health Disorders

Older persons are at greater risk of mental health disorders and associated health inequities, including chronic depression, anxiety disorders, delirium, and suicidal tendencies. Age discrimination directed against these individuals—including discrimination related to the built environment—occurs as well, resulting in the violation of older persons' basic human rights. The COVID-19 pandemic became superimposed on prior decades of deep-rooted ageism of this type, creating deplorable conditions for institutionalized older people in RLTC settings with mental health issues, including the problematic absence of proper physical distancing space and over-crowded bedrooms with four (and sometimes more) residents per room.[7] As for the suffering associated with depression and related psychological disorders, unipolar depression globally occurs in 7 percent of the general older population, accounting for 5.7 percent of the years lived with disability among persons aged 60 and older. Depression, however, often remains undiagnosed and untreated, its symptoms often overlooked because they can occur concomitantly with other health and social problems frequently encountered by older individuals. Nonetheless, persons exhibiting such symptoms tend to experience poorer overall functioning, compared with those suffering from chronic medical conditions such as hypertension or diabetes. In one recent study, older persons who had been diagnosed with a mental health condition experienced more than twice the number of acts of discrimination against them as individuals without this type of clinical diagnosis.[8]

Older Persons with Cognitive Deficits

Dementia is generally associated with the later stages of life, and the risk of developing Alzheimer's disease—a major cause of disability among older persons—increases significantly with age. Currently, more than 55 million persons in the world suffer from some form of dementia, with over 60 percent living in low- and middle-income countries. With the total number of cognitively afflicted older people increasing by the day, this number is expected to rise to 78 million by 2030 and 139 million by 2050.[9] Individuals diagnosed with these cognitive deficits come from virtually all social classes, racial and ethnic populations, and walks of life. Although only 5 percent of persons over 65 are affected, this number increases to 25 percent among those aged 85 and older. Unfortunately, these individuals are frequently stigmatized, and this, combined with ageism, can become too burdensome. Despite such difficulties, more than two-thirds of persons diagnosed with moderate to severe dementia continue to live independently in their long-time home or apartment, with only roughly one-third ever actually relocating to a 24/7 long-term care custodial setting, despite the fact that one in three individuals aged 65 and older will die with this clinical diagnosis, based on current demographic projections.[10]

Cognitive decline often is accompanied by feelings of loneliness, depression, and lower self-esteem, resulting in a tendency to withdraw from others—a condition gerontologists define as social disengagement. Individuals with dementia do not choose to have this disease, and they certainty do not deserve to be dismissed, ignored, or negatively stereotyped. Yet, because it remains a misunderstood occurrence in many societies, it is easy to overlook the day-to-day needs of these individuals.[11] The World Health Organization recognizes age-related stigma directed against persons with dementia is widespread; its corrosive effects are far reaching.[12] No successful, widely accepted medical treatments for dementia and related cognitive disorders yet exist, and this has direct impacts on the role and efficacy of architecture in the overall socioenvironmental supports equation. Without accompanying medical treatment, architecture is thrust into a perfunctory role not entirely unlike its delimited role in the bygone era of the insane asylum, prior to the advent of psychotropic drugs for clinical treatment of a wide spectrum of mental health disorders.[13] The onus is therefore still on successful advancements in medical science and public health policy, in tandem with the provision of supportive, age-appropriate architecture.[14] In this broader equation, architecture and the total built environment are prosthetic support mechanisms capable of fostering a heightened degree of well-being and healthfulness.[15]

OLDER PERSONS AND RELOCATION

Over a period of decades, Soviet authorities diverted rivers that flowed into the Aral Sea in Uzbekistan, using its water to irrigate cotton and other crops elsewhere. As a result, the world's fourth-largest inland body of water—an area about 15 percent larger than Lake Michigan—gradually shrank, triggering an immense ecological and economic domino effect, a calamity not dissimilar from catastrophes befalling other environmentally fragile places globally, due to gross resource mismanagement.[16] By 2007, the Aral Sea's surface area shrank by about 90 percent, leaving the formerly waterfront city of Muynak a mere landlocked waystation. Visitors now come to marvel at this newly created ecocide disaster zone. It has become a place where tourists take selfies near rusting ship hulks, perched high and dry in the midday sun, sprawled across a seemingly endless toxic sand bowl. This former expanse of the Aral Sea is a now blighted realm called the Aralkum Desert. Over the decades, it had been contaminated by pesticides and myriad other toxins long suspected of causing high levels of birth defects and other chronic health problems that had manifested in the surrounding area for decades.

As the Aral Sea died, this region's once-rich pastures and forests became ecologically degraded, its once-thriving biodiversity having entered a spiraling doom-loop freefall. Salty dust blown about from the parched seabed severely impacted the surrounding agricultural fields and crops, and the region's population precipitously fell as people migrated elsewhere in an unmanaged retreat. An entire natural and human ecosystem was destroyed. Tragically, Soviet authorities knew full well what was happening, yet economic interests apparently were the far more urgent priority. Interestingly, many political and economic experts note how ecological hardship related to this sea's demise greatly contributed to the region's current political volatility. A truly frightening aspect in all this is how such ecological catastrophes are being replicated across the world. Refugees flee from now-uninhabitable homelands, from bitter conflicts over dwindling resources and land disputes, from cities and regions threatened by rising seas. In the US, Lake Mead and the Great Salt Lake are shrinking, and nearby cities (including Las Vegas, Phoenix, and Los Angeles) are bracing for a severely water-restricted future. The widespread unchecked depletion of groundwater aquifers, combined with fracking and excessive irrigation for agriculture, is a looming national and international crisis. Drought and water scarcity are fast becoming symbols of humanity's environmental hubris, with vulnerable older persons frequently, increasingly, among those segments of the population disproportionately bearing the brunt of the calamitous environmental consequences.[17]

As these ecological disasters exponentially multiply, older persons with cognitive and physiological deficits are being placed at more and more risk.[18] As we age, our thermoregulatory system does not function as efficiently as earlier in life, and the inability to adroitly respond to heat waves and intense cold spells can adversely affect human mortality.[19] In addition, the reduced ability of older persons to eliminate pollutants from the body, combined with decreased lung capacity, can result in a greater risk of respiratory and heart disease. When combined with diagnosed depression, anxiety, or post-traumatic shock disorder (PTSD), it becomes ever more complicated. The physiological impact alone can adversely affect a person's well-being and mortality. Socioeconomic factors—poverty, low educational level, or the absence of family and social networks—further heighten vulnerability to excessive environmental conditions. In India, the rapidly growing need for air conditioning is accelerating global increases in temperature due to increased greenhouse emissions.[21] Currently, between 8 and 10 percent of that country's 300 million households—a country with a population of 1.4 billion people—own or rent an in-home personal AC unit, although this number is expected to explode to 50 percent by 2037, according to governmental projections. Air conditioning in India traditionally was a luxury commodity only for the wealthy, but no more. It is now a necessity for survival.

Recent research in the field of gerontology seeks to better understand older persons' vulnerability to rising temperatures and other environmental adversities attributable to a changing climate.[20] These impacts are being studied cross-culturally, including research conducted in the Nordic region,[22] in mainland China,[23] in Hong Kong,[24] and in New York City,[25] as well as in research on environmental stress experienced by older persons in extreme cold and hot conditions within residential buildings in São Paulo, Brazil.[26] A recent methodological study in Auckland, New Zealand, focused on older persons' self-assessments of their private homes after climate-related adaptations were made in order to better insulate the dwelling against extreme temperatures.[27] In a study on the impact of the type of housing construction (wood siding versus brick, in this case), it was found that for homes in the study sample (thirty, all occupied by older persons), the indoor mean ambient temperature was significantly hotter *indoors* during a summer heat wave compared with the mean outdoor ambient temperature.[28] And non-brick constructed homes were identified as the primary cause of the hotter indoor temperatures. Overall, poorly insulated dwellings, combined with nonexistent housing options, can contribute to increased health inequities among older persons.[29] As Gaia Vince writes:

> A great upheaval is coming. It will change us and our planet. Over the next fifty years, hotter temperatures combined with more intense humidity are set to make large swathes of the globe lethal for 3.5 billion. Fleeing the tropics, the coasts and formerly arable lands, huge populations will need to seek new homes. This migration has already begun—we have seen the streams of people fleeing drought-hit areas in Latin America, Africa, and Asia where farming and other rural livelihoods have become impossible. Climate-driven change is adding to a massive migration already underway to the world's cities. The number of migrants has doubled globally over the past decade, and the issue of what to do about rapidly increasing populations of displaced people will only become more urgent.[30]

In the architectural profession the alarm was sounded in 2005 in the book *Adapting Buildings and Cities for Climate Change: A 21st Century Survival Guide*. Among the topics addressed was one chapter signaling the plight of people and places most vulnerable to the adversities inflicted by forced migration.[31] More broadly, alternative diplomatic channels, cross-border negotiations, cooperative ecological pacts, and innovative built environment, policy-driven strategies in the planning and governing of existing cities will be required. High-risk cities and regions, due to their known history of and future heightened susceptibility to disaster, are attempting to transform themselves. In the extreme, some urban areas will need to be entirely abandoned in the future. With every degree of increased temperature, roughly 1 billion people are being pushed outside the global biological comfort zone in which humans have lived for thousands of years. In the Anthropocene, particularly vulnerable populations—especially children and older persons—will require relocation to new and at times entirely unfamiliar places in a world, experiencing twice as many days where temperatures exceed 50°C compared with thirty years ago. Population increases, expected to peak at perhaps 10 billion by the 2060s, will disproportionately occur in tropical regions, with their tendency to be worst hit by climate catastrophes. Paradoxically, Americans continue to migrate south straight into harm's way in high-risk locales, such as Florida and Arizona.[32]

Northward and southward migration away from the equator, by contrast, is still mainly viewed as a cultural, political, and economic disaster among countries experiencing rapid in-migration. As for the role of the climate crisis, it is a threat multiplier, with those most adversely impacted already experiencing a debased level of well-being. Ecologically degraded, denatured built environments foster income instability, causing a further-degraded ability to prepare for the next disaster. This is exacerbated by no access to health care resources, inadequate sanitation, insufficient governance structures, and a lack of collective civic agency, all of which might otherwise help improve dysfunctional conditions. The coming shocks and stresses will cause the most harm to those with the least individual and collective resiliency—the very young and the very old. Currently, most of the world's population is clustered around the 27th parallel, traditionally the latitude where the most comfortable climates and fertile land exist. On average, climate niches around the world are moving poleward at a pace of 115 centimeters per day, although this is occurring far faster in some places, such as the Bordeaux region of France. Relocation to a new home has been a time-tested solution through the millennia and can help in mitigating health and built environment inequities, architecture notwithstanding.[33]

ARCHITECTURE, RELOCATION, AND HEALTH EQUITY

It is daunting to leave the dwelling and community where one has resided, perhaps for many decades, for a new place, whether nearby or far away. The transitioning process can seem insurmountable. Health-promoting architectural supports are critical on the receiving end and along the way; their inequitable distribution can bring severe consequences and, in the extreme, death. For internally displaced persons, economic hardship migrants, and wartime refugees, the two basic types of relocation are *voluntary* and *involuntary*. Research in gerontology provides a lens through which to view this phenomenon. More specific to architecture, the involuntary relocation of institutionalized older persons has been a source of controversy since the 1970s, stemming from research in the field of environmental gerontology. This research has fairly consistently revealed the adverse consequences to health and well-being by involuntarily relocating an aged person from a private home or apartment to a nursing home, including a higher rate of occupant mortality post-move. Involuntary relocation from one nursing home to another also continues to be a source of concern from health policy, broader built-environment, and architectural perspectives, because this practice has been revealed to result in higher mortality rates post move.

Voluntary Relocation

When a resident and one's family agree to a move *a priori*, this usually consists of three phases: the anticipatory phase, the actual relocation itself, and a settling-in adaptation (or maladaptation) phase. A recent policy review essay found that once the move occurred, small-scale RLTC facilities are preferred more by residents and families, and by caregiver staff.[34] Among older residents with dementia, place attachment pre-relocation is critically important. Paying close attention to the critical details pre-move can effectively prepare the resident for what is to come. This has been repeatedly shown to help ensure a more successful overall relocation experience.[35] It is therefore important to engage the resident's family during all three phases of the move. Educational preparation meetings throughout the relocation process have also been found to be helpful, with, for example, the resident and family having a say in the size, the floor plan layout of the residential unit, and the total number of beds at the new facility.[36]

Relocation from a 24/7 long-term care custodial facility to an acute care hospital has also been studied. Here, thoughtful pre-move protocols can also help ensure a smoother outcome. This can occur as an intervention, with nursing staff involving, informing, and preparing the older person and family beforehand.[37] Pre-move education has been shown to reduce frail residents' self-reported loneliness post-move, thereby lessening the negative psychological and social impact of the transition.[38] In general, in situations lacking pre-move educational workshops, adverse outcomes, including a higher mortality rate post-move, are more likely to occur.[39] In addition, a local eldercare advocacy organization or local health council, working in concert with the facility's administration and caregiving staff, can also be beneficial when the resident is relocated from one building to another on the same campus. In short, effective pre-move educational preparation measures, together with a supportive architectural environment, can make the difference between life and death post-move.[40]

Involuntary Relocation

Relocating residents against their wishes (or those of the family) to a new, unfamiliar facility is stressful.[41] If the involuntary move is to a higher-quality architectural setting, however, then an adverse physical or mental health outcome is not nearly as likely to occur. Among one group of older residents involuntarily relocated to a smaller-scale skilled care/memory care unit within the same larger long-term care facility, no significant decline in their socialization activities or related behaviors was recorded among the study's twenty-two participants, all of whom had dementia.[42] In a related study conducted in Japan, the community's infrastructural range of amenities already in place was found to be key in older persons' successful adaptation post-move from a private apartment to an unfamiliar *nearby* setting, because it was at least in the same area of the city.[43] Their successful post-move outcomes were attributed to having previously known their new neighborhood. Involuntary uprootedness can result in a greater incidence of post-move falls among those with and without a prior history of falling. In one study, 76.9 percent of study respondents fell post-move, compared with only 51.2 percent having fallen during the pretransfer period.[44] In this same study, residents' cognitive performance declined, the incidence of clinically diagnosed depression increased, and interest in social engagement with others declined significantly.

In related research, the administration of antipsychotic medications was significantly lower among an untransferred residential cohort, compared with the group involuntarily relocated to a new 24/7 long-term care custodial facility.[45] This evidence-based research points to the reality that as we grow older, we tend to become more attached to our longtime home and local community. In post–Hurricane Katrina New Orleans, older persons involuntarily relocated from one 24/7 long-term care custodial facility to another experienced a higher rate of ulcers and a greater incidence of mortality post-move, with the new facility cited as having had a strong negative influence.[46] Another recent study found a significant post-move decrease in mood, outlook, physical functioning, and cognitive performance among the involuntarily relocated respondent group.[47] Related research in Japan found older residents who voluntarily engaged in the process, pre-relocation, through educational workshop sessions (referred to as the "acceptance cohort") proceeded to self-initiate the personalization of their bedroom at the new facility more enthusiastically than those in the "non-acceptance cohort" post-move.[48]

The Critical Role of Family

The role and agency of the family as a support modality is important in the success or failure of relocating older persons in need of 24/7 long-term custodial care. Family members can help ease the transition to a new, unfamiliar architectural setting, whether the move is involuntary or otherwise.[49] When genuinely consulted pre-move and throughout, both families and staff caregivers in general expressed a preference for aesthetically attractive, homelike—residentialist—physical surroundings.[50] When the family is involved, additional built-environment–related quality of life benefits can accrue, including heightened self-dignity, enhanced personal autonomy, lessened agitation episodes, improved sleeping patterns, increased overall nutritional health, and even stabilized physical weight level. The involvement of the family and significant others functions as a built-environment prosthetic support modality when, for example, this constituency advocates for the new architectural setting to be designed with enhanced acoustical control building materials, to minimize what would otherwise be an excessive noise level at the new residence.[51]

MANAGED RETREAT

Migration, whether within a country or across borders, is increasing. Just how many people will need to move in the coming years remains an open question—and a matter of increasing urgency. Since 2000, the World Bank has modeled anticipated future climate migration patterns globally, concluding much will be unmanaged, although out of acute need more and more will be government-mandated managed relocations.[52] In Fiji, one village has been relocated, with another thirty to forty on the waiting list, and this is happening concurrently in many other nations. In the US, the first managed retreat in this century was authorized for a tribal community in South Louisiana.[53]

> In 2016, the federal government awarded the State of Louisiana a $48.3 million block grant to assist with the Isle de Jean Charles Tribe's [now called the Jean Charles Choctaw Nation] community relocation. For three years, an unproductive back and forth transpired between the tribe and the State of Louisiana as to how best use the funds. In 2019, fed up with how discussions were going, Elder Naquin abandoned negotiations, claiming that the State had hijacked the funds and had no interest in keeping the Tribe's members together as part of the reloca-tion effort in honor of the Tribe's vision. "If you believe that the reset-tlement of Isle de Jean Charles was successful, you're headed in the wrong direction," he said during a conference on the status of the initia-tive. The State has been making improvements to roads on and around the rapidly disappearing island, and it appears to be planning on turning the island into a recreational area, despite the protests of the Tribe. . . . It is heartbreaking. . . . Instead of becoming an example of its members exercising their right to self-determination, it ended up becoming a tool that the state used to advance its own agenda. . . . This is no guide for correctly addressing the climate crisis.[54]

In 1957 this island covered 35 square miles. Now less than 1 square mile remains, and the island's remaining population is mostly French speaking. A previous relocation scheme for the tribe, headed by the US Army Corps of Engineers, failed some years earlier, as it required 100 percent buy-in from the residents, which was not forthcoming, This was mainly because most of the tribe's elders were against the move on cultural grounds. This second effort, however, did not require total buy-in. In 2016, an outreach needs assessment commenced. Many community consultation meetings occurred, followed by the establishment of a committee to identify a suit-able relocation site, encompassing between 300 and 1,000 acres, with-out direct flooding risks. A 515-acre site near Houma was soon purchased in Terrebonne Parish, forty miles inland. The relocation effort has been plagued by fits and starts, and many problems remain.

The political and economic focus in the US has only recently turned to the relocation of entire at-risk communities. State and local governments are taking notice, with some beginning to act. Managed retreats of communities are in the planning stages in Alaska, New Hampshire, Washington State, and New Jersey. Between 1989 and 2017, the Federal Emergency Management Agency (FEMA) funded more than 43,000 individual property buyouts across forty-nine of the fifty states, as well as in Puerto Rico, Guam, and the Virgin Islands.[55] The problem with this top-down governmental managed relocation policy is that it is being enacted too slowly and nearly always *after the fact*, rather than as proactive pre-move policy. In the case of Isle de Jean Charles, more than six years after the grant was awarded, only twelve homes had been built on the 515-acre site purchased, and many of the tribe's elders who had resisted the move were dead. Did the stress associated with this debacle contribute to their demise? We will never know for certain. Meanwhile, critics questioned spending $48 million (USD) to relocate thirty-six households for what, at the outset, was simply to be a model case study.

These scenarios will play out across North America from the Artic Circle to the southernmost parts of the continent. Villages in the Far North region will be relocated, because the permafrost is melting. This makes it impossible to use the frozen pathways and overland truck routes once called "ice roads" to get to and from these communities. Their fishing and hunting seasons are already radically altered, due to biodiversity losses and extreme ecohabitat destruction. In the far southern parts of the continent, excessive heat is destroying agricultural land and, in the process, annihilating farmers' livelihoods. As people in the Far North and Far South seek to migrate, where will they go? In practically every case most likely to nearby cities: Yellowknife, in the Northwest Territories in Canada; Anchorage, in Alaska; Guatemala City and Panama City, in Central America. Will these cities be able to handle unprecedented in-migration from surrounding rural regions? Time will tell. Regardless, the major share of these migrants will be the parents and grandparents of the displaced. Will they opt to stay behind?

This is where the intergenerational bonds that tie families together, which have done so for millennia, will be tested unlike ever before. Is it too much to expect governments to be entirely responsible for fully underwriting and coordinating the scale of the managed retreats that lie ahead? This is doubtful without new types of public/private partnerships. Will government alone be capable of securing the scale of public and private investments necessary to build the types of housing so acutely needed by older persons in these new places—including long-term-care, 24/7 custodial housing for those aged unable to continue living independently in intergenerational households?

Based on a United Nations estimate, each year over 20 million persons—a number that includes over 5 million older persons beyond age 65—are forced to leave their homes worldwide due to extreme weather events. By the end of this century, somewhere in the range of between 3 and 6 billion people will be left outside the human climate niche that best supports our species' continued existence, as we know it today. Many vulnerable populations will be in desperate need of access to sustainable, predictable, resilient relocation options, or else face their demise.[56] Geographic displacement from place A to place B (and beyond), combined with the impact of ecological degradation, are deeply rooted in cultural, political, economic, and health inequalities.

What precisely is organized, or managed, retreat, and how does this phenomenon pertain to the forced relocation of older persons in the climate crisis?[57] *Managed retreat* is the coordinated movement of people from places with actual environmental risks, involving the orderly (or disorderly) relocation of individuals, groups, entire communities, and, perhaps, even their physical infrastructures. Communities in disaster-prone areas are typically at the geographic epicenter of managed retreat initiatives, with the specific type depending on the particulars of the environmental threat. Managed retreat consists of voluntary (or involuntary) property acquisition, asset demolition, and relocation to a less-at-risk community—sometimes nearby, but often much farther away. Based on this discussion, infrastructural determinants, including architectural factors, to ensure a successful relocation experience among older populations in later life are presented in figure 5.2. These determinants are presented as a set of questions, or concerns, across six thematic categories.

Public Health Policy Redundant Cueing

Public health policies informing well-planned, properly funded government-managed retreat initiatives, whether voluntary or involuntary, will greatly mitigate their adverse impacts on vulnerable elderly populations. For those with reduced cognitive and physical abilities, during the pre-move phase, the use of multiple (redundantly formatted) educational media and other modes of policy-driven communications and strategies—from the very beginning of a managed retreat to its conclusion—is important in instilling greater personal control and self-confidence in the to-be-relocated population, benefiting the individual, the family, and significant others. Compassionate public health policies, especially policies involving the family (in conjunction with eldercare advocacy organizations), can help instill

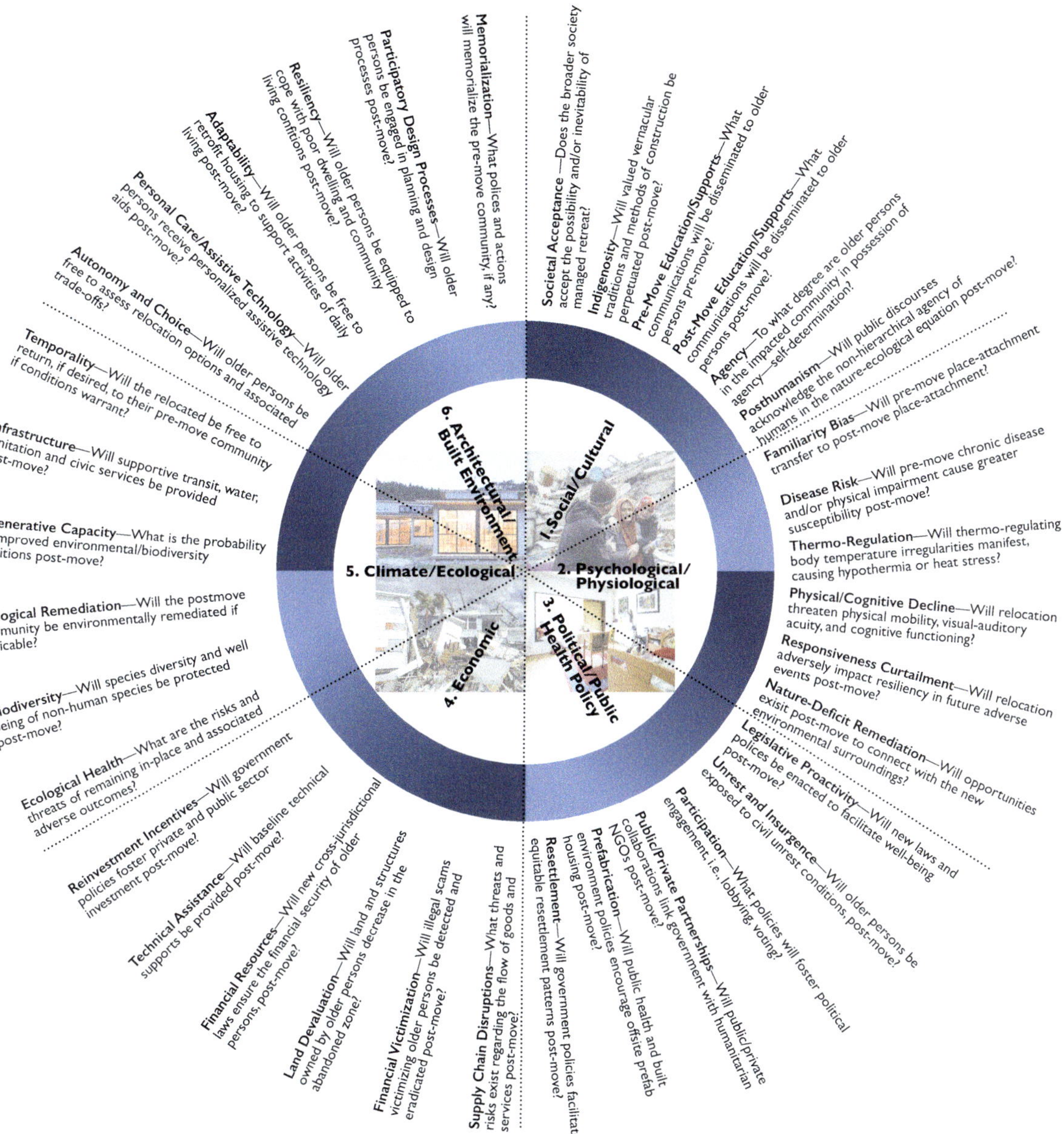

Figure 5.2. Managed retreat determinants impacting older persons. Diagram by Stephen Verderber and Lucas Siemucha.

enhanced cognitive clarity and comprehension in the impacted older persons regarding what is about to happen. Redundant cue-driven health education policies may consist of embedded educational cues, beginning in the pre-move phase, combined with best practices on how to acclimate the individual pre-move to their future home.

Built-Environment Redundant Cueing

This architectural design strategy calls for architects, landscape architects, industrial designers, engineers, and allied designers to collaborate with health policy experts and health care providers to *build redundant cues directly into* post-move places and buildings to be inhabited by older persons. Interventions should be carefully keyed to the five sensory modalities—particularly to sight, sound, and the kinesthetic experiences of movement—and based on the actual habitation and use of interior architectural spaces and exterior immediate environs. Built-in messaging, or encoding, of an architectural environment is extendable beyond the building and immediate site environs into the community, such as a nearby park or nature walking trail. The aim is to instill a sustainable level of cognitive ability, personal safety, and personal control over one's physical surroundings. Architectural redundant-cued features improve the navigational amenity of circulation paths, including contrasting flooring, walls, and ceilings. Also, embedded instructional triggers will sound a "message" if one should accidently open an emergency door, encounter a potentially hazardous staircase, or attempt to leave the building or grounds through an unauthorized exit.[58]

For the medically underserved who must relocate due to disaster, regardless of age, managed retreat may function as a road out of poverty, and frail older persons with physical and cognitive impairments are especially vulnerable (fig. 5.3). They are disproportionately impacted by exposure to harmful air and groundwater pollution, a scarcity of fresh water, flood-prone zones, overcrowded living conditions, increased noise, litter, dilapidated buildings, few or no public transit options, drought, and food deserts. These environmental factors, or eco-stressors, render an individual further incapable of coping with a sudden injury (e.g., a fall) or illness (e.g., pneumonia or cancer). Although persons aged 75 and older comprised only 6 percent of the total population of New Orleans in 2005, they accounted for 50 percent of those who died due to the catastrophic conditions caused by Hurricane Katrina. In Northern California's 2018 Camp Fire, seventy-one of the eighty-four identified fatalities were persons aged 60 and older. When Hurricane Sandy struck the New York tristate area in 2012, nearly half of all fatalities were persons aged 65 and older.[59]

Design Considerations

In response to these and other threats frequently encountered by older persons, fifty design considerations are presented in appendix B. This compendium pinpoints key architectural design and landscape issues for 24/7 long-term custodial residential facilities as a specific building type. (Due to space limitations, independent living settings are not addressed per se in this appendix.) Also addressed are urban ramifications of these considerations, such as site selection, transit options, access to civic amenities, and intergenerational living arrangements on shared sites. Each design consideration is, in

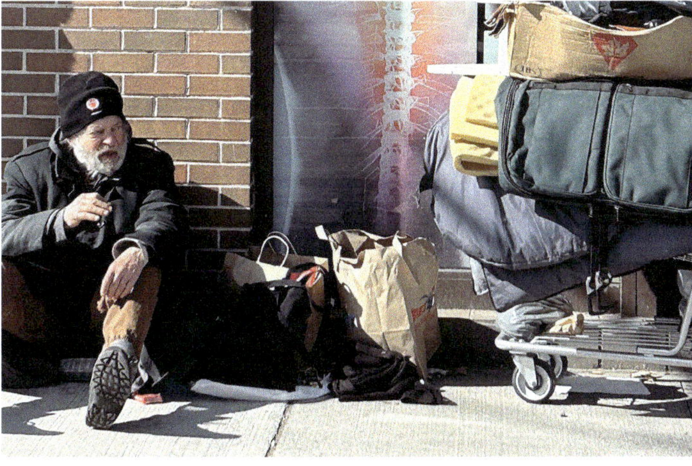

Figure 5.3. Unsheltered older person, Toronto, 2023. Photo by Stephen Verderber.

a sense, a *hypothesis* for further testing and application in renovations, new additions, adaptive uses, and new construction. With increasing pressures to build structures more resiliently, and *faster*, an underlying theme is modular prefabrication. It is becoming more widely seen as a viable alternative to current conventional building methods. This compendium is presented according to eight thematic categories:

1. site context and spatial organization,
2. private realm,
3. shared realms,
4. biophilia and nature connectivity,
5. circulation and navigation,
6. support amenities,
7. sensory and environmental supports, and
8. prefabricated housing for long-term care.

The fifty design considerations are particularly directed to health care and medical professionals; gerontologists and related social scientists; architects; landscape architects; interior designers; urban planners; engineers; health care administrators and their boards of directors; local, state, provincial, and federal governmental agencies with oversight authority in the design and construction of these built environments; private philanthropic foundations; grassroots eldercare advocates; elected officials; and public health policy specialists in the public and private sector.

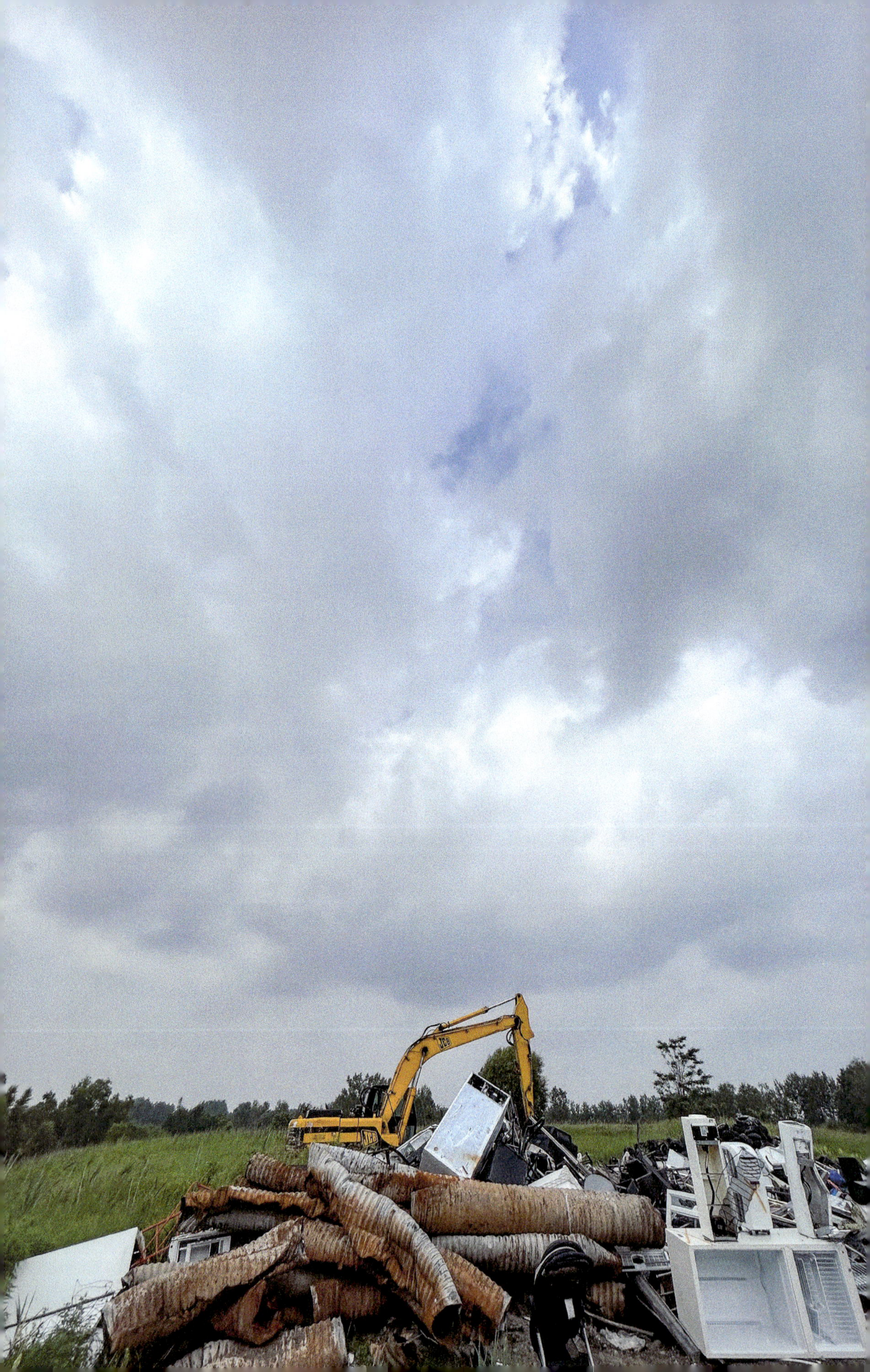

Posthumanism, Architecture, and Health Equity

The earth that humans have taken for granted for millennia as the natural environment no longer is independent from our existence. From this point on, we are inseparably linked with our ecological surroundings. The age of cheap, abundant, infinitely "consumable" commodified nature and landscapes, or N-L, is in the rearview mirror.[1] Theorists and researchers across a broad swath of disciplines—including sociology, geography, anthropology, psychiatry, public health, gerontology, literary theory, art, architecture, and planning—are critically reexamining the possibilities of a posthumanities. This reappraisal represents a profound shift beyond traditional concepts of *humanism* and the humanities themselves, generally defined as the period of history dating from the Age of Enlightenment to the present.[2] Today, as the earth's nonrenewable reserves are being drained, burned, depleted, poisoned, exterminated, or otherwise exhausted, the Anthropocene marks the end of a *refugia*—that is, any semblance of an untouched utopia where we could be entirely free from the consequences of the debacle we created. We must now face the harsh consequences of our actions, which are already reshaping our everyday lives in large and small ways (fig. 6.1).[3]

Figure 6.1. Landscape desecration in the Anthropocene, Havilock-Methune Transfer Station, Havelock, Ontario, 2023. Photo by Stephen Verderber.

Posthumanist perspectives, in opposition to classical definitions of the humanities, are tied to a perceived reality where we humans can no longer afford to think and act as an exceptionalist species, free to carelessly think and act without regarding the planet, other life forms, and inanimate entities (or "things"). Too much has and continues to go very wrong for the status quo to persist. Humans' long dismissal of nonhuman life forms, the earth, and inanimate things has led us to where we are. *Posthumanism* is inclusive and refers to our species' capability to view ourselves as being *no greater in any way* than our nonhuman surroundings, other living species, and inanimate entities. Posthumanist thinking and subsequent actions, framed as more-than-human arguments with respect to ecological planning, design, and stewardship, have come to the fore in the Anthropocene— perspectives whose theoretical and pragmatic underpinnings allow a transcendence beyond the anachronistic classical perspectives that previously drove intellectual life for centuries.

Give-and-take transactionalism between the environment and human health has been of some significant concern in medicine since Galen's theory of the humors sought to explain disease as a dialectical relationship between one's bodily constitution and environmental and societal hazards.[4] The rise of germ theory and medical models of sickness and disease would later undermine this dialectic, with public health emerging as a separate discipline in the Victorian era and the retention of "humoralist" concerns— that is, awareness of the deleterious impact of toxic factory towns on the public's health, and the rise of epidemiology as a health discipline.[5] In the Anthropocene, particularly in the fields of geography and sociology, important new questions and narratives are being triggered on how to genuinely coexist with nature, frequently drawing from Indigenous narratives and lessons to be learned from rural communities that, across generations were able to successfully sustain mutually rewarding connections with nature, while simultaneously remaining cognizant of evolutionary codependencies.[6] The Indigenous societies in Canada's Far North region stand out as one such example of this sustained interrelationship.[7]

Within the academic discipline and practice of architecture, the Anthropocene would seem contentious, even threatening. Fundamentally, posthumanism accepts a future of uncertainty and unpredictability, conditions in many ways contradicting the premeditative art and process of creating a building. A structure is presumably built to be predictable, standing the test of time, space, and place. For centuries, builders have operated from the fundamental premise of being in control of the physical world within which they live and construct objects. Planners and architects are taught early on to make a better future, a future premised on the vision that things will be better in the times ahead than they are at present or previously were—a vision practicing professionals aim to perpetuate through what they design and see constructed in the real world. In stark contrast to these assumptions, any tacit acceptance of the uncontrollability of extreme climate events and the consequences of adverse ecofeedback loops—potentially occurring anywhere, with varying degrees of ferocity—challenges the basic premise of architecture. In the Anthropocene, the aim of "improving" the quality of the built environment for the enhancement of human health alone seems quaint. The question now is whether this uncertainty contradicts, or even entirely negates, the core traditional assumption that architecture is able to contribute something of permanence.

The urban and regional planning profession, like architecture, has retained a nearly entirely human-centric—or *anthropocentric*—exceptionalist view of the physical world. For the same reasons cited above, this operative assumption now warrants a critical reframing to more inclusively embrace a city/nature nexus, or interface, while also ethically and pragmatically embracing all nonhuman species and "things of all kinds."[8] This much-broadened perspective also advertently embraces the relational, codependent, bioresponsive forms of posthumanism. It similarly emphasizes the fallacy of humans' ecological dominance and sense of somehow being exempt from the new normative assumptions. This exceptionalism is socially fabricated, constructed, and codified all around us.

To posthumanist theorists in the traditional humanities, this is where it dovetails with feminist movements, which seek to empower the previously unrecognized voices of women in political discourses through a systematic dismantling of essentialist categorizations of gender as a historical criterion or reference point for past exclusions by gender. When viewed collectively, racism, sexism, ageism, and political marginalization have been male-driven phenomena throughout recorded history. By contrast, the feminist ideal of radical inclusivity, when coupled with posthumanism, now compels us to embrace animals, insects, plants, cells, and bacteria as legitimate "voices" to be heard. Rosi Braidotti, a leading theorist in posthumanist thought, has argued that such broadened perspectives are currently spawning entirely new fields of transdisciplinary knowledge, while also fueling a basic rethinking of increasingly archaic definitions of the classical humanities.[9]

Within these now-reshaping disciplines, qualitative health researchers are exploring posthumanism with respect to the meanings, place attachments, and far broader identities individuals and populations associate with their health, illness, and the type and quality of the health care they receive.[10] This approach differs from long-standing positivist traditions in health services research, which are squarely focused on identifying precise determinants (causes) of disease, illness, and access (or a lack thereof) to appropriate health care resources. Conventional emphasis has been on how humans—and humans alone—tend to rationalize experiences and then try to comprehend their own health, apart from all other living species and inanimate "things."[11] This *relational humanism* in public health has also been grounded (similar to the built-environment professions) in a concomitant devotion to classical humanism—phenomenology, existentialism, idealism, and hermeneutics—particularly in the fields of medicine and nursing.[12] At present, these two approaches uneasily coexist, although much attention in health research is currently being devoted to biosocial and neurosocial studies, new mobilities, and animal/human relations studies These are among the many health-related fields now being impacted by posthumanist, largely qualitative research methodologies in the health disciplines and professions.[13]

Against this backdrop, this chapter first and foremost aims to review certain narratives with respect to why architects, allied designers, planners, and health care providers might now consider posthumanism and its relationship to health equity as a promising alternative theory and method versus conventional, static, mainstream narratives, such as *sustainable* or *resilient design*, and *sustainable health*—both highly anthropocentric movements/strategies generally seeking to merely protect that which remains on an already environmentally degraded planet. Sustainability, in particular, has dominated the discourse on the built environment for nearly forty years and now appears to have run its course, even though many invaluable contributions have been made along the way.[14] The second aim of this chapter is to examine the justifications for why posthumanist perspectives are distinct and potentially meaningful from here on, to the point where those with the prescribed agency to plan, design, and provide health care physical built environments should pay special attention to them.

Specifically, these two aims, taken together represent an attempt to acquire a more precise, inclusive understanding of how posthumanism can guide future efforts to plan, design, and construct more-than-human, inclusive, and far more fully equitable built environments for health. To this end, three case studies, based on building types introduced in the previous chapters, serve as vehicles to demonstrate how this perspective might become an integral part of thinking and acting in an imperiled world.

As Ihnji Jon writes:

> For a long time posthumanism has been associated with "new age" counterculture movements, often dismissed as minority sentiments or not taken seriously enough to be integrated into mainstream political arguments. However, upon the arrival of alarmingly frequent climate irregularities and extreme natural disasters, more and more policy-oriented academic communities have started engaging with more-than-human ecological discourses . . . although [it is] yet to be "popularized" enough to be accepted by mainstream practitioners who juggle different priorities that often eclipse long-term ecological concerns. . . . The beginnings of posthumanist or more-than-human thought can be traced back to 19th century philosophy where political geographers explored the influence of physical [territorial] environments on social evolution, recognizing the role of non-human forces greater than human will in constituting a society. Especially in the disciplines of critical geography and anthropology, there have been important discussions on the significance of the "Anthropocene" in our time and its potential promise.[15]

In urban and regional planning, as is simultaneously happening in numerous other disciplines, posthumanist perspectives center on what is referred to as *new materialism*. For the past thirty years, planning, as a profession, had been preoccupied with policymaking and quasi-economics at the expense of a real concern for the physical fabric of actual neighborhoods, cities, and regions. Ironically, this de-emphasis on the physical materiality of the built environment took planners away from being in a position to directly impact real, tangible physical environments. This policy-obsessed, quasi-economic focus resulted in disconnects from actual networks of nonhuman surroundings or things. Mainly drawing from Bruno Latour's widely cited actor network theory, or ANT (discussed further below), new materialist philosophical positions have moved to the forefront.[16]

ANT emphasises network associations and connections between diverse actors and their respective agency while concurrently questioning the lead, or centralist, role of the planner. Within a broadly redefined distribution of agency— policymaking or decision-making authority—planners often are no longer the lead actors in planning processes, because decision-making processes are constantly in flux, ever changing in new and often unpredictable ways, due to myriad externalities in the climate crisis, which consist of far-more-than-strictly-human forces—ecological, procedural, legal, and political.

It is becoming much more about collaboratively working in tandem with heterogeneous societal elements in a variety of smaller or more incrementalist ways, and doing so more inductively, aiming to convince collaborating actor-mediators into coexisting or, at a minimum, stabilizing assemblages of concern and physical reality so resultant changes can be generated—yet with little absolute certainty as to what that change (or its outcome) might actually be.[17]

Especially since the 1990s, planners were anthropocentrically preoccupied with how to accommodate conflicting procedural agendas brought on by seemingly irreconcilably different human actors with divergent viewpoints, aims, and degrees of agency. This human-centricity typically concentrated on leading a series of dull and rather perfunctory meetings and workshops, with the fundamental goal of getting people to arrive at some point of agreement on something. The planner could then go off and execute the decisions that were made, while leaving the majority of material planning—that is, the organization and construction of, for example, a highway-widening project through an historic neighborhood—to the architects, landscape designers, and others, with the "voices" and agency of more-than-human "things" in most cases being entirely undervalued if not completely ignored.[18]

I witnessed this dysfunctionality firsthand in the aftermath of Hurricane Katrina in New Orleans in fall 2005. The uptown neighborhood where my house was located flooded, as did 80 percent of the city. Next, some weeks later, the city hurriedly brought in a prestigious planning firm from Philadelphia to organize and direct a series of (highly controversial) post-disaster neighborhood "recovery workshops" across the city's highly diverse neighborhoods. This planning process was cleverly dubbed "Bring Back New Orleans." The city's entire footprint was carved up into individual planning districts, and each ad hoc neighborhood organization was instructed to organize itself and then attempt to meet informally at someone's house, at a local school, or somewhere else on a weekly or biweekly basis, beginning in January 2006. My neighborhood's planning group and others like it were tasked with developing and agreeing on a single agenda—or strategy—for the recovery of our own ruined parts of the city.

What happened next was most unfortunate. The out-of-state planning team brought in huge base maps and proceeded to hang them up on the wall in the basement of an elementary school cafeteria, for us to peruse as the reference point for our meetings. The goal (or hidden agenda) appeared to be getting us to agree on something—*anything*. This would justify the hundreds of hours the planning firm was collectively logging in our flood-ravaged city. Audaciously, we were told to *dream big* without due consideration of budgets or any physical, materialist implications. We eventually agreed on some prioritized, wholly human-centric, completely unrealistic goals for our neighborhood recovery planning district that very soon fell by the wayside, since there was no investment money available anywhere in the city, let alone in our neighborhood, to implement any of our "big" ideas. Tragically, this abortive planning effort would result in death threats received by the planning team, along with local politicians and Mayor Ray Nagin especially from the angry, displaced residents of the city's Lower Ninth Ward, after the planners advocated the entire abandonment of that part of the city.[19]

A key lesson from this debacle for urban and regional planners (and their architects) is what is now known as *tactical urbanism*. This method is grounded in critically, tactically working in harmony *with* people, nature, and environmental ecosystems—in short, thinking and acting beyond defunct classical concerns that for centuries had politically positioned the so-called leaders (humans) at the center of the this inequitable universe.[20] Can we continue to be singularly focused on controlling, suppressing, or harnessing nature, as we did in the past? Similarly, the vast levees built by the US Army Corps of Engineers in the twentieth century along the lower Mississippi River were an attempt to freeze-frame this powerful river in place without thoughts of much else, either ecologically or sociologically.

Post-disaster planners and architects in New Orleans and elsewhere are, it might be hoped, wiser now, having recognized the true ecological free agency of both human and nonhuman entities—lakes, bayous, rivers, rainfall, animal species and their ecosystems—with an unprecedented emphasis on green infrastructure, urban climatology, and the preservation of endangered species and habitats. This *assemblage thinking* encourages planners and architects to recognize that humans do not exist apart from the total ecological world we live in. Moral responsibility must be equitably redistributed from here on, far beyond the narrowness of how humans previously acted—solely in their self-interest.[21] Alternatively, visionary urbanists and architects are drawing inspiration from posthumanist perspectives. More-than-human(ist) ecological planning acknowledges that, as a species, humans have to now be humbler than ever. By acknowledging the deep codependencies between human and nonhuman agents, we now become capable of creating genuinely diverse multispecies communities where humans, native and nonnative animals, birds, insects, plants, soils, fungi, and microbes are all equal participant-actors, each with equivalent agency in shaping health-promoting built environments.[22]

Bruno Latour, in *Politics of Nature*, asserts we must stop considering Nature with a capital *N* and, therefore, disregarding it as having nothing to do with our everyday lives.[23] He refers to this as "externalizing" nature, where Nature has no direct connection with our economic obsession in exploiting it. To us it appears idle and inactive (passive), merely serving its core function as a background or stage for unabated human consumption. He argues that we must cease persisting with such useless human/nonhuman dichotomies. By questioning these prosaic categorizations, Latour posits that our emphasis should not be on nature as a physical entity alone, but far more on those whose voices have been left out of discourses in the political arena—not only humans, but also nonhuman living beings and "things." To this point, and drawing on scientific evidence from developmental biology, Donna Haraway notes that the reexamination of species coevolution across animals, humans, and bacteria underscores how the development of all living, material "critters" are profoundly intertwined.[24]

In her influential writings, Braidotti has argued once we abandon our habitual ways of categorizing, through sexism, racism, ageism, and the like, humans will finally be able to see the role of other stakeholders—entities that have been unjustly muted or entirely ignored in the past—in shaping the planet's present and future.[25] Latour, Haraway, Braidotti, and others strongly advocate for previously excluded nonhuman actor-entities to have their interests meaningfully considered in the realm of *ecopolitics*. Posthumanist ecopolitics assigns equal agency to every single organism that has shaped our existence. The New Materialists refer to this prerequisite function as *distributive agency*, highlighting how human agency is to be perceived relative to nonhuman actors. Humans run a real risk, however, of disempowering themselves by not acting fully affirmatively to create positive environmental change within this broadened, myriad set of actors. In other words, humans must be humble to an unprecedented extent, but without relinquishing their will and ability to act on behalf of all the entitity-actors who cannot speak for themselves.

In the Anthropocene, this translates into taking responsibility for both previous and ongoing widespread environmental degradation. It is about a collective survival strategy for negotiating cascading calamities concurrently and dealing with their ramifications for humans' complex entanglements with nonhuman entities. Yet to truly recognize their importance, we must first reimagine a world without humans, and the planet Earth even before human civilization existed:

> What becomes clear . . . is that non-human critters (nature) do not need us; rather, it is we who need their support for our survival. . . . It is not the trees, forests, and biome that need us but we who are utterly dependent on them. And only when we account for the Anthropocene (or the end of "refugia")—that ultimately underlines human species' dependence on other non-human beings—can the idea of "entanglements" have meaningful normativity in environmental politics. We must first wholeheartedly embrace what we cannot walk away from—environmental degradation—because our lives are entangled with all other beings and things on earth—[and] the normative agenda for posthumanism will be to "stay with the trouble" . . . because caring for something involves more than merely a moral stance; it involves affective, ethical, hands-on agencies of practical and material consequence . . . care ethics, as opposed to top-down, hegemonic, *a priori* ethics. . . . This requires each of us to acknowledge our inevitable self-*in*sufficiency.[26]

POSTHUMANISM, ARCHITECTURE, AND HEALTH EQUITY

These arguments resonate within architecture and its inextricable relationship to health equity. The traditional way we assess a building, and the manner in which buildings have been critically viewed throughout the course of architectural history, are at the root of the current crisis. A building is first objectified and analysed in its *static*, isolated moment, beginning from the time of its creation. It is not grasped transactively—that is, as a dynamic entity in constant interaction with its creators, its inhabitants, or even in relation to its environmental surroundings. Latour and Yaneva, among others, argue buildings are not static objects but moving *projects*, long after their completion, as they age and are transformed by their occupants.[27] They are continually modified by everything that happens inside and near them, and by how they adapted to change and were altered over time, including by the forces of nature. A major problem in the way hospitals, clinics, and the like have always been conceived and built is that we always picture them, at least aesthetically, in this static way (by default) as islands—fixed, stolid structures, for one moment's unfettered depiction in a glossy magazine, usually without showing people or any other real signs of occupancy.

Instead, what is needed is a dynamic reconceptualization of health and health care structures as a continuous time/space flow accepting of and embracing this province of specialized buildings as fluid and ever changing. The current mode—where architects have to get the "right" photos of their newly completed health care projects in one *perfect* isolated moment, and somehow capturing the "life" of the building and its environs—is absurd. It is as if the structure is always to be an isolated work of sculpture, to be recorded as uncontaminated by human occupancy or any other "adverse space/time forces." It is incredible that this practice still stubbornly persists in the face of what is happening on this planet.

Euclidian space and the way buildings were always depicted *a priori* through drawings (and later photographs) are seen as a main cause of this misconception of what a building really is and truly represents in the Anthropocene. This failing always falls back on Euclidean space as the only justifiable way to capture what a building is and what it means—and afterward fostering complaints that too many dimensions of reality were missing. To consider and document a building merely as a static object at one moment in time and space is, in Latour and Yaneva's words, like "gazing endlessly at a gull, high in the sky, without being able to ever capture how it moves." They call instead for blurring a building's objective reality as an object solely for human use. Instead, it should include broader subjective relationship(s) with nonhuman entity-actors and the full agency of N-L. This calls for no less than the abandonment of the critically important lacuna that has, up until now, artificially isolated the purely objective from the subjective (or subjective-objective) in architecture:

> It is paradoxical to say that a building is always a "thing" that is, etymologically, a contested gathering of many conflicting demands [while] being utterly unable to *draw* those conflicting claims in the same space as what they are conflicting about. Everyone knows that a building is a contested territory and that it cannot be reduced to what it is and what it means, as architectural theory has traditionally done. . . . A building is a *navigation* through a controversial datascape . . . a changing and criss-crossing trajectory of unstable definitions and expertises, of recalcitrant material and building technologies, of flip-flopping users' concerns and communities' appraisals . . . concentrating flows of actors and distributing them so as to compose a productive force in time-space . . .

composed of actors, data and resources, links and opinions, all in orbit in a network, and never *within* static enclosures. . . . "Context" is this little word that sums up all the various elements that have been bombarding the project from the beginning: fashion spreads in architectural magazines, clichés burned into the minds of clients . . . entrenched zoning laws, static building types taught in art and design schools by professors, visual habits. . . . A building project resembles much more of a complex ecology. . . . Biology offers much better metaphors for speaking about buildings. Instead of explaining the assembly building in Chandigarh with economic constraints or with the trivial conceptual repertoire of LeCorbusier's modernist style . . . we should better witness the multifarious manifestations of recalcitrance of this building . . . [in] resisting breezes, intense sunlight and the microclimate of the Himalayas . . . and earthly accounts of buildings and design processes. . . . [The] new task for architectural theory: inventing a new vocabulary that will finally do justice to the "thingly" nature of buildings, in contrast to their tired old "objective" nature.[28]

This critique castigates the practice of viewing a building, designed and built for health care or something else, as a collection of static cultural meanings and symbols. Latour and Yaneva specifically call out mid-twentieth-century postmodern architects and theorists Robert Venturi and Charles Jencks, among others, in this regard.[29] As for the human body, rather than treat illness, disease, and healthfulness as narrowly defined causal relationships, it is perhaps far more insightful to position health and illness as dynamic, emergent expressions of distinct sociomaterial assemblages. This builds on the insight that subjectivity and agency are relational capacities distributed across assemblages of diverse bodies, forces, signs, and cause-affects. Posthumanist medical and public health researchers note how health itself may be treated as an emergent quality, distributed in this same way. Accordingly, human bodies should not be classified according to their static health status, but rather as broader time/space assemblages of both human and nonhuman determinants. For example, studies of obesity and addiction provide useful insights by pointing to the ways myriad externalities shape desires and appetites. Bodies, marketing, fashion, culture, politics, and media intersect in the emergence of an "obese" or "addicted" patient.

This level of analysis elevates the requisite agency of the actors and network forces involved in the emergence of epidemics like obesity and addiction. It recognizes how nonhuman actors and forces variously and fluidly contribute to any state of healthfulness. A key insight is to understand how these encountered determinants affect one another within health assemblages and, by extension, within *health-equity architectural assemblages*. Therefore, for posthumanist health researchers or practitioners, these assemblages, rather than any one actor alone, are best suited as the focus of their analyses.[30] This requires the ability to engage in assemblage thinking. It involves identifying and tracing the components of assemblages as they reveal themselves through the active contributions they make in the process of a human becoming either more or less healthy. This can occur, however, with or without any direct relationship to the built or natural environment.[31] First, it is essential to identify and track the specific local actors, their degree of agency, and associated network force determinants. This follows from Latour's 2005 assertion that forces near and remote, distant and proximate, are critical in helping shape these assemblages and their ripple effects into wider networks of efficacy.[32]

A New Lens

Hybrid conceptualizations in the Anthropocene of the more-than-human and related constructs—such as a focus on the nonhuman, multispeciesism, and the decentralization of the human—hold the promise of expanding humans' awareness of the ecological world that must remain healthy enough to support our continued existence. Multiple agencies, codependencies, entanglements, and conundrums that constitute our imperiled world cannot be ignored or sidestepped any longer. This reconsideration of humanity's role in ecological degradation and its attendant social upheaval, and the ways in which these changes are reshaping humans' place in the world, call for applying these ideas relative to architects' design methodologies, applying and redefining them in ways to make things fairer and more equal in this world. The hope is that by becoming open to this type of relearning, far more equitable ways of doing things will result. For example, the Whanganui River in New Zealand has recently been granted the same legal-rights status as a human being after a local Māori tribe unsuccessfully fought for its recognition as an "ancestor" entity *for 140 years*. This tribe had continually been claiming this river should be re-regarded as a viable living entity, rather than a controllable resource for mere human ownership and (mis)management. By granting the river its legal rights, or ecological agency, future crimes against the river can be treated in the legal system as crimes against the tribe itself.[33] This new way of understanding and revaluing the natural environment allows it to acquire greater recognition and higher social status than ever before.

Actor-network theory is premised on humans' understanding of the relationships between networks and assemblages of human and nonhuman actors. In the above case, water (the river) now shares equal agency as a full participant in the shaping of local land use and related environmental policies. Such nonhuman entities and their relationships with humans compose assemblages of living and inanimate "things," shaping the interweaving ways in which scientific knowledge and technology are materialized. What happens if a local population post-disaster denies the installation of a portable field hospital on their tribal land, because doing so will destroy their local water supply? How do these people reconcile their urgent need for localized medical care with its traditional land use rights? What if they have historically been highly skeptical of outsiders' intrusiveness, even if only temporary, such as in a public health emergency? Are not local populations chronically suffering from being medically underserved or cut out of the health equation entirely fully entitled to be skeptical of "outsider" building technologies and unfamiliar building types?

As adverse built and natural environmental impacts of the climate crisis deepen and social/technological changes occur more rapidly than ever before in recorded history, architects who design for health will increasingly need to develop new ways to make sense of its complexities and contradictions. Human and nonhuman stakeholders—their perspectives, agency, and subjectivities—deserve full engagement. But how will an architect plan new initiatives, communicate them, collect information, and test prototypes? Importantly, how and why is posthumanist design excellence critical to well-being and survival in an imperiled world? Three examples of what might be possible are discussed below, all three of which were the focus of individual previous chapters in this book.

An Infectious Disease Treatment Hospital

In 2022, the World Health Organization initiated its "Infectious Disease Treatment Module" project (WHO-IDTM). This was the first time in recent history it commissioned a direct architectural response to a health care crisis (COVID-19)—in this case the need for an adaptable, redeployable, state-of-the-art health care facility (see chapter 3). An iterative, team-based participatory design protocol was established, drawing together numerous specialists from Europe and North America (including this author), with the aim of applying an essentially human-centric lens to the task at hand. Throughout the WHO-IDTM design process, the overarching goal was to create a transportable structure to effectively mitigate transmissible diseases while treading as lightly as possible on its immediate ecological site and associated landscape—in other words, as if this structure were to appear to float, hovering slightly above the ground without needlessly or recklessly harming the installation site's ecological agency. It is designed to be installable on diverse sites in infectious disease hot zones for a period ranging from a few weeks to up to six months. A second goal was to scale up from a single prototype module to an installation comprised of nine to twelve modules. This international team of designers, engineers, physicians, and internal WHO team members served as actors within a network of interpersonal actor-network transactions. The team collaborated for nine months on the stage 1 (1.0) prototype.

The prefabricated module's design and a technical schematic analysis were performed virtually, with some exceptions. Communications were fluid throughout, with the design process in constant motion—never static—as new actor-agents were added into the design and prototyping manufacturing equations. The module's design evolved rather quickly, with changes visually documented, at times contemporaneously during design team meetings. Feedback was provided from the team's *human* actor-participants and their collective agency—physicians, nurses, and public health administrators at local, regional, and national levels and staff based at WHO headquarters in Geneva. Unfortunately, no nonhuman actors—neither the earth, nor any nonhuman species—were directly considered at this stage in the design and prototyping processes. Ecologically, however, the stated aim was to cause minimal disturbance to an installation site's intrinsic agency. This was important, although how this would specifically occur was beyond the stated scope of the project, as human health needs were the first and foremost priority. Was this enough, in light of posthumanist concerns? In retrospect, it was not. This transportable field hospital is ostensibly for the treatment of human illnesses and diseases, even though infectious diseases that attack humans are often zoonotic viruses transmitted from nonhuman species—further proof of the profundity of human–non-human interspecies codependences (see chapter 2). Nonetheless, consider for a moment the possibilities of rapid-response architecture for post-disaster mitigation if it were to be designed anthropocentrically, for the equal benefit of all impacted nonhuman species and "things." In parallel, is it now time to design redeployable modular trauma hospitals dedicated spe-cifically to the care of *nonhuman* species? This goes beyond talking about the typical animal hospital in North America, which is designed for routine, normative veterinary care. In an imperiled world is it any longer justifiable to place human health that high above or apart from the ecological health of impacted assemblages of affected nonhuman species and "things"? These, without a doubt, are provocative questions.

Conventionally designed portable field hospitals, for their part, histori-cally had to function as fluid, adaptable, ever-shifting structures. The most prosaic tent hospitals the American Red Cross deployed since the late nineteenth century ably assisted in civilian disasters, dating from the mas-sive Thumb Fire in Michigan in 1881; the Johnstown, Pennsylvania, flood in 1889; and many US disasters since then. These "tent cities," as they were sometimes called, grew and expanded in size, based on the unpredictable needs of the disaster's victims, local political realities, and climate. These structures were not designed by architects. Perhaps their impermanence and basic functionality accounted for why architects, architectural histo-rians, and theorists have consistently overlooked this building type (see chapter 3). In the case of the WHO-IDTM and similar transportable archi-tectural structures for health, standardized protocols are needed, taking full cognizance of posthumanist "spokesperson" concerns at the local level of deployment, such as water management resource conservation, wildlife habitat protection, forest management factors, and so forth. In a rapidly changing, uncertain world, might the time have come for humans to be decentered from their traditional role as the dominant, all-controlling spe-cies, even in disaster response? Perhaps this will change in the name of achieving real, holistic health equity for humans as well as for nonhuman living species and "things" that fall victim to disaster.

Maggie's Centres

Multidisciplinary posthumanist literature prioritizes the primacy of sen-sory and bodily experiences over abstract representations of nature and landscapes in the everyday world.[34] This is also a main tenet of theraserialization—dematerializing the barriers that traditionally isolate a building from its site context for the mutual betterment of building occu-pants and the external ecological realm (see chapter 4). It is about a pro-cess of sensitization to the adverse impacts of human network-actors and awareness of the therapeutic affordances of N-L. But it is not about humans blindly bending and altering nature, such as attempting to change weather patterns through the now-trendy practice of cloud seeding, as if nature were some abstract construct for geoengineers to toy with. Latour argues that humans must become *earthbound* by listening to biofeedback loops and subsequently adjusting human actions based on the whole ecological system versus any subset of its constituent parts. For purposes of the present discussion, this ethical obligation to protect and revitalize nature is, similarly, much more than a top-down moral imperative—it is a survival strategy. It is about using our senses to feel the consequences of our actions through a complete awareness of our immediate surroundings and the specific territory (or territories) we occupy.

This quality is what many of the Maggie's Centres have achieved, both architecturally and ecologically (see chapter 4). Their soft-spoken architecture does not place humans above nature and landscapes. Instead, the most architecturally noteworthy Maggie's Centres have been conceived and constructed to be quite the opposite—thoroughly, humbly, embedded in *nature* almost to the point where the building itself recedes or merges with its N-L context(s). In Manchester, UK, a 1960s asphalt parking lot, which once covered the entire site of the current Centre, was demolished and the area returned to its previous natural state before any new construction would begin. The Maggie's Centre in Oldham, UK, was built on a reclaimed site on an old hospital campus with the building elevated on pilotis (columns), as if to celebrate the humility of architecture by means of its volumetric dematerialization. The building reads as intentionally yet ironically, anti-heroically *not even there*. In the case of both the Oxford and Oldham Maggie's Centres, the architects, by raising these structures up on pilotis, succeeded in revealing and honoring the agency of these sites' intrinsic natural ecologies—a realm for equal use and continued existence by human as well as nonhuman actor-species and "things." At Oxford, three portal windows are in the floor of the main circulation space nearest the front door/reception area, inviting the visitor-occupant to look down onto the diverse affordances of N-L visible directly beneath, as if looking through to the ocean floor from a glass-bottomed boat.

The Maggie's Centres cited here (also see chapter 4) are in a way heroic yet humble reactions to external forces deeply out of balance within the health care industry, especially in highly developed countries. In their aim to *recapture* nature and landscape through sensorial rebalancing and architectural ingenuity, they hold the promise of reaffirming the legitimacy and essential importance of nonhuman living species and "things" by acknowledging the full agency of a broadened array of actor-agents. In architecture for health, this rebalancing requires a blurring of the human/nature/culture dialectic, which can only be achieved by convincingly advocating for the validity of impacted nonhuman "voices." Second, by "staying with the trouble" in terms of striving to interweave N-L with architectural space, posthumanist design strategies simultaneously acknowledge and support more-than-human concerns. Third, by emphasising immediate empirical sensory experiences, political/environmental activist frameworks can arise in support of more-equitable health-centric architecture. When visiting these Maggie's Centres, I was struck by the extent to which the *spirit* of Maggie Keswick and the continued activities of her foundation permeate every aspect of these physical settings. It is based in her strong conviction that the modern medical system and its technocratic architectural apparatus utterly failed to treat her cancer with compassion or a genuine ethics of caring.[35]

To Latour, adherents clinging to modern architecture's minimalist aesthetic biases even in the Anthropos continue to hold a belief in human exceptionalism, whereas the best of the Maggie's Centres that have been built exhibit a posthumanist respect for intimacy, quietness, and repose. They are humble buildings, in many cases sited so one barely sees them, having to look carefully even to locate the front door. This deferential design strategy takes into consideration far more than human actor-agents. It seeks to celebrate salient assemblages, highly unique for a health care facility in this or any Western culture. In stark contrast, too many medical center hospitals and other conventional health care facility typologies are architectural "screamers"—that is, they strive to be technologically heroic, bold, totally dominating their ecological surroundings. They are usually overtly self-referential, architecturally inhuman in scale, and visually opaque in terms of their navigability. These attributes were *not* in evidence at the Maggie's Centres I visited in Oxford, Manchester, and Oldham in the UK, as well as in many of the others I have become acquainted with. Instead, these places express the logical evolution of Maggie Keswick's original concept, beginning with the first freestanding Maggie's Centre built in Dundee, Scotland, and designed by Frank Gehry (1996).[36]

Residential Environments for Older Persons
Gerontology is an interdisciplinary field especially well-suited for posthumanist reassessment, given how pervasive technological interventions

have become in treating and preventing illness and disease. These advancements are recalibrating the definable essence of an aging human body. An emerging paradigm embraces connectivity, independence, social engagement, and well-being, with older bodies becoming enmeshed in more-than-human networks of externalized assemblages. This recognition of human with nonhuman biologic materiality not only accounts for the aging process and its experiences, but also for the material influences all impacted actor-agents share within the same level or plane of existence. All deserve a voice with equal agency in health care. In this context, an assemblage provides a vehicle to more narratively (and ecologically) explain aging as a chorological and biological process—as a life-stage construct:

> Posthumanist gerontology involves a decentering of the older human body in favor of a broader sweep of actors and forces. Without ignoring them altogether, it shifts the focus of attention away from physiological and biological changes in the body (the conventional scientific and positivist understanding of aging) and subjective opinions and judgements about the body (the humanistic understanding), towards the wide origins and character of the social, affective, and material expression of bodily aging. . . . Biologically aging human bodies are recognized as assemblages of matter and energy, open to change and realizing their potential through their encounters. . . . For example, rural aging has been studied as an embodied affective and atmospheric experience . . . big skies, open spaces, fresh air, brisk walking, and everyday encounters. . . . This emerging work reveals the processual, powerful "pushes" of aging. That is, it reveals something of both the affective dimensions of aging (how important *affect* is to aging), the affective force of aging (the influence of *affective* social aging in social life), and particular human and non-human entities and their interdependencies.[37]

Exclusion from cultural discourses on the basis of age, gender, race, or ethnicity is an advocacy point for posthumanist theorists and practitioners across a growing number of scholarly disciplines. Proponents argue that new narratives are needed, recognizing the necessity of shifts to more holistically satisfy the unmet health needs and aspirations of the disempowered, the medically underserved, and Indigenous peoples, with older persons often haphazardly falling into these categories. This is not a new phenomenon. Traditionally, developed societies have chronically stigmatized aged individuals with physical and cognitive deficits as being less than fully human, negating the actor-agency of older humans—of their material interdependencies with associated nonhuman living species—despite the reality of these related "things" being fully capable of sensorially improving the well-being of older persons' lives (see chapter 5). Gerontological research that pushes beyond conventional theory and methodologies can, it is hoped, disentangle these subjectivities that have allowed discriminatory ageism to persist. Architecture for health can be a positive influence/force in this disentanglement.

Unfortunately, for the past half century, nearly every long-term care home in North America was minimalistically programmed, designed, constructed, and administered over its lifespan. Many RLTC homes are still being constructed to cram too many beds (up to four, and sometimes more) into a single bedroom, rendering it nearly impossible to provide the personal distancing and nature-engagement affordances so therapeutically essential in mitigating the high airborne transmission rates that occurred during the coronavirus pandemic.[38] One example of this misguided bureaucratic public health policy response to the crisis unfolded in Ontario, Canada. In mid-2020, the provincial government boldly proclaimed by 2030 it would construct 30,000 new long-term care beds across a province with a population of 14.3 million. With over 38,000 persons on the waiting list for a bed in 2024 (portrayed as a scandal in the media at the time), the sum of $1.75 billion (CDN) was budgeted to begin this process.[39] In the abrupt rush to build *fast*, anywhere, land parcels were haphazardly purchased and cleared, with little regard for any potential adverse impacts on either the future materialist well-being of the residents of these places or the health of the disrupted environmental assemblages. A top-down bureaucratic narrative was hastily formulated to achieve this ambitious goal, which was ill fated from the outset, especially from a posthumanist perspective.

As is well known, ageism is often wielded as an institutionalized weapon, allowing societies to tacitly remove older persons from the social mainstream and carelessly relocate them to age-segregated "nursing home warehouses" on remote sites with few, if any, connections to urbanity, friends, and loved ones. The COVID-19 pandemic in many ways further compounded this complex discriminatory trend of isolated segregation and segmentation. A disproportionately high number of fatalities occurred among the aged in isolated, overcrowded, institutional residential care homes, many of them dating from the 1960s and 1970s and often built on the outskirts of town (see chapter 5).

With societies aging at such a rapid rate the status quo is no longer tenable. Long-term care residences no longer need be solely minimalistically driven—as nearly always has occurred. Socially equitable, health-centric architecture need not be anti-ecological, either. It can reclaim abandoned sites that previously were paved over or otherwise neglected for decades. Concrete-encased, abandoned shopping malls offer much promise for being returned to their prebuilt (natural) state, with long-term care residences then added, nondisruptively, as part of a *returned*, regenerated, redistributive natural site. Similarly, this type of architecture can reclaim abandoned unbuilt green parcels, such as in Dallas, Texas, with its 6,000-acre Great Trinity Forest.[40] Affordable housing, geared to socially and racially marginalized older persons, could be built on its edges. This forest is one of the largest urban woodlands in the US, with its expanse of mature hardwood trees, and ponds, swamps, and meandering creeks evolving freely. In these examples, the benign neglect of the past is being reinterpreted as a source of inspiration, potentially for the benefit of all impacted, including underrepresented older persons who often are denied their rightful agency in self-determining their own living options.

COMPASSIONISM AS HEALTH POLICY

Actor network theory is premised on the belief that traditional ways of making buildings (including for health care) are now out of step with the world we live in. As for architects and their clients, determinants that previously drove "health care architecture," especially in the 1975–2000 period, generally dismissed the growing importance of sustainability or ecological concerns. The old ways of thinking about buildings for health care were limited to static, self-referential narratives, as if every new hospital was an island unto itself. Sadly, the vast majority of health care facilities built worldwide are still unimaginatively conceived and constructed in this archaic way. For decades, the architectural profession consistently beat the drum about how technology always should drive health care architecture, resulting in extensively mega-technological facility apparatuses housing CAT scanners, MRIs, and the like, continually driving the pulsating narrative forward. By contrast, first and foremost, ANT calls for addressing the fluid *spirit* of a place or building and its essential materialist ecologies. What is the essential spirit of a redeployable field hospital, a Maggie's Centre, or a 24/7 residential care home for older persons? It is pointless to continue to obsess on narrowly defined concerns when designing a hospital or other built environment for health or health care purposes—because how it looks objectified in a glossy magazine matters less now than ever in an imperiled world.

Static Architectural Objectivity Is Dead

In the Anthropocene, the road ahead will be daunting as we become ever more dependent on complex ecosystems created over the millennia by non-human entities and their collective, distributive agency, long before medicine, public health, or architecture (as we know them) existed. The reality of our material dependency on threatened ecosystems and their myriad code-pendencies requires us to be more responsible for our actions than ever before, especially when the extinction of plants and animals is occurring at such an alarming rate. Sadly, human interventions entirely destructive to these species continue to dishonor their longstanding right to existence in the imperiled world we now live in, in turn jeopardizing our own existence.[41] We need to now pay very close attention to nature's feedback mechanisms. The interconnected concepts of *repair* and *return to a previous state* are critical in redefining what architecture can be (and yet isn't) in the Anthropocene. *Repair* denotes reconnecting with and improving a preexisting place or ecology through the removal of some anachronistic or outright destructive force, object, or influence. It calls for a commitment to revealing, or uncovering, prehuman anthropocentric legacies. *Returning*, for its part, denotes removing something once constructed by humans, together with regeneratively restoring places and ecologies to their prehuman, unbuilt, natural condition and, in so doing, simultaneously nurturing their becoming new/old reclaimed buildings and places. As such, in a resynthesized human-built environment dialectic, such as the Maggie's Centres, acknowledging Latour's emphasis on "feeling the repercussions of our actions" becomes the basis for ecopolitical policies and actions by rejecting worn out, obsolete, top-down, human-centric moral imperatives.[42] Human-centric thinking (humanism), which muted and silenced the "voices" of nonhumans, is ending. Now, the feedback channels emanating from the ecologically historically underrepresented need to resonate louder than ever:

> Posthumanist ecology . . . fundamentally questions the essentialist division between human/non-human and culture/nature . . . so intertwined

> though our co-development (or "becoming-with") processes. The story of how we came to become what we are today cannot be told without the roles of non-humans; our material being itself is a product of historical evolution from microorganisms [to] our everyday decision-making agency, often influenced by non-human agents . . . [ranging from] atmospheric weather patterns to the digital gadgets we interact with from the moment we start each day. Second, posthumanist ecology does not impose environmentalism on us as an essential moral imperative; rather, it focuses on demonstrating . . . our dependency on ecosystem [precursors] who render possible the material world. . . . Our destiny is entangled with the destiny of other species on the brink of disappearing precisely because of our irresponsible intervention. Posthumanism's pragmatic empiricism emphasizes the importance of our sensory experience with our immediate surroundings. . . . This implies that "love for nature" starts with caring for our everyday interaction with [our] most local surroundings.[43]

The colonialist imperative imposed by European military and economic powers on other cultures was, by and large, a ruthlessly materialist, unethical, culturally debased enterprise. It was fundamentally supported by the enforced separation between humans and animals, carried out on the backs of people native to Africa, Asia, Australia, and the Americas. It was this separation that fostered the enforced dehumanization of Indigenous cultures and their subsequent racialization by their colonial rulers.[44] Danielle DiNovelli-Lang examined the material, racist quest of conquering colonial powers for land, labor, and control over the disenfranchised that fostered the exploitation of animals in warfare and as prided symbols of political power.[45] The denigration of animals has been essential throughout the history of racism. In this context, the "post" in posthumanism and the "post" in postcolonialism are very alike in questioning the central, critical role of animals and their persistent historical abuse for the associated purpose of human-over-human domination: "*Treat them like animals.*" For this reason, much of the recent research on animals in sociocultural anthropology has centered on the materialist reality they *are* our others, and that animal species, as innocents, have been thoroughly intertwined with, yet debased by, colonialist societies and abusive human-animal dialectics.

Still other theorists view posthumanism as a vehicle by which to frame transhumanism:

Posthumanism, as generally defined, is the current, perhaps unavoidable, perhaps inevitable turn toward technology as the dominant paradigm of the future world. As such, the posthuman, i.e., transhuman, is a new phase in human history that necessitates a redefinition of what it is to be human given our increasing power to manipulate, change, and perhaps recreate the world, nature, and eventually, humanity itself. The provocations and implications of posthumanity thus require a reassessment of not simply traditional definitions of human beings, humanity, etc., but of nature, the animal, and ultimately, God. . . . It admits its evolving nature . . . mirroring our contemporary cultural situation . . . crucial for understanding the opportunity that posthumanism provides for a seamless exchange between science and the humanities . . . the notion of knowledge as *coding*. . . . Digital code is literally the conduit of virtually all information, and the translation of human genetic code. . . . Its manipulation [is] arguably the most singular scientific pursuit today. . . . As creatures, humans have the blessing and the curse of reappraising memory and history . . . what we did or didn't do . . . [via] the theoretical architecture of a new humanities through posthumanism.[46]

Regenerative Designs for Health

In human-centric, traditional Western architecture, questions about the negative impact of buildings on environmental health and public health have largely been conceptually absent or theoretically externalized. Historically, architects have considered *nature* as an inexhaustible resource that could never be fully consumed, while homeostasis, or *good health*, has been taken for granted. The reawakening of the architectural mainstream to its practitioners' unsavory role in perpetuating large-scale adverse ecological and human health impacts is creating a significant crack in the foundations of architectural theory—engendering a growing tension between the theoretical mainstream and the core tenets and protocols of architecture's humanist traditions. At the center are questions of its role relative to other-than-human externalities. When such previously unwelcomed externalities begin to boomerang back on architects, the concept of decoupling—a term developed by economists—comes to the fore.[47] In theory, *decoupling* presumes it is econometrically possible to detach behaviors from consequences or, in this case, material culture from the physical, ecological environment. To resolve the outcomes of economic growth, decoupling should, it is presumed, allow humans to decrease their materialism and waste generation while continuing to increase their unabated, continuous economic expansion. While there was initial enthusiasm for economic decoupling, research in the past decade has revealed that countries identified as "decoupled" are, in fact, rapidly outsourcing—exporting—their environmental waste removal and associated public health problems to other countries.

The dilemma of how to decouple architecture for health care from its adverse health impacts manifests itself in the techno-economic realm whenever a new, so-called sustainable building, material, or technique is marketed with the promise of reducing our carbon footprint without noticeably disrupting the mainstream practice of architecture. For example, in the illogic of sustainability, we may continue to pave over paradise, but at least we have now invented a new type of concrete that minimizes the release of greenhouse gases. Innovative solutions to the problem of unsustainable greenhouse gas emissions remain decoupled from the vexing belief in human exceptionalism—humanity's seeming right to entirely dominate nature. We still see this happening everywhere, including where cities (including Miami) seek to "harden" their threatened shorelines from the effects of rising sea levels and land subsidence. Moreover the term *resilience*, as in "a resilient architecture for health," has come into popular usage in the past decade.[48] But it, too, suffers from similar anthropocentric shortcomings, signifying the mainstream profession's continued vacuous excuses for settling for attaining merely a *sustainable* architecture for health.[49] Meanwhile, human exceptionalism persists at all scales of development, even in the case of the United Nations, which continues to reinforce policies of decoupled economic growth without limits and thereby risks worsening already adverse ecological feedback loops.[50] Curiously, the term *sustainability* still holds sway in both public health and architecture, although attempts to supplant this concept with more-progressive concepts, such as *regenerative design* or *circular design* (in health-related structures), are now gaining some momentum. While both of these terms, or concepts, have merit, they are synonymous neither with one another nor with sustainability. It is feared these concepts, too, will fall prey to the political forces of unchecked hypercapitalistic societies globally. As Matthew Dalziel writes:

> Bill Reed, a key voice in the regenerative movement, explains the problem by using an asymptotic curve, where sustainability understood as zero impact equals infinity. In other words, the closer we get to our sus-

tainability goals, the harder they are to achieve. Zero impact is a human concept that does not exist outside anthropocentricism. A regenerative design practice therefore requires an ontological leap . . . where humans are not non-player actors but rather become positive actors within a diverse set of ecosystems. Far from being a romantic notion, this is a position in nature where we have many good role models, ranging from fungi to beavers. These are understood as keystone species . . . helping define the entire ecosystem they contribute to. . . . When we move into a fully regenerative mode . . . [we] depart from any familiar touchstones of ecological thinking for here we must address the cultural issues at the heart of ecological questions allowing us to become one with nature, or rejoin nature.[51]

Is it any longer justifiable to think of human health equity as distinctly apart from—or, social status–wise, *better*—than the health equity of other living species and environmental ecologies? Is it acceptable to bring portable trauma centers into the Amazon rainforest to combat the latest plague or pandemic, without any real consideration for the well-being and health of other living species and inanimate "things" in the same geographic vicinity? Is it equitable, as a society, to ignore the acute housing needs of older persons who suffer from cognitive and physical impairment, and then to add ecological insult to injury by economically and politically decoupling the issue by building a facility in a pristine wetland without due consideration of its deleterious impacts? Is it equitable to do so without fully considering the effects on all impacted actors and the agency they bring to the discourse? Or are the economic and political pressures simply too great? Must we expediently rampage onward to build new long-term care housing for elders *anywhere* without any real ecological concern?

Fertile rewards await those who employ imaginative strategies to promote posthumanist health and health equity for *all species* and *all "things"* in this imperiled world. Posthumanism in architecture for health, unfortunately, still tends to conjure sci-fi narratives and aesthetics of AI bots that will perform the tiresome, mundane activities of daily living for us. Nonetheless, critical posthumanist health-equity theory and practice hold the potential to transform both the definition of the subject (what really *is* architecture for health?) and its modes of knowledge production (what really *is* evidence-based research and educational pedagogy?). The challenge is to reconceptualize our failed ways of thinking and doing and move beyond merely servicing human exceptionalism. First and foremost, this can be centered on expanding our ethical duty regarding health care concerns to promote the health of *all matter*, both *animate* and *inanimate*. To paraphrase Braidotti, a posthumanist architecture for health asks what it means to serve the public's health, safety, and welfare in an era at once more than human and less than human—that is, more than human in its technological advances (transhumanism and artificial intelligence), and less than human in the continued inhumane, careless, harmful impacts of thoughtlessly rationalized built environments randomly imposed on the planet (see chapter 1).[52]

If posthumanist architecture—including architecture for health—is capable of fostering the necessary ontological leap forward toward equitable, regenerative health for *all*, is it any longer sensible to dismiss it? A redefined subdiscipline of *architecture for health equity* is about much more than human health alone. It embraces the entirely of all ecologies in which humans live and coexist. Because of this, the very concept of healthfulness in relation to architecture requires full-scale redefinition. What is healthful and what is unhealthful? To whom? Where? And to what ends? It isn't as if we can simply return to the late-nineteenth-century town-planning principles of Ebenezer Howard's Garden City movement, the public health–inspired urban parks in North America designed by Frederick Law Olmsted, the mid-twentieth-century health-promoting American residential architecture of Richard Neutra, or the bright and airy TB sanitoriums of the period, such as Alvar Aalto's Paimio Sanitorium in Finland (see chapter 2). Despite their creators' laudable intentions, these advancements are long past.

Regenerative built environments for human health call for innovative ideological and strategic paths forward. In the Anthropocene, if we are to survive regeneratively and with equanimity, healthful planning, design, construction, and ecological stewardship of the built environment are essential. We must see, sense, and interact in an iterative cycle of learning, relearning, and doing. We need to redefine how humans learn, think, and act without drawing some arbitrary (theoretical) line or boundary of concern, ignoring that which lies just beyond it. The survival of all nonhuman actors and "things" is highly entangled with our own survival. What will posthumanist urbanism and architecture for health look like? This question is answerable only through a process of empathic, ethically grounded caring, compassion, and work to *become more than we are now*. The challenge is to *decenter*.

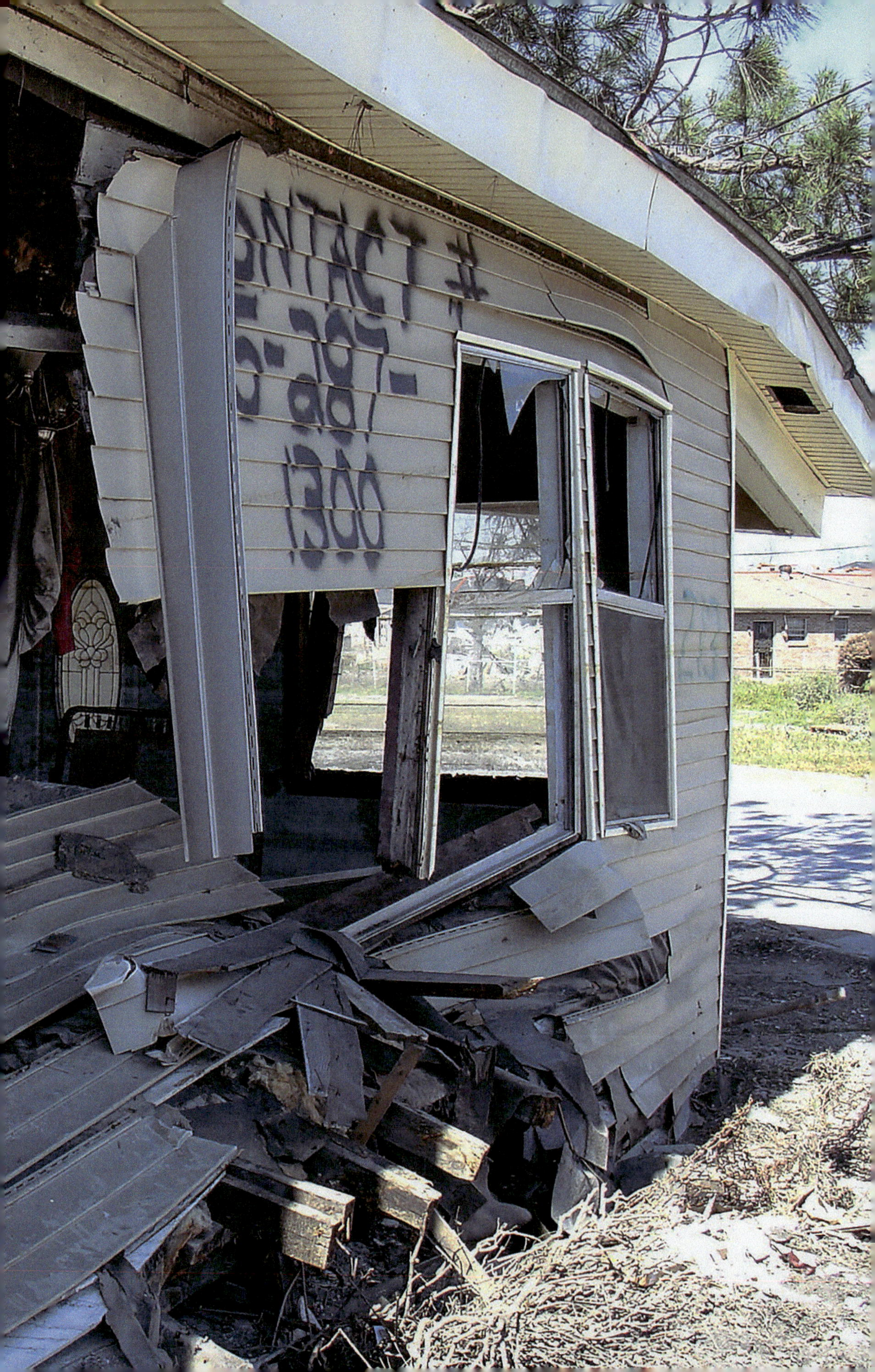
ONTACT #
5-787-
1300

Architecture for Health Equity

2050 and Beyond

META-HEALTHSCAPES (EPOCH 6)

Synopsis: The Anthropocene, widely considered to have coalesced scientifically and philosophically post-2000, signifies that planet Earth has entered a new epoch. The human species radically intervened in the planet's ecological well-being, with the stage set for a likely series of cascading calamities with increasingly severe impacts on all living and nonliving things. Earth's atmospheric chaos is further exacerbated by the continued burning of fossil fuels, with the nations of the world unable to agree on how to abate this urgent threat. As the climate crisis fully blooms, it manifests in Black Swan events and previously unforeseen natural disasters, with the hope smarter-than-human AI bots will take a leadership role in saving the planet (and humanity). This exigency dovetails with artificial intelligence and its transformative impacts, a duality with profound consequences for all living species and inanimate objects. The downsizing and redeployment of health care services expresses a pattern of functional reconstitution—the re-centering

Figure 7.1. Hurricane Katrina destruction, New Orleans, 2005. Photo by Alex Verderber.

of care with the risk anti-globalization will lead to widening health inequities between have and have-not populations. Hospitals continue to be the health care setting of last resort for the sickest of the sick as more and more care is distributed and received virtually, anytime, anywhere. Access to proper health care as such remains haphazard, with poor, medically underserved populations struggling to attain and maintain relative healthfulness. Continued destruction of the ozone layer, assaults on previously unspoiled natural landscapes, regional water wars, and ecosystem collapses are accelerating on an increasingly populated planet. Public health policy, medicine, and the health sciences struggle to keep abreast, as health care provider organizations are pressured to become ever better ecological citizens—stewards in promoting the well-being not only of humans, but of all living species and inanimate "things" within a posthumanist medical care framework. By 2050, hospitals and health care systems provide care for all living species, no longer singularly caring for humans. Global public health challenges give rise to well-structured, politically empowered patients' right movements.

***Architects' primary focus**: As new interdisciplinary fields emerge, architecture for health care strives to expresses posthumanism, the therapeutic affordances of nature and landscapes, anthropomorphism, multisensoryism, and correspondingly redefined building types.*

***Predominant building types**: Diagnostic and treatment settings incorporating knowledge transference from prefabrication technologies applied to inpatient and ambulatory clinical care, primary and tertiary medicine, behavioral health, physical rehabilitation, field-based healthcare in pre- and post-disaster contexts, refugee and migration centers, palliative care, nature immersion/reimmersion, and intersections between AI and built environments for health care.*

Since the late nineteenth century, the fields of architecture and public health have evolved from a primary emphasis on applied professional practice, in time becoming much broader disciplines—a deliberative process involving the continual search for professional relevancy to society while seeking to establish autonomy within the community of professions, with their associated scholarly disciplines. The operative assumption was relevance and autonomy together would hold greater stature and prestige than either one or the other alone. This has proven to be the case as evidence-based knowledge in medical and epidemiological research has demonstrably fueled the progress and elevation of entire societies in global contexts. By comparison, in architecture systematic research advancements have occurred in relatively slow motion, in a comparatively muddled series of fits and starts. While evidence-based innovation does take place, albeit haltingly, it often has occurred at a snail's pace. As a result genuine disciplinary-based contributions to new knowledge in architecture tend to remain in their infancy for far too long. This problem persists both from the standpoint of positivist, empiricist foundations and in an inability to definitively elevate the profession and discipline, similar to what generally occurs in public health and medicine.[1] Nevertheless, evidence-based knowledge in architecture for health care has recently impacted the health professions' view of the legitimacy of the disciplinary side of the equation, despite architecture continuing to be unfocused and therefore unprepared to rapidly, adroitly, respond to disaster emergencies (fig. 7.1).

Architectural theory, for its part, evolved from a traditional reliance on pure historical precedent to a position informed to a large extent by methodologies adopted from scientific inquiry. It tends to borrow from diverse disciplines, including the social sciences, engineering and, in the following discussion, the health sciences. It remains anthropocentric, however, and this bias unfortunately continues to drive most mainstream discourses in architecture. As a consequence, posthumanism and its relationship to evidence-based physical planning, architecture, landscape architecture, and construction in the realm of health care remain oblique.

In this chapter, thematic prognostications for the year 2050 and beyond are put forth—including alternative care settings to traditional hospitals; the significance of community-based preventive care; prefabricated modular architecture for health capable of rapid deployment and adaptation in pre and post-disaster contexts; the incorporation of posthumanist perspectives; the transformative influence of AI in our everyday lives; and the responsiveness of architecture in future public health emergencies. In the following discussion, *transhumanism* is defined as phenomena associated with and centered on the human body. By contrast, *artificial intelligence* is defined as those phenomena associated with beyond-human-body technologies and their associated sociological and cultural ramifications in our daily life. Eight themes presented below seek to extend the narrative established in the previous six chapters (although additional themes could have been included, space permitting). An attempt to visually illustrate these trends projected outward to the year 2050 is depicted in figure 7.2.

Theme 1

Transhumanism dematerializes the physical space between the human body and the physical environment. Posthumanist architecture increasingly expresses anthropomorphic and multisensory therapeutic affordances.

Astounding technological developments will transform humans' relationship with our evolutionary past. Technology will matter far more, impacting all living species and "things" in the physical environment. New interdisciplinary fields coalesce around the concept of transhumanism. This thinking dates from the 1960s as depicted in science fiction, where humans are decentered from traditional roles of supremacy in the universe. *Trans-humanism* —a condition of hybridity in both theory and practice—is a the-oretical stream within *posthumanism*. Biotechnological advancements will rework our species into something beyond its present configurations.[2] This altered state of existence for humans as well as other life forms will bear a strong resemblance to cyborgs or chimeras.[3] To its advocates, it will sig-nify a cultural shift, aiming to revolutionize, empower, and improve human beings as a species, both physically and intellectually, through the *techno-sciences* of so-called human enhancement—genetics, regenerative medi-cine, hibernationary theory, robotics, agelessness methodologies, and the insertion of subcutaneous microchips into humans. To its cheerleaders, this futurist hybrid condition involves the insertion of prosthetic enhancements into the body without obviating the human body altogether, since transhu-manism is fundamentally utopian in its assumptions and expectations:

> Prior to 1990 the term "posthuman" was rarely used and even though science fiction and futuristic philosophies of technology conjured up numerous visions of new humans, the idea of radical change in life conditions and essential traits of the species did not set a broader agenda. Since 2000, however, it has become a thriving subject where very different approaches and visions intersect and where science and medicine as well as philosophy, law, art, literature and psychology contribute with unique perspectives. It is a field that deals with both imminent uses of new technologies and longer-term conjecturing on the human species. In both cases . . . it tests the limits of what is considered ethical. . . . Are individuals with a higher dignity possible? Or is it that

human dignity will be corrupted by biotechnological enhancement of the human body?[4]

What will it mean to be an "uploaded" human in the future, inhabiting a technologically enhanced, health-centric building? Will the dystopian prognostications of Aldous Huxley's *Brave New World* (1932) come to pass? Recent developments present a range of bewildering ethical questions, certain to become ever more intractably challenging in the future. In advanced genetic engineering and in medicine, these progressions may engender better health and longer lives. Concomitantly, they may result in far less access to diagnoses and treatment among non-uploaded individuals and populations, further exacerbating existing health inequities perpetuated by the persistent digital divide. Regardless, human/machine and animal/machine transactions will increase, enhancing transhumans and transanimals (God forbid!) with spare body parts far beyond today's benign surgical insertions of artificial knees and hip replacements. The goal will be to strengthen the human species, with the widely accepted caveat this may foster myriad adverse unintended consequences, further separating the "haves" from the "have-nots" in societies globally. Will a society with huge differences in life expectances be acceptable, where some live to 150, while others die prematurely at age 60 or younger? How much of a cyborg will we allow a human (or an animal) to become? Nature has proved to be adroit at cloning itself, but should humans also do this? Who shall decide? Immanuel Kant's three questions—What can we know? What ought we to do? For what may we hope?—personify the inner profundities embedded in these dilemmas.[5]

Over the past 10,000 years, human societies' integration of technology resulted in the rapid evolution of our species' capabilities. Because cybernetic organisms synthesize the organic (living, naturally evolved beings or substances) with inorganic machines (nonliving, artificial, invented objects) to create a modified entity through vaccinations and biocomputers, it will be incumbent on us to take ownership of our increasing cyborgness. In other words, we bear the full responsibility for our continued evolution toward our species' indeterminate future. For better or worse, the present growing dependency on the informational vagaries of social media will be integral in this process, as part of a reconfiguration of both knowledge production and political control of this knowledge.[6] Uploading our brain's memory to a microchip will likely enable us to experience any architectural environment, situated anywhere, from any period in recorded history. Brain scanning enables the mapping of interconnections between the brain's complex networks of neurons and synapses, thereby allowing the transference of our analog brain to our AI bot assistive devices.

Futurologist Ina Pearson maintains that at some point in time, it will be considered commonplace to create a transhuman mind by linking the analog mind with biochip insertions.[7] One result may be that immortality will be assured, in theory at least, since an uploaded mind will not experience a conventional physical death—having achieved virtual agelessness—where some mode of ongoing "survival" is made possible by continually upgrading to the latest hardware and software iterations (e.g., a 125.0 or even 195.0 software update). These new beings may mentally travel at the speed of light with enhanced memory functionality, ending memory loss as we now know it, which is a serious aspect of declining health among increasing numbers of older persons.[8] Transhumans will experience therapeutic environments virtually, including multisensory walk-throughs in nature and landscapes—places that connote positive recollections from the past, such as that memorable vacation spot in the English countryside some thirty years ago. But will this advanced technocratic apparatus actually help combat diseases, aid in healing, or enable the maintenance of wellness? Who and how many will have access to these transhumanist technologies? And what populations will inequitably be left behind?

Theme 2
The digital divide perpetuating health inequities will lessen yet remain persistent. Regardless, inequalities between developed and developing nations' health care systems will decrease as a result of a trend toward more universally distributed telemedicine infrastructure.

At the 2022 B20 Summit (the business arm of the G20 Summit) held in Bali, CEOs and political leaders from around the world struck an upbeat tone when discussing growth opportunities, new partnerships, and collaborative alliances regarding the role of emerging digital technologies in helping close the persistent global divide between the world's digital haves and have-nots. Yet in 2024, 2.7 billion people around the world had no access to the internet. This lack of connectivity persists, despite the slight uptake in broadband access that occurred during the COVID-19 pandemic. At the pandemic's outset, worldwide governmental lockdown orders included quarantine restrictions and shutdowns with people virtually everywhere suddenly forced into isolation. The interruption to everyday life drove individuals in many places toward telemedicine, virtual classrooms, social media outlets, and other alternative sources for their health care. According to the United Nations, a 10 percent increase in the penetration of mobile broadband services increases a nation's GDP by 1.5 percent.[9] With AI optimistically projected to deliver double-digit GDP growth globally, AI's value and extended reach will be somewhat restricted. This is because only 60 percent of the world is currently online to any degree, and private corporations as well as government at all levels will confront this widespread challenge. As more people are connected to one another through this technology, the greater the opportunities to learn and hopefully prosper—which opens the door to exploitation by multinational megacorporations.

The *digital divide* is defined as a techno-cultural condition where individuals and populations experience chronically *unequal* access to broadband and satellite-based digital technologies. It is increasingly associated with dystopic health inequalities in many countries. In the 2010–2017 period the number of US hospitals utilizing telemedicine technologies increased from 35 to 76 percent.[10] This infrastructural non-capability separates highly developed from developing economies, further magnified by ageist stereotypes and racial and gender discrimination. It has allowed new billionaires under age 30 to emerge, while it holds many millions down in abject poverty. In an era where health infomatics and communication technologies eclipse traditional manufacturing as the basis for economic growth, the lack of predictable access to the internet remains problematic—and likely will remain so unless dramatic public policies are enacted. The places and people remaining shut out are, in effect, cut off from democratic processes, work advancement opportunities, new knowledge, emerging social trends, and political movements.

Advantages of telemedicine/telehealth include its cost effectiveness, its ability to extend access to previously underserved locales, and a potential to mitigate looming nurse and physician shortages in medically underserved parts of the world. Disadvantages include the continued unavailability of predictable, robust digital connectivity in rural regions and many urban centers; persistent political threats as a result of the unethical confiscation or duplication of confidential patient data; and continuing technical challenges and inconsistencies associated with performing even basic patient examinations and medical procedures online. By 2050, the most empowered patients—those wealthy enough to afford being diagnosed and treated in person—are most likely to obtain the best health care available. The sheer volume of health-centric information procurable by then, however, will have elevated the technologically "privileged" patients to unprecedented advantages in terms of available care options. By contrast, fewer possibilities will be available in poorer societies without public health policies enacted to rectify these critical gaps in access to health care. The digital divide will only be eliminated once and for all through the empowerment of all communities, everywhere, with fully predictable and robust internet access.

Theme 3

Posthumanist architectural theory and practice embraces humans and all living species and ecological "things." Obsolete hospitals are reinvented as new building types emerge and inpatient and outpatient care evolve into species-inclusive health care delivery systems.

The behemoth medical centers built in North America and elsewhere in the late twentieth century were virtual mini-cities.[11] A self-serving attitude of institutional exceptionalism among the builders of these citadels of high-tech medicine provided them with virtual carte blanche to execute their techno-utopian visions. These mega-facilities often looked like military fortresses or automobile factories looming over their surroundings not entirely unlike their medieval precursors—the large open-plan chapel ward hospitals run by religious orders (see chapter 2). But what would a posthumanist hospital look like, and how would it function? Will it reject conventional building types in seeking to recapture the multisensory therapeutic affordances of nature, ecology, and landscape? In the Anthropocene, existing hospitals and their associated outpatient clinics and urgent care centers will be out of sync with prevailing climate realities unless they adapt. Their reinvention expresses a new functional imperative. In so doing, they are more broadly redefined, in recognition of the agency of nonhuman living species-actors and inanimate "things" within an expanded ethics-of-care framework that embraces the benefits of providing multispecies holistic care on-site. This shift is predicated on decentering the human species, as opposed to currently accepted ethics-of-care standards where humans are squarely positioned at the top of the species-survival pyramid. This redefinition assumes the legitimacy of the vital role of nonhuman species-actors and their "voices" (agency) in helping maintain and improve the quality of life for all species and ecologies, including nature, landscapes, and architecture.

In the Anthropocene, a much-broadened manifold of compassionate caring necessitates redefining the role and function of the hospital as a place that salutogenically expresses the *spirit* of health and wellness in its every aspect. It requires first acknowledging and then working to rectify the failures of the modern health care industrial complex, its highly contradictory technocratic underpinnings, and subsequent health inequities perpetuated worldwide. As for apologists who cling to techno-utopian, machine-for-healing, worn-out anthropocentric biases, they remain anxious to tightly grip an obsolete belief in human exceptionalism. Similarly, nonrenewable resource consumers will be the last to relinquish fossil fuel–guzzling vehicles. The new spirit, and its antecedent attitudinal expressions in built environments for health care, symbolizes human *decenterdness*—constituting the core aesthetic ethos and functionality of the posthumanist hospital, its allied health care institutions, and their associated network of geographically dispersed outpatient clinics. Soft-spoken, *humble* architecture does not elevate humans above ecological concerns and priorities. These structures are conceived, designed, constructed, and administered across their useful lifespans by being ecologically *embedded in nature* at the same time as their formerly heroic physical presence physically and symbolically dematerializes. These institutions no longer aggressively dominate their site and local ecologies, instead visually and functionally blending harmoniously with all that is around them. This imperative is about projecting less ostentatious, non–traditionally defined imagery in a new era of antiheroism in health care architecture. In other words, the posthumanist hospital and its allied health care institutions compassionately embrace their immediate site and broader ecological contexts, while wholly philosophically and physically rejecting any semblance of a forbidding, domineering scale of formal imagery (see chapter 4). These hospitals and their health care architectural networks of service sites exhibit due respect for the virtues of intimacy, aesthetic humility, functional appropriateness, and resonant ecological communality with nonhuman species, inanimate "things" and the intrinsic affordances of nature and landscape.

Theme 4
The professions and disciplines of architecture, landscape architecture, urban and regional planning, and the health professions and health disciplines coalesce into an interdiscipline that transcends anthropocentrism. This and allied ecologically based disciplines will be brought to the fore to improve the healthfulness of societies.

To its critics, the profession and discipline of architecture has become rather sclerotic. In the US, many complaints are currently being lodged against the American Institute of Architects, the principal professional organization representing nearly 122,000 licensed architects in the country as of 2022. Similar complaints are being waged against university-based programs in architecture offering professional degrees in the field and the North America-based Association of Collegiate Schools of Architecture. Currently there are 175 National Architectural Accrediting Board–accredited programs offered by 139 institutions of higher learning in the US and abroad. More and more, prominent practitioners and academics in the field are openly admitting an inconvenient truth—architecture as a profession is at risk of losing its societal direction and is in need of change. In 2024, there were only about 2,500 licensed architects in the US who were Black (2 percent). Its critics argue that, in the context of the profession's long-held legally mandated charge to protect the public's health, safety, and welfare, and aside from the issue of race per se, too many self-aggrandizing architects remain insular by choice, rather disinterested in overtly providing culturally, socially, racially, or ecologically attuned work for rapidly changing societies globally. A case in point is the ill-fated Make It Right public interest architecture foundation in New Orleans, founded by Oscar-winning actor Brad Pitt in 2007 in the aftermath of Hurricane Katrina's devastation of the city's Lower Ninth Ward:

> This program invited firms, most of them avant-garde, to design housing for poor New Orleanians whose homes were destroyed by Hurricane Katrina. The architecture world was exhilarated: the initiative was to showcase how the best contemporary design could improve lives. The predictable result was weird, sometimes discomforting, houses of non-native motley futuristic design with virtually no relation to one another or the beloved historic architecture of the city. A story in *The New Republic* called these 90-some houses a waste of money and a distracting sideshow. The homes were expensive to build ($400,000 on average) and their high-tech fabrication made them expensive to fix; mold has grown on the untested experimental materials and the eco-wood decks and stairs are already rotting. The neighborhood remains a wasteland—the failure of urban planning to reconnect residents with social networks and public services.[12]

This cautionary tale illustrates how architects have tended to remain preoccupied with the wrong issues. For example, the renowned Dutch firm MVRDV designed one Make It Right house that looked like a travel-trailer home broken in half. The resulting piggy-back scheme strangely resembled one new house seemingly haphazardly (but intentionally), carelessly thrown atop another new house, all on a very small lot. Insider architectural jokes?[13] The profession tends to perpetuate existing power structures that, sadly, range from gender and race stereotyping to the sanctioned misdirection of private and public investment capital. Even in the specialized arena of professional practice widely known as *architecture for health*, the notion of a building—first and foremost—as fashion or an aesthetic statement stubbornly persists (although somewhat less now, compared with other specialized areas of practice), as if that newly opened hospital or ambulatory care clinic is about to stroll down the runway in the latest designer evening attire. What the overall profession needs most is a *new humility*, as opposed to more egocentrism. The architect of the future is an interdisciplinist, an excellent collaborator, a keener listener than current practitioners, and a better orchestrator of seemingly incompatible viewpoints transcending prosaic anthropocentric ideologies and attitudes in favor of *inclusivity* over *elitist exclusivity*. This attitude no longer excludes others from concern on the basis of racial identity, gender orientation, or income level. It is collaborative versus tediously individualistic. To foster this new attitude, an entirely new interdiscipline emerges to supplant traditional, shopworn conceptions of architecture. This interdiscipline in the Anthropocene will be about *health ecotecture*, the synthesis of architecture with its allied disciplines, including landscape architecture and industrial design, and new close alliances with public health and epidemiology, medicine, medical research, and their associated health disciplines.

The 2023 Venice Architecture Biennale, titled "Laboratory for the Future," opened on the same day the leaders of the G7 industrialized nations met in Hiroshima, Japan. Lorenzo Marsili, writing in *The Guardian*, pointed out how the profession of architecture is the most globally homogenized of all the arts. But is anything new here? Erecting International Style copycat buildings in far-flung locales was the staple of European-centric colonialist policies in the twentieth century and even up to the present day. In financial capitals worldwide today, the current generation of ubiquitous-looking glass/steel skyscrapers appear interchangeable from one country to the next, because they were conceived and built with scant attention to place specificity. The Biennale in 2023, however, critically reassessed this one-world narrative. According to Marsili, the International Style has historically been "a singular, exclusive voice, whose reach and power ignores huge swathes of humanity."[14] Exhibits included a reassessment of Brazil's capital, Brasilia, as having signified the colonial invasion of the Indigenous vernacular traditions of central Brazil. In this worldview, non-Western countries and the entire Global South should now be free to reshape their own architectural agendas. The risk is great, however, that authoritarian nations will establish newly undemocratic—even fascist—built-environment traditions, including in health care, that foster human and ecological oppression, furthering health inequities among the medically underserved and medically non-served.

Theme 5
Artificial intelligence redefines the human species' role as stewards of the planet. If misdirected, health-promoting built environments become inaccessible, further exacerbating health inequities, especially among the medically underserved and the poor in disaster-prone communities.

The coronavirus pandemic jarred humanity out of its complacency and in so doing caused widespread conniptions. The public skepticism toward technoscience's inability to combat contagious disease spilled out into full view. Despite this, recent advancements in machine-based learning are elevating the visibility of technoscience to an unprecedented degree. The rapidly accelerating fields of AI and robotics (see transhumanism, above) are garnering headlines daily. Their ethical and moral imperatives are questionable, however, and this narrow "code of self-responsibility" to self-establish the necessary guardrails for the industry to proceed into this unknown territory has become a matter of grave mainstream concern. This concern revolves around the relative relationship between science, ethics, and the future independence of scientists worldwide to freely pursue AI and robotic avenues of inquiry, even if they do not fully comprehend or approve of what the endgame may be. A glimpse of this occurred in 2023 with the confession of Gregory Hinton, widely seen as a pioneer in machine learning, who astonishingly admitted to being frightened by the potentially uncontrolled abuses of AI in everyday life. Will AI bots of the future be in favor of the human species' continued existence? This concern raises myriad further questions of the ethics of *scientism*, which still defends the unconditional value to society of AI and advanced robotic technologies, as opposed to its critics who support *antiscience*'s ethical viewpoint of restricting scientific applications in this deeply important matter.[15]

An intermediate, somewhat more optimistic viewpoint accepts that the technosciences will improve the human condition in myriad ways, but with humans continuing (and still allowed by the machines) to occupy a central, intermediate level of control over AI bot and related machine-trained technoscientific innovations. Will this human control be tacitly supported by the machine-trained AI bots in a world where the machines have become integral in our everyday life? Will so-called enhancement devices be surgically inserted into our brains as extensions of the human body? For instance, will AI-guided augmented reality eventually directly challenge the notion that "real experiential exposure" to nature is always and unconditionally *better*, or preferred more by humans, compared with representational simulations of nature (see the discussion of nature surrogation in chapter 4). Assumptions such as this will be challenged, given the propensity of humans to continuously seem compelled to forcibly dominate external ecological nonhuman species and "things" that are perceived threats to humans' healthfulness and survival.[16]

In this transhumanist world, the real and the artificial continue together down the path of full integration. If a true crisis appears on the horizon, the question becomes, How can we wisely manage AI, so it does not blossom into a profoundly deep threat to the very survival of the human species? Six windows of thought regarding this anticipated (or real) threat are discernable in this relationship—the unthinkable, the radical, the acceptable, the sensible, the popular, and any eventual legal parameters in public health policy. But at the end of the day they are likely to result in an increasing acceptance of the AI-driven technosciences. That which, in the beginning, is initially unknown and generally considered incomprehensible starts to arouse our curiosity, later becoming fashionable (and attracting theorization), then quickly reaching the stage of formal legitimacy. Just as countless routine and nonroutine jobs are already disappearing due to AI, so, too, will some traditional human-occupied building types disappear. As nonsmart health care systems and institutional structures fall by the wayside due to their declining societal agency, health-centric building types with new types of agency will take their place. Yet the risk is great these will only be available to the technocratically elite and the wealthy. Without an equitable distribution of fiscal resources, the medically underserved and the poor will experience little access to health care of any kind, especially in high-risk disaster strike zones.

Theme 6
Disasters—including droughts, mega-wildfires, flooding, and wars—result in mass geomigrations and exert unprecedented pressure on public

health care systems to address the worsening plight of the poor and medically underserved populations.

Poor and medically underserved populations face great risk of harm from climate-induced disasters on a denatured, resource-depleted planet. Many governmental ministries of health and allied health agencies worldwide are hard pressed to develop effective policies, and nonprofit humanitarian organizations struggle to alleviate gaping disaster preparedness disparities. As for post-disaster recovery interventions in hard-hit strike zones, rapid-response resources are increasingly stretched thin (see chapters 3 and 4). New types of public/private sector partnerships are, of necessity, established to respond to acute survival needs of the most highly vulnerable, including persons living on low incomes, racial minorities, individuals lacking formal education, and persons over age 65 (see chapter 5 and appendix B). Among adversely impacted groups, the politically disempowered are particularly prone to live in places that will, in many cases, be most adversely impacted. Hurricane Harvey in Texas in 2017 took a severe emotional toll on its most vulnerable victims:

> The first thing Dana Jones, 61, tells you to do when you enter her grey-blue house in Melrose Park [a Houston inner neighborhood] is to walk across her warped flooring. And Jones, too, feels warped, five years after Hurricane Harvey forced her to wade through waist-high water that came too fast. It took her a month to find somewhere to live so she lived out of her truck. The thing she fears most is having to flee her home again. When it rains, she cries. She hyperventilates. She can't sleep. . . . The wood siding is deteriorating and has dark water stains and the mold is black. She tries to keep it at bay with bleach . . . and says there are still so many people still hurt by this [disaster] and property owners can no longer safely occupy or afford to fix their homes, as thousands remain in limbo. Others moved on, selling for far less, having been deemed ineligible for federal or state aid as a result of discriminatory federal rules.[17]

Disasters take an increasing toll on their victims' economic and mental health. Hurricane Harvey produced more than 60 inches of rain across Houston and the southeastern Texas region in the US. It caused dramatic flooding, with many area residents still harboring post-traumatic stress disorder years after the actual event. New descriptive terms are being coined to describe this phenomenon—disasterphobia, ecotrauma, ecogrief, to name a few—in an attempt to capture dimensions of the incontrovertible trauma and related adverse behavioral impacts being magnified by the worsening climate crisis worldwide. In 2021, the International Society for Traumatic Stress Studies published a report documenting the dramatic adverse psychological impacts that lie ahead.[18] In the US, African Americans are estimated to be 40 percent more likely than non–African Americans to live in areas with the highest projected increases in mortality rates due to elevated extreme temperatures alone. This dire warning is magnified by the inequitable histories of populations who live in disaster-prone places. Those who continue to be politically and socioeconomically marginalized— African Americans in particular—face socioeconomic factors historically relegating them to living in substandard housing conditions in environmentally hazardous communities. This was the case in New Orleans' flood-ravaged Lower Ninth Ward, resulting in living conditions that further worsened after Hurricane Katrina in 2005 and persist to this day.. Two relevant examples in Louisiana, the state where I lived for twenty-two years, involve the environmentally toxic zone situated along both banks of the lower Mississippi River's petrochemical "Cancer Alley" that lies between New Orleans and Baton Rouge and the aforementioned Hurricane Katrina catastrophe.

Cancer Alley is an 80-mile stretch of the Mississippi River that is lined with toxic petrochemical and fertilizer plants, with many poor communities located literally next door to the entrances of these enormous industrial plants. The annual cancer death rates in this part of Louisiana are among the highest in the entire US and, in some cases, the entire world.[19] Along Cancer Alley, a pattern of *environmental racism* was virtually unnoticed— and therefore remained unchecked—for generations. In Hurricane Katrina, the most deaths by drowning (out of a total of more than 1,800 who died) occurred in the low-lying Lower Ninth Ward, a neighborhood nearly 100 percent populated by Black residents. In the case of Cancer Alley, multinational corporations, with their industrial footprints firmly entrenched in this unhealthful, beleaguered zone, audaciously (but not surprisingly) mounted an all-out campaign in 2023 and 2024 to discredit local environmental-civil-rights advocacy groups seeking remediation and compensation for the many well-documented health problems these communities have disproportionately endured for so long.[20] Natural disasters do not discriminate, although human responses to them often do. This is especially true when the lingering effects of structural racism hamper emergency relief activities and longer-term compensation efforts. An organization called the Institute for Diversity and Inclusion in Emergency Management now deploys equity assurance teams into the field before and after a disaster to aid local community organizations and to help ensure that social and health equities are present in all facets of public policy and direct disaster relief aid efforts.[21]

In 2020, the US Federal Emergency Management Agency's advisory council finally acknowledged the need to address these persistent health inequities on an official policy level.[22] Also, the US Centers for Disease Control and Prevention, together with the Agency for Toxic Substances and Disease Registry, recently launched the "CDC/ATSDR Social Vulnerability Index." Working together, these agencies now compile data, based on sixteen variables/metrics, to assist in-the-field emergency planners and public health officials in identifying especially vulnerable communities before, during, and after an industrial/ecological disaster event. At the local level, these determinants include the poverty rate at the time of the disaster event, a lack of access to effective transportation resources, a lack of access to health care facilities, and the poor quality and unaffordability of the local housing stock.

Nonetheless, the process of seeking federal disaster assistance in the US is predicted to become ever more demanding and time consuming. Proving need will require ever more extensive pre-condition documentation of losses, making it highly burdensome for the displaced poor to apply for assistance and then sit idly by and wait for months, if not years, while their lives continue to be uprooted as they struggle to live and care for their families.[23] Databases and maps generated from these disaster events will, in the future, help estimate and pre-position the anticipated required supplies on-site and staged nearby, as well as determine emergency aid personnel needs (including redeployable trauma care facilities), best-practice emergency evacuation protocols, and the number and type of post-disaster emergency housing units required.[24] Despite future polices to keep victims of disasters in their longtime communities, many governments will have no option but to initiate managed retreats from repetitively disaster-stricken zones. How can evidence-based architects and health care specialists contribute in a compassionate and creative way?

Theme 7
Water wars erupt in regions with severe drought, and coastal regions and cities struggle with rising sea levels as both experience population displacements. Modular off-site–built health-centric buildings aid these and other places in need of rapid response disaster architecture.

The climate crisis will cause population dislocation. Regions and cities are already being pitted against one another over how to best manage their precious dwindling water supplies as carbon dioxide levels further drift in the wrong direction, such as what is occurring in the Colorado River basin in the US.[25] In 2023, the increase in global CO^2 levels was the largest on record, and the current amount of carbon dioxide in the earth's atmosphere is now 50 percent higher than it was before the dawn of the Industrial Age. Meanwhile, policymakers around the world face pressure to commit to ever more aggressive plans to reduce greenhouse gas emissions.[26] If this upswing in CO^2 levels continues, the Arctic Ocean will be totally free of summer ice as soon as 2030, even if humanity somehow immediately manages to drastically scale back its greenhouse gas emissions.[27] By 2050 another trend—dramatically rising sea levels—could affect three times as many people as previously predicted and threaten to erase a significant number of the world's coastal cities. Based on current and projected satellite data, roughly 150 million people currently occupy land that will lie below the global oceanic high-tide line by 2050.[28] The climate crisis is environmentally pressing these coastal zones, with more places being flooded more frequently, creating adverse effects for agriculture and countless other industries.

China will be home to sixteen of the twenty regions of the world most vulnerable to the climate crisis, according to the Intergovernmental Panel on Climate Change.[29] In Shanghai, one of Asia's most important economic engines, water will threaten to consume the heart of that mega-region, along with dozens of smaller yet economically important nearby cities. Climate-risk specialists XDI recently examined more than 2,600 regions worldwide—using climate forecasting models, together with weather patterns—to assess the economic damage rising temperatures will likely cause by 2050, asking the question, Which regions and cities will adapt most defensibly, and which will need to be abandoned in due course?[30] This study was based on a 3°C (5.4°F) increase in temperatures by the end of this century. The Chinese coastal province of Jiangsu, which currently accounts for one-tenth of China's total GDP, was ranked the world's most vulnerable territory. Outside of eastern China, Florida is the second-most-vulnerable region to rising seas, and the US government's National Oceanic and Atmospheric Administration does not expect these adverse trends to reverse themselves.[31] Rising temperatures will cause intense rainfall events, along with longer, more severe periods of drought and flooding.

How will public health and other health care specialists (namely, physicians), architects, landscape architects, urban and regional planners, private foundations, and public policymakers address the health consequences of a dramatically changed climate? One promising strategy is to design ecologically in support of healthy communities including living on water instead of next to it. Aquatecture communities will actually float atop the water. A new floating island city is currently being constructed in the Indian Ocean in a lagoon ten minutes by boat from Male, the Maldivian capital.[32] The Maldives, an archipelago of 1,190 low-lying islands, is highly vulnerable to the adverse impacts of the climate crisis. Eighty percent of its land mass is less than 1 meter above present sea levels and, based on current projections, nearly the entire country will eventually be inundated. Yet this island nation is opting to be a climate innovator, rather than a country with ultradependent climate refugees forced to seek new homes elsewhere. Its floating community will eventually be large enough to house 20,000 people. Designed anthropomorphically to resemble a coral reef, it will consist of 5,000 floating housing units and associated infrastructural amenities (scheduled for completion in 2027). It is a joint venture between developer Dutch Docklands and the Government of the Maldives, adopted as a practical policy solution to a changed reality. The community's off-site–built modular structures are being fabricated in a local shipyard, then towed to their installation sites. Once positioned, their components are anchored to a massive underwater hull, attached to the sea floor with giant telescopic steel stilts that allow the massive platform to gently move atop the waves. Coral reefs surround the site, providing stabilization and functioning as an urban breakwater.

This aquatectural community was designed by the architectural firm Waterstudio, founded in 2003 and based in The Netherlands. The firm is dedicated to building atop the water worldwide and, to date, has designed more than 300 floating homes, offices, schools, and health care facilities around the world. The Netherlands already is home to several floating constructs: parks, a dairy farm, housing, and a commercial office building. Other current floating projects include its Oceanix City in Busan, South Korea. The goal of these oceanic communities is self-sufficiency, including hospitals and other health care facilities. But it is equally likely many such threatened cities and regions will be deemed unfeasible sites for this floating aquatecture, either due to local topographic limitations, excessive construction costs, the lack of local and federal political will, or because it may otherwise prove unfeasible to construct certain types of complex structures (such as a hospital) on stationary piers above the high-water line while being able to ensure their continuous operation during major emergency events. Instead, a hybrid equation will emerge, composed of a mix of water-borne and interconnected land-based communities, encompassing key civic and emergency-response building types. Effective design strategies will include the widespread use of off-site–built modular health care facilities, including those with rapid redeployment capabilities. As sea levels rise worldwide, a given clinic or hospital will be able to be anticipatorily disassembled and transported; perhaps relocated in its entirety; or, at a minimum, become a prosthetic "architectural appendage" at an entirely new site on higher, safer ground nearby—or, if water-based, perhaps to a lagoon or harbor more resiliently shielded from direct storm surges and sea level rises.

Theme 8

Contagious diseases will continue to occur in the meta-healthscape. The COVID-19 pandemic alerted the world to the perils of zoonotic pandemics. Anticipatory, redeployable rapid-response architecture and associated prosthetic design interventions mitigate the adverse impacts of public health and environmental emergencies.

The functional deconstruction of hospitals will continue, as it has in recent years, with multiple decentralized "spokes" radiating outward from centralized motherships. These architecturally autonomous building types will include specialized and increasingly self-sufficient outpatient health centers and microhospitals, with the latter in many places housing a smaller compliment of inpatient beds (50–100) compared with today's typical community hospitals containing 300 to 500+ beds. These networks will emphasize the provision of preventative care, coordinating the transference of health data within and between various regional health care networks as the planet continues to experience Black Swan events. In 2005, James Howard Kunstler, in his insightful yet unsettling book, *The Long Emergency*, predicted multiple types of adverse events likely to occur in the coming years, including the coronavirus and other pandemics.[33] Adverse health events, such as COVID-19 and the recent Ebola outbreak in West Africa, demonstrated how forced lockdowns helped stem the tide of local community contagion. In the case of Ebola, the populations of many villages became so fearful of their local hospital that they did all they could to avoid any contact whatsoever with it. These "infected hospitals" subsequently were literally abandoned because they themselves had become virulent disease transmitters.

As for COVID-19, 645 million cases and 6.64 million deaths have occurred, at this writing. Early on, governmental ministries of health partnered with many urban medical centers (including in Israel, Italy, and New

York City), springing into rapid-response mode. The Chaim Sheba Medical Center at Tel HaShomer, in the greater Tel Aviv area, expediently set up an underground, forty-five-bed COVID-19 ICU surge hospital unit in its parking garage in just 72 hours. In Spain, two expansive halls of Barcelona's Olympic Vall d'Hebrón municipal sports center were repurposed into a temporary 132-bed surge hospital (see chapter 3). Since the 1960s, an organization called Public Interest Architecture has sought to eradicate the unmet shelter and health care needs of the poor and the marginalized globally. Unfortunately, during the COVID-19 pandemic, relatively few architects and firms globally were pre-positioned to step up quickly and offer their services in assisting the public health sector. This did not occur to any widespread, direct, consistently impactful degree anywhere (see chapter 3). This widespread general lack of emergency preparedness on the part of architects was not surprising, however. Advocates for helping disease and disaster victims in need had been arguing since at least 9/11 to rally this profession and discipline to no longer remain on the sidelines in times of emergency, in light of the urgent need for rapid-response capabilities and impactful short- and longer-term architectural design solutions. With capitalism being what it is, most architects and firms still find it most assuring to provide their services to wealthy individuals, corporations, and other prominent institutions. These clients, who may represent polluting industries (e.g., hospital systems), can afford to pay full professional fees and receive in exchange highly tailored professional services.

Fact: professional architects/firms design only 2–5 percent of all the buildings constructed annually in North America. Meanwhile, the United Nations expects that by 2050, the number of medically underserved persons worldwide will reach 2 billion in a world with 9.7 billion inhabitants.[34] Moreover, populations will dramatically increase in Asia and Africa. In a world experiencing such massive demographic shifts, combined with sudden dislocations caused by the climate crisis, advocacy-based architecture for health care is urgently needed. The coronavirus pandemic alone clearly demonstrated how *architecture for health* will need to partner with public health and the medical professions in mitigating, for example, a recurring cholera outbreak stemming from a sanitation crisis in the slums and shantytowns of an overcrowded city in the developing world. Unless architects and allied designers with foresight become far more creatively proactive, the engineering professions, alongside massive multinational corporations who predatorily are awarded no-bid contracts from governments whenever a disaster strikes, will continue to dominate this burgeoning field of "disaster capitalism." Meanwhile, architects/firms who remain immobilized in this regard will continue to be relegated to the sidelines and continue to be labeled by the engineering community and other first-responder professionals as impractical artists/dreamers.

Off-site–built modular buildings for health care will be more commonplace in the future (see chapter 3). They will coalesce, achieving aesthetic and functional sophistication on a level rather comparable to the types of prosthetic devices worn by humans/transhumans. This prosthetic architecture is to become highly advanced, constructed in nearly fully automated factories. It will be made of sophisticated eco-friendly materials, with modular components and subassemblies produced by means of highly efficient, repetitive manufacturing processes. These components and larger modular assemblies will be highly adaptable, malleable, and resilient in the face of rapid change and, as warranted, of blunt force impacts to their structural integrity. These buildings and their componentry will be capable of returning resiliently to an approximate yet acceptable previous functional state of equilibrium, as predetermined beforehand. And, as is possible with a human-worn prosthetic device, these redeployable structures will be designed to maintain their functional integrity should one major component, module, or wing (e.g., a limb or an inhabitable system module) go down or offline even temporarily for a few hours. Finally, next-generation prosthetic architecture for health will be outfitted with sophisticated on-board intelligence capabilities, allowing these new building types to adroitly maintain their baseline operations (intelligence quotient) in highly diverse topographic, climatic, cultural, and political contexts.

For these reasons, compassionate, aesthetically appealing, and salutogenic off-site–built prefabricated building types for health will be deployed in response to more and more public health and humanitarian emergencies.[35] Why? Rapid responsiveness, more than ever, requires a profound commitment to the timeless Vitruvian precepts of commodity, firmness, and *delight*. This is why aesthetically high quality, salutogenic design must not be overshadowed or somehow relegated to a secondary priority. Similarly, this architectural paradigm for health care will reflect technical and caregiving advancements in the relationship between architecture, medicine, and public health. The first two Vitruvian precepts (commodity and firmness), when considered alone, will be insufficient architecturally. But when inventively incorporated with the promise of interprofessional collaboration in the Anthropocene, much can be achieved in compassionately addressing health inequities.

LIVING ON A HOTTER PLANET

In Greek mythology, heat was controlled by Ankhiale, the goddess of warmth. Throughout the centuries, heat, as an energy source, has been culturally defined and redefined—although we have never lived on a planet this hot. Scientists have concluded heat waves around the world are becoming hotter, more frequent, and longer lasting. The 2018 *National Climate Assessment*, a scientific report authored by thirteen US federal agencies, noted that the frequency of heat waves in the US jumped to six per year by the 2010s, from an average of only two per year in the 1960s.[36] This situation is growing far worse in urban centers, and 2023 was the hottest year, globally, in more than 120,00 years. As Jeff Goodell states in writing about this urban heat island effect:

> On a scorching day in downtown Phoenix, when the temperature soars to 115 degrees or higher, heat becomes a lethal force. Sunshine assaults you, forcing you to seek cover. The air feels solid, a hazy, ozone-soaked curtain of heat. You feel it radiating from the parking lot through your shoes. Metal bus stops become convection ovens; flights may be delayed at Sky Harbor International Airport because the planes can't get enough lift in the thin, hot air. At City Hall, where the entrance to the building is emblazoned with a giant metallic emblem of the sun, workers eat lunch in the lobby rather than trek through the heat to nearby restaurants. On the outskirts of the city, power lines sag and buzz, overloaded with electrons as the demand for air conditioning soars and the entire grid is pushed to the limit. . . . As the mercury rises, people die. As the climate warms, heat waves are growing longer, hotter, and more frequent. Since the 1960s the average number of annual heat waves in 50 major U.S. cities has tripled. . . . Ice sheets are melting, seas are rising, hurricanes are more intense, rainfall patterns are changing, but extreme heat is much more likely to kill you directly if you're poor, sick, old, or homeless. It doesn't have to be this way.[37]

Since the earliest projections (dating from the early 1970s and even earlier) of global climate change, the scientific community has been remarkably prescient in predicting the rate of global temperature and sea level rises. For decades, climate change worsened in accord with these scientific projections.[38] The World Health Organization predicts that heat stress linked to the climate crisis will cause 38,000 extra deaths a year worldwide between 2030 and 2050.[39] As the earth's temperature gradient flattens, Rossby waves tend to bend, so the jet stream is more likely to get stuck in place and, in the process, trap weather systems inside massive heat domes. In the summers of 2021 and 2023, intense heat waves gripped the western US and British Columbia in Canada, where hundreds of heat records were broken and nighttime "lows" (still high temperatures) shattered all-time records.[40]

Every day now, it seems like a natural or human-made disaster strikes somewhere, with the repercussions having an impact far beyond the immediate strike zone. What is most important is how we anticipate and prepare for them. Of course, we are powerless to prevent certain adverse environmental events, including earthquakes and volcanic eruptions. But even the risk from major earthquakes can be mitigated through adoption of more-progressive seismic building codes. The inhabitants of a city located on the banks of a flood-prone river cannot prevent the rains, but they can better prepare for them. Similarly, we can better protect communities against the threat of massive wildfires (such as what happened on Maui in Hawaii in 2023) through better early warning systems, improved building codes mandating fire-resistant building materials, policies requiring flammable underbrush to be cleared from nearby structures, and sufficient funding sources to ensure local top-notch and adequately staffed fire departments. Finland offers an instructive model in many ways of best practices in emergency preparedness.[41] After its harsh experiences during World War II, the national government immediately established an interdisciplinary panel of experts that has met monthly since 1946. Its task remains to consistently maintain a sense of civic urgency, or what might be referred to as "constructive paranoia," in its response to hypothetical disaster event scenarios, as well as in methods to mitigate an adverse event when governmental agency response may go awry. Unsurprisingly, Finland remains unusually well prepared for adverse disaster events, as was proven once again recently in the COVID-19 pandemic.

THE NEED TO SWITCH OUR EPISTEME

In the Anthropocene, this may be the most important challenge we face as a species, because the future is here. We need to be aware of our delimiting, historically anthropocentric biases in the way we see and perceive the world around us and in how we talk to our children, our parents, our families, and our friends. We must explain to them and others why we need to adopt a post-anthropocentric worldview.[42] It will be hard—as is anything important and worthwhile in life. At the macro scale, developing countries will face soaring debt payments to their wealthy-country moneylenders. If little is done to reduce this massive rate of indebtedness, the world's poorest governments will continue to spend grossly disproportionate amounts of their federal budgets annually on these repayments. The biggest potential losers in this unfolding economic and political scenario will be the citizens of the developing world, who will continue to be denied basic public services because their government remains saddled with unsustainable fiscal debt. These fiscal resources would otherwise be diverted by governments in developing nations for earmarked investments in their schools, hospitals, clinics, and other civic, urban, and public health infrastructures. With increasingly disappearing available physical land resources for development/redevelopment in many cities, and the majority of the world's population already living in these overcrowded urban enclaves, there is exceedingly little margin for error in the future. The climate crisis cannot be allowed to deteriorate into a downwardly spiraling competition for increasingly dissipating resources—with the survivors unwittingly becoming the unlucky ones.

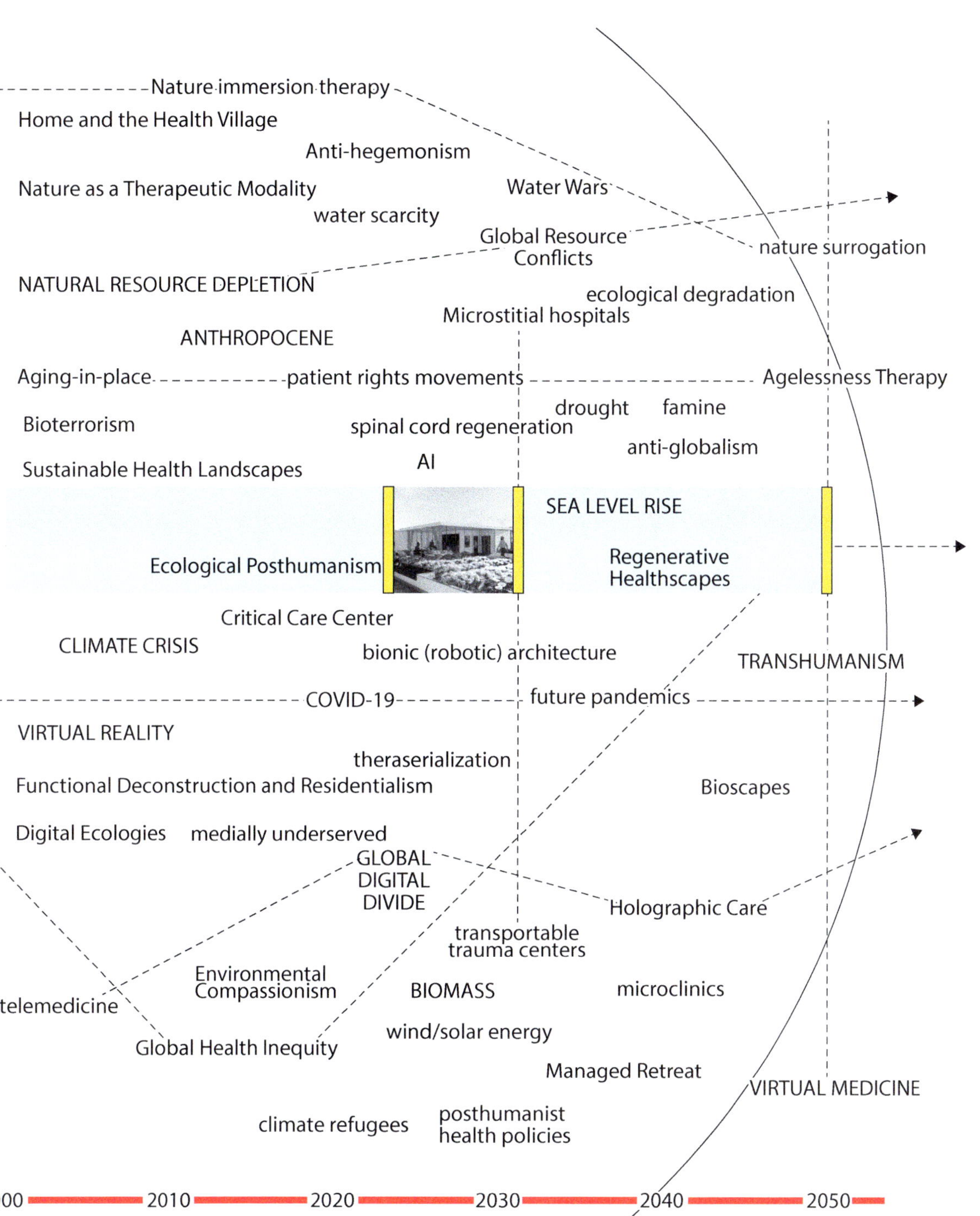

Figure 7.2. Architecture and health equity in an imperiled world, 2050 (epoch 6). Photo by Stephen Verderber.

Design Considerations for a Nature Immersion Center

MISSION STATEMENT

In chapter 4 of this book, the concept of a nature immersion center (NIC) is presented and argued for as a new type within the typology of health care architecture. The NIC is visualized as a calm, welcoming, therapeutically designed built environment for persons experiencing symptoms of nature deficit disorder (NDD), seasonal affective disorder (SAD), individuals suffering from chronic health inequities, and populations who live/work in medically underserved communities where direct engagement with the therapeutic benefits of nature and landscape (N-L) are minuscule, in decline, or entirely absent. A host of physically restorative activities and treatments are prescribed—particularly geared for adolescents and adult cohorts—in helping individuals/populations endeavoring to cope with sustained personal disengagement from N-L, subsequent nature-related sensory deprivation symptoms, and the broader general adverse psychological impacts of ecological denaturization. These places for clinical treatment of these conditions are visualized therein as providing a menu of pertinent therapies, chosen in consultation with professional assessment and guidance (as such, this aspect of the NIC is beyond the scope of this discussion). For instance, nature-related sensory deprivation is becoming more widely viewed by medical specialists as symptomatic of psychological disconnection from long-time lifestyle preferences and physical places of long-held importance. The focus of NIC activities and treatments would be to clinically attend to these symptoms, as facilitated by a host of prescribed N-L immersion activities and therapies. The goal is to renew the human spirit, help restore the patient's personal autonomy and self determination, instill coping strategies to enable one to independently seek out N-L immersion exposure in the everyday milieu, and pre-position oneself to maximize overall self-empowerment.

This behavioral health treatment would eschew overt pharmacological interventions. Rather, the overarching aim is to provide individually attuned dosages of real and representational simulations of N-L immersion. Activities and prescribed associated therapies might include meditative therapy, individual and group counseling, N-L immersion workshops, field trips, art and music therapy, virtual reality simulation, hydrotherapy/heliotherapy, and horticultural therapy. These clinical settings are visualized to function as a distinct breakaway—total physical separation—from the sources of environmental stress commonly associated with NDD, SAD, and related sensory deprivation behavioral health disorders. They are visualized as safe places—bold, confident, hopeful, supportive, upbeat—not unlike those qualities intrinsic to Maggie's Centres (chapter 4).

A Maggie's Centre is an entirely nonclinical alternative to a hospital. It is not a medical "clinic" at all, because no physicians, nursing staff, and related clinical staff are based on-site and, therefore, no clinical treatment is provided. The NIC, in contrast, is visualized as a medical/behavioral health clinic, whether an inpatient facility, an outpatient facility, or both. Similar to a Maggie's Centre, this vision of the NIC rejects the institutionalism, impersonality, and architectural complexity of mainstream hospitals and mental health and substance abuse rehabilitation facilities, places where the patient too often feels little more than a small cog in an immense technocratic "machine for healing." This is a critical distinction. The following fifteen design considerations are an initial attempt to capture the essence of this new building type as a proposal to address a main challenge to our survival as we confront our species' future in the Anthropocene.

1. ENVIRONMENTAL CONTEXT

1a. Community Context

As a child, Andrea Martinelli (now age 62) was able to experience nature by walking in the wooded area near her family's home. Raised in a midsized town in southwestern Ontario, she was never far from nature—whether a creek, wooded area or one of the nearby hills overlooking broad vistas of surrounding farms. After living in a large Canadian city for three decades, something seemed to be lacking in her life. It was becoming more and more difficult to access nature in the ways she did in her earlier life, a separateness exacerbated by rampant overdevelopment of the few remaining unbuilt land parcels near where she lived, a sensory deprivation condition worsened by seemingly random suburban sprawl. Developers were now targeting her residential neighborhood for highrise condo towers under the guise of transit-oriented development. Meanwhile, it had become necessary to drive two hours and more from her urbanizing neighborhood in order to reencounter nature.

In order to support persons who live in urban neighborhoods lacking N-L immersion opportunities, locate the NIC near public transit systems, so one need not drive an excessive distance or through artery-clogged, stress-inducing traffic in order to reach a destination where N-L immersion is attainable—a large park with hiking trails, perhaps a creek, a ravine, a mountainous area, and the like. Recent evidence-based N-L research underscores the importance of being pre-positioned to sustainably access mass transit and thereby avoid undue traffic congestion in one's everyday routine, as this can contribute to fewer diagnosed mental health disorders among urban dwellers. This was a key finding of a recently conducted survey in eleven cities in Latin America.[1] This survey was conducted with over 5,000 residents in Latin America.

Long daily commutes were linked with an increase in clinically diagnosed depressive symptoms. For example, mass transit users, unlike drivers, were 4.8 percent less likely to screen positively for clinical depression. Among respondents, not having a transit stop within a ten-minute walk from one's home was found to have a similarly adverse impact on individuals' mental health. The mounting evidence supports the view that medically underserved populations will likely benefit, due to nature deficiencies and various health inequities they experience on a daily basis in their communities, such as a lack of urban tree canopies, heat island effects, and few or no parks or residential neighborhood green spaces. This pattern is exacerbated, and decidedly more pronounced, among urban populations who have resided for generations in undernatured communities and neighborhoods, such as is the case in low-lying parts of New Orleans in the US. (see chapter 4). These places are subject to poor or nonexistent tree canopies, few green spaces, and a paucity of immersive N-L experiences with the recreational affordances of water. Not surprisingly, urban populations such as these tend to already be medically underserved and therefore particularly vulnerable to the symptoms of NDD and related sensory deprivation disorders (fig. A1).

1b. Campus Context

The strategy to build each of the 26 Maggie's Centres near or directly on the periphery of the campus of an affiliated hospital/medical center has been a general success. This proxemic relationship with a nearby hospital's diagnostic and treatment services has proven successful. The patient has access nearby to a nonmedicalized (no fee) respite from hospital-based conventional medical treatments. In addition, it functions as a recuperative waystation between hospital and home both during and after one has completed treatment. As such, the local Maggie's is typically viewed as conveniently located in an already known place in the community. In the

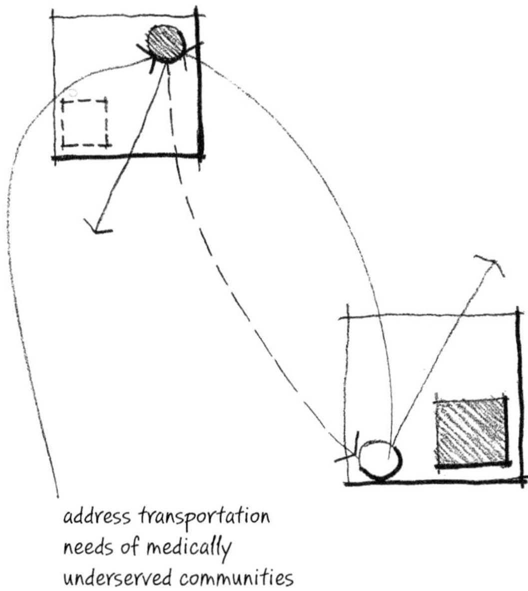

Figure A1. Community context. Drawing by Stephen Verderber.

NIC (as visualized), patients are diagnosed and treated for anxiety disorder, depression, or related NDD and sensory deprivation symptoms. These diagnoses will provide the foundation for the types of treatment offered. It is anticipated the majority of patients will likely be referrals from a local or regional community hospital or psychiatric facility. Some patients may return to the referring community hospital, psychiatric hospital, or mental health/substance abuse rehabilitation facility for follow-up care, perhaps while simultaneously attending the NIC. The referral of individuals from these 24/7 facilities to the NIC can occur more fluidly, due to its geographic closeness.

Ideally, the NIC (as visualized) is constructed on an open site, vegetated with trees and with some degree of informationally rich views of nature and landscape. Is it counterproductive to locate the NIC in a dense urban setting? Not necessarily. But such sites should offer the potential to be *reclaimed* (especially if currently an underutilized, bleak asphalt parking lot or the like), proactively renaturizing them by planting trees and restorative plant species. This offers opportunities to re-create green spaces and provide prospect-refuge–behavior N-L experiences for the patient on-site. The provision of one or more green terraces, at grade level or as upper level terraces, can be effective if insufficient open space exists at ground level due, to site restrictions. Similarly, providing a screened, out-of-sight place to park a vehicle can be problematic. In situations where a parking lot is a necessity, minimize its visual impact and seek innovative strategies to screen vehicles parked on-site from direct view from the NIC. In visually and auditorily shielding an adjacent parking area or other unsightly view, incorporate earthen berms, trees, and various plant species; accept topographically irregular sites; and employ inventive landscape design strategies, as this will simultaneously renaturize the site. These measures will help transform a former liability into an aesthetically desirable *place*. Accordingly, it is counterproductive to select a site too restrictive in size or excessively urban, as this makes it all that much more challenging, if not impossible, to create a therapeutic exterior environment (fig. A2).[2]

1c. Equitable Community Engagement

Hospitals, psychiatric treatment centers, and substance abuse rehabilitation programs are potential sources of patient referrals for the NIC, although not exclusively. Perhaps medical referrals would not always be a prerequisite condition for admission. Either way, the NIC's menu of nature-immersive therapies would be developed to diagnose and treat symptoms of NDD and related sensory deprivation, including SAD. The community where the patient lives provides a primary backdrop, impacting the specific types of treatment regimens prescribed. In addition, this backdrop would influence the types of activities prescribed, not unlike patient-dreamers receiving treatment at the ancient Greek Asklepion (chapter 2). In this regard, connections between the patient's everyday life and the amenities at the NIC, including its garden, the greenhouse, and winter garden, would all play a therapeutic role. The local community would, ideally, be proud of and support its local NIC, such as what occurs at Maggie's Centres. It is anticipated the design, construction, and operation of the NIC facility and its grounds would be funded through a private nonprofit organization or a public/private partnership. As in the case of Maggie's Centres, private local fundraising, in collaboration with philanthropic foundation support, is recommended. The local affiliated health care referral institution may elect to help coordinate the fundraising campaign because of its prior experience in such endeavors. This assistance may include donating the land for construction and supplying hospital foundation staff to aid in fundraising. Community engagement amenities might include a playroom and adjacent outdoor play space for toddlers and children. In building community support for the NIC, fundraising guidelines and corresponding downloads should be developed at the outset of the planning process. This can include donor/

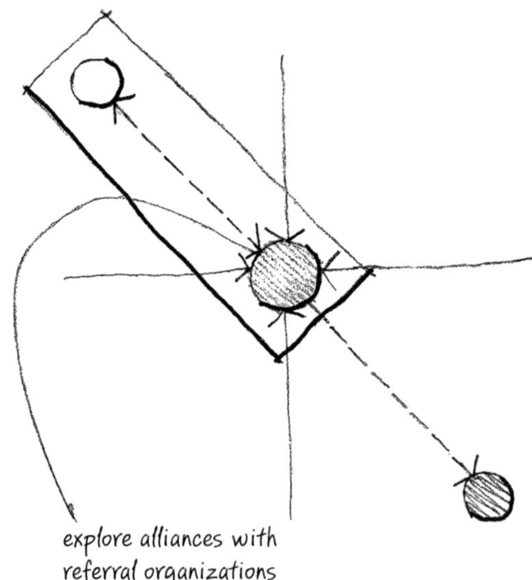

Figure A2. Campus context. Drawing by Stephen Verderber.

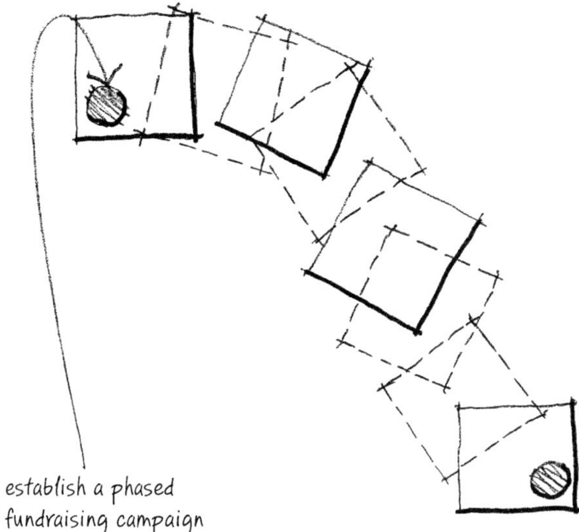

Figure A3. Equitable community engagement. Drawing by Stephen Verderber.

sponsor profiles, press release templates, fundraising poster templates, a description of the proposed governing structure of the NIC, the profile of the center's initial advisory board, and a donor/sponsor contribution form. This information should be systematically archived and updated. It is of the utmost priority to formulate the vision for the NIC, as careful formulation *a priori* will help tremendously in attracting broad interest from potential donors. Everything begins with the mission statement, supplemented in the early stage of fundraising with, perhaps, renderings and a scale model of the proposed center (fig. A3).[3]

2. ARRIVAL AND IMAGE

2a. Serialized Arrival

The architectural and landscape design vision for the NIC is anti-institutional, insofar as an individual's first encounter should not be a parking structure or the affiliated hospital and medical center complex. Avoid at any cost the dehumanizing experience of being forced to walk through a dark parking garage or across a vast asphalt expanse, weaving through row after row of vehicles to eventually reach the front door of the NIC. Carefully, compassionately designed, human-scaled serialized arrival paths direct the individual to the front door and interior of Maggie's Centres. Similarly, establish serialized spatial experiences—multiple inventively designed nodes and pockets along a path. These elements draw one toward the front door, with the building itself set in repose on the site and effectively set back from busy nearby streets and other urban distractions. A landscaped front courtyard or path can function as a transitional device in this regard. Serialization of the arrival sequence can establish a multisensorial atmosphere, helping the individual break away and mentally shift from the everyday milieu. Along the arrival sequence, provide opportunities to sit and rest, if one so chooses, while establishing lines of sight to vistas near and afar. Reinforce a perception where one has arrived at a very *different* place—welcoming, unique, quite in opposition to the highly rigorous, technocratic ambiance of the nearby affiliated hospital or psychiatric treatment center. In creating an attractive, welcoming N-L experience for an arriving patient, the path functions as a portal to a retreat beyond, quite apart. This can be further achieved by inventively incorporating level changes or a footbridge, allowing one to view undisturbed nature below and to either side of the NIC while remaining on this serialized arrival path. Inventive landscape design strategies can render this serialized arrival path as quasi-residential in scale and feeling, not fully viewable from any single vantage point.

Numerous Maggie's Centres employ this design strategy to establish and accentuate the sense of having experienced a visual and psychological break from the surrounding everyday milieu (see chapter 4). The Maggie's Centre in Nottingham, UK, looks like a treehouse, with this type of meandering path leading to the front door and its parking area obscured from direct view (fig. A4).[4]

2b. Appropriate Imagery

A prudent architectural and site-planning strategy is to establish an inviting, *residentialist* image. Place priority on the spaces immediately viewable upon entering the front door of the center. The front door opens onto the reception/arrival area and a sign-in/admissions desk or adjacent workspace alcove. A main waiting room is in close proximity, and one or more subwaiting rooms are located down a natural daylit corridor within the clinic area and its exam/consult rooms. An adjacent kitchen and informal countertop area is provided in the center of the building, with seating for up to twelve with barstool-height chairs and tables for additional seating, all located in proximity to the main reception area. The center's resource library should

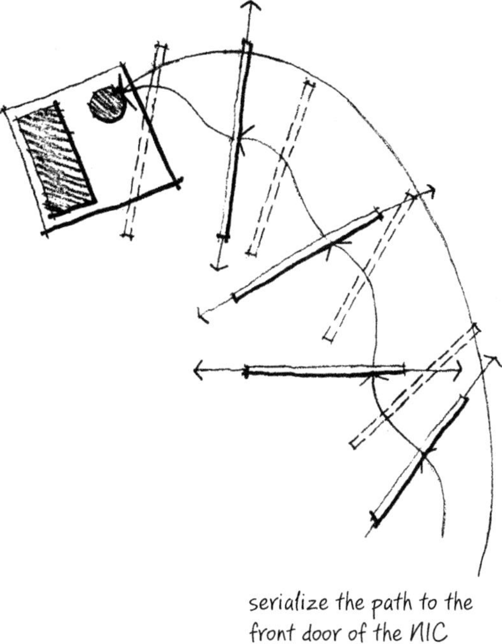

Figure A4. Serialized arrival. Drawing by Stephen Verderber.

be close to the reception/arrival area, not unlike the network of twenty-six
Maggie's Centres. The reception area and these associated spaces should
be inventively configured to collectively convey the message, "We're glad
you're here." The main waiting area should be welcoming and comforting,
not at all like most hospitals. Perhaps include a fireplace and surrounding
seating in close proximity. Include a full-service kitchen with a pantry. Provide full views of the outdoors and invite natural daylight into interior spaces.
Daylighting is a high priority: a blend of natural and artificial task-ambient
natural light types. Establishing a residentialist aesthetic is highly important
and should be inventively reinforced throughout. This is the NIC's defining
architectural quality and defines its non-institutionality—part art gallery, part
neighborhood branch library, part large contemporary residence—basically
anything other than a banal, all-white-walled health care clinic dominated
by windowless rooms and drab corridors with little to no direct N-L multisensory engagement.. The staff and the patient should feel comfortable
here. Color palettes, physical scale, variable ceiling heights, room shapes,
and materiality (materials of construction) are important. Wherever feasible,
draw on local indigenous vernacular building traditions. Balance natural
tones and accent colors with adjoining shadowed and partially shadowed

wall surfaces, with varied flooring types, wall textures, and interior finish materials. Color-code surfaces to enhance occupants' "readings" of the NIC's physical setting and immediate site environs, without relying on intrusive directional signage. The center's immediate site environs should foster an informal, inviting atmosphere, functioning as theraserialized extensions of the interior: for example, the building-as-vegetated-planter metaphor of the Maggie's Centre in Leeds, the treehouse metaphor of the Nottingham Maggie's, and the homelike metaphor of the Maggie's in Oxford and Manchester (all in the UK). Above all, the recommended architectural and landscape design imagery is one of *domesticity* versus institutionality (fig. A5).[5]

2c. Integral Artworks

The origins of contemporary visual art are traceable to early Paleolithic cave art.[6] The installation of works of art in hospitals dates from at least the fourteenth century, a period when virtually all hospitals were operated by religious orders. The dying would be positioned in their beds so they could view paintings, which frequently depicted religious scenes of human salvation versus damnation. At the Hospital de Jesús Nazareno (1456) in Mexico City, numerous large murals were meticulously painted with each

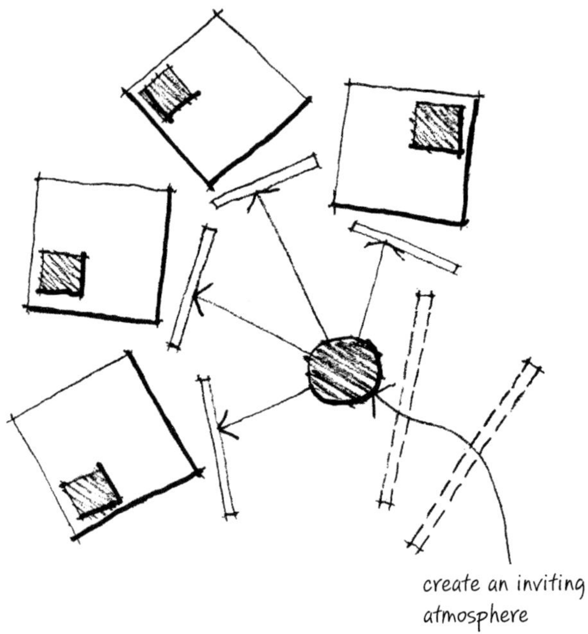

Figure A5. Appropriate imagery. Drawing by Stephen Verderber.

scene portraying the arrival of the European colonialists. These impressive works of art still line walls of this hospital's beautiful cloistered courtyard.

For centuries, patients and caregiver staff have been able to see and sometimes themselves touch various artworks in health care settings—artworks adding to the dignity and aesthetic ambiance of these physical settings, which therapeutically contributed to patients' health status. This was a repetitive theme in the writings of Florence Nightingale (see chapter 2).[7] One viewer of Claude Monet's masterful *Water Lilies* described his personal experience with art: "When viewing the *Water Lilies* series [1897–1899] in my present condition [vision loss from glaucoma] I slip into a sense of completeness. Surface, depth, and reflection converge as past, future, and the present moment become one. And I've realized I've lost nothing. I feel no anxiety or dread. I simply luxuriate in the joy of color and celebrate it. This to me this is the healing power of art." Neuroscientists, working with somatic practitioners, therapists, psychiatrists, educators, and mindfulness instructors, have recently systematically examined the ways in which art is therapeutic, exploring its healing effects on the human psyche. But this is not to imply merely looking at a work of art or making art oneself somehow holds intrinsic curative powers for the patient. Creating an architectural environment where art can be meaningfully experienced is far more than merely something to tick off on a checklist.

Art effectively functions as a positive psychological distraction. For these reasons, an increasing number of hospitals and other types of health care facilities are initiating healing art and art therapy programs, as well as musical performances, and are including art galleries on- site to host installations of local and regional visual artists' work. The NIC is a platform for weaving together architecture, art, and landscape. Throughout the building and its immediate exterior environs, this will a yield positive therapeutic amenity for the patient. Include paintings, sculpture, and interactive art installations as personal immersive activities for individuals of all ages. Specialists in the acquisition and installation of artworks frequently work with the architectural team from the project's design inception. For additional information regarding this key experiential dimension of the NIC, the nonprofit Center for Health Design provides a free resource: its *Guide to Evidence-Based Art.*[8] Nightingale is often cited as a strong advocate for the therapeutic functions of art in hospitals in her pioneering *Notes on Nursing* (1860). Nightingale extolled the importance of exposing patients to the aesthetic value of art, music, and nature, because this not only nourishes the mind, but also the body (fig. A6).

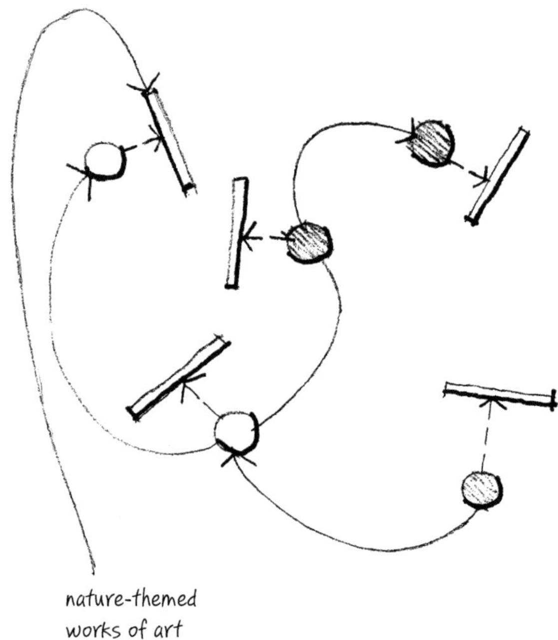

Figure A6. Integral artworks. Drawing by Stephen Verderber.

2d. Compositional Clarity

While a graduate student in architecture and environmental psychology at the University of Michigan, I first acquired appreciation for the concept of *smallness* in the built environment. At the start of the term, Stephen Kaplan, the well-known environmental psychologist (and my doctoral dissertation coadvisor) had us read E. F. Schumacher's *Small is Beautiful*.[9] Schumacher's core thesis expounded on the inability of humans to clearly see the full ramifications of the harmful world we had constructed around us. Overlapping environmental, social, and economic forces, such as the 1973 energy crisis and the popularization of the then relatively new concept of globalization, would later bring this book to a wide general audience in the 1970s and ever since (a second edition was published in 1999). In 1995, the *Times Literary Supplement* ranked *Small is Beautiful* among the 100 most influential books published since 1945. In applying the small is beautiful thesis to human transactions with the built environment, Schumacher advocated for *sustainable development, appropriate technologies*, and the virtues of what he referred to as small-scale *village culture*—all unfamiliar terms at the time—as offering a far more viable future path for society's further advancement in a resource-constrained world. His thesis advanced the virtues of appropriately scaled and, by extension, grassroots-focused public health polices and other best practices in public health, highlighting the *individual* as the core unit within any aggregate population, superior to the ethos of "bigger is always better" and related top-down policymaking philosophies. This flew in the face of the accepted best practice (at the time) of urban and suburban hospitals in North America—being built to house more and more inpatient beds—in what would soon become a singularly misguided facility-expansion arms race. By contract, the NIC holds the promise for appropriately expressing the virtues of smallness, spatial comprehensi-bility, and low-level eco-friendly technologies in treating the symptoms of NDD and related sensory deprivation psychological disorders. Make these places comparatively small in scale (as opposed to what may likely be a gigantic affiliated hospital nearby) and easy to navigate from a wayfinding perspective. Experiment with evidence-based inventive design strategies to enhance occupants' spatial comprehension while underscoring and extending the physical setting's *residentialist* aesthetic and its ambiance throughout. In their scale and inventive informality, the Maggie's Centres succeed in this regard. As for Schumacher, who passed away in 1977 while on a train during a European lecture tour, he likely would have endorsed the Maggie's architectural concept, as well as the NIC concept (fig. A7).

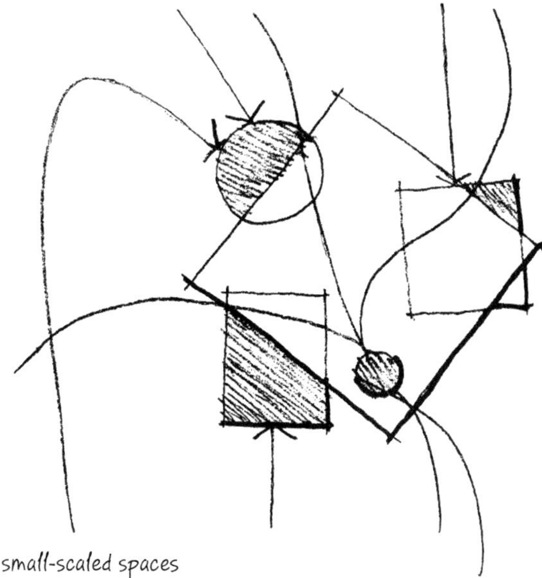

Figure A7. Compositional clarity. Drawing by Stephen Verderber.

3. CLINICAL TREATMENT REALM

3a. Multifunctionality

The counseling and treatment functions in the NIC clinical setting support the diverse aspects of multisensory therapy, including music and art therapy, nature immersion therapy, hydrotherapy and heliotherapy (a hot pool, cold pool, tepidarium, and solarium), and quiet rooms to encourage prospect-refuge therapeutic activities experienced either alone or in small group sessions. These spaces allow the individual patient to take in intrinsically interesting views of nature and other activities within the NIC and its grounds from a safe and protected viewing station. The recommendation is to provide a minimum of six to eight medium-sized rooms in the clinic, with windows that overlook nature or otherwise therapeutically interesting views, in support of counseling and stress-reduction treatment sessions. Nature immersion therapy has proven an effective treatment for stress and related anxiety diagnoses. These therapies may be either passive (actual versus live), active, simulated (surrogate-based) or hybridic (active with live simulation). This multiplicity of exposure and exposure rate modalities are, ideally, adaptable to changing diagnostic and treatment protocols, tailored to each individual patient. Multifunctionality denotes readily modifying a given room's functional purpose, guided by a change-as-a-constant design strategy. For example, the art therapy room is easily convertible into a group counseling room and then a space for an evening yoga class two hours later, all in a single day. General support functions for these spaces and their amenities include male, female, and gender-neutral restrooms, showers, and locker rooms; housekeeping facilities; staff breakroom; lockers for storage of personal items; and a screened outdoor semiprivate patio. Of course, provide a separate service entrance for deliveries and trash removal. As for safety and security considerations, all key exterior and interior spaces should be CCTV monitored, with perimeter screening and security buffers provided (as necessary),while not inadvertently creating an unaesthetic image or hospital-like institutional appearance. Incorporate smart building technologies, activated via on-site security systems to achieve greater spatial flexibility in support of spatial multifunctionality. Devote particular attention to theraserialization: moveable walls and partitions, foldaway sliding doors, indoor-outdoor retractable roofs, transparent lift-up garage doors, and shaded patios and terraces. Skylights, clerestories, varied ceiling configurations, color-accented wall surfaces, multiple lighting options, and natural materials and finishes are recommended. All are beneficial in the creation of flexible, adaptable indoor-outdoor treatment/counseling spaces (fig. A8).[10]

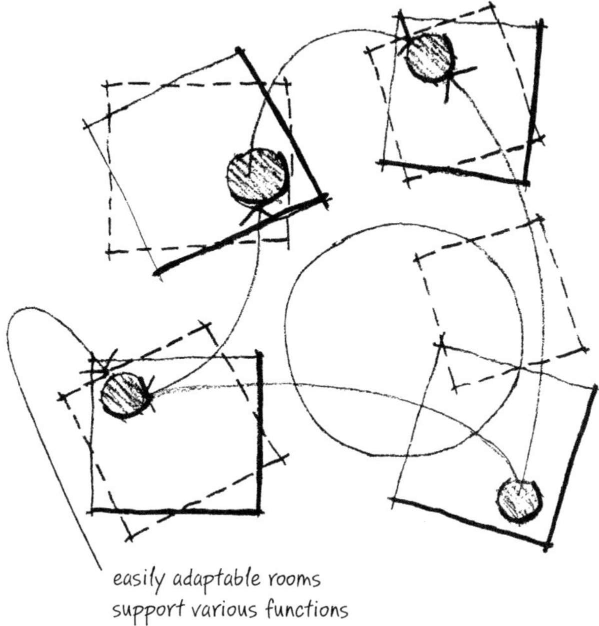

Figure A8. Multifunctionality. Drawing by Stephen Verderber.

3b. Water and Sun-Based Therapy

Hydrotherapy

Hydrotherapy involves the prescriptive use of water (in liquid form, in the form of ice, or steam) for treating varied diseases and illnesses through temperature modulation, pressurization, impact duration, and its applications to localized areas of the body. These naturopathic treatments were used widely in ancient cultures and have since been employed in modern wellness and health care treatments at contemporary mineral spas and natural-spring rural retreats from the late eighteenth century.[11] In designing hydrotherapy pools, adequate door widths, ramps positioned for wheelchair users, and clear informational signage is essential. Locate these pools at grade whenever possible, avoiding the need to construct universal access ramps. In the case of pools with variable depths, their entrance steps should be at the shallowest end. Two main types of pool installations are *deck level* and *semiraised freeboard*, with nearly all pools now built as off-site prefab manufactured assembly kits, transported to the construction site for installation. Contemporary spas/retreats (including the network of day-use-only Nordic Spas in Canada) make extensive use of these indoor and outdoor hydrotherapy pools.

Heliotherapy

In Western recorded history, heliotherapy—the systematic treatment of disease and illness utilizing therapeutic applications of natural sunlight—was first practiced by Hippocrates (generally considered the father of Western medicine). He advocated for practical applications of daylight-as-therapy as a medicinal intervention. Bright-light therapy was also practiced in ancient Chinese, Hindu, and Egyptian societies over the past fifteen centuries. The first modern clinic in the West to use heliotherapy for systematically treating tuberculosis opened in 1903 in Leysin, Switzerland. This method in the treatment of TB continued to be practiced in Europe and throughout the Mediterranean region in subsequent decades.[12] Heliotherapy is currently used to treat skin disorders, as well as symptoms of seasonal affective disorder (SAD). Other treatment applications include as a prescribed outdoor rest activity for patients with neurologic, endocrinologic, and psychiatric disorders, and in indoor sessions using ultraviolet filtered-light therapy technologies.[13]

3c. Prospect-Refuge Affordances

The psychological recharging and restoration of the patient's cognitive equilibrium through nature-immersive prospect-refuge therapies requires a seamless continuum between interior and exterior realms within the NIC. This positive outcome can be further advanced by the visual and sensorial cueing of seasonal change when choreographed with the ebb and flow of N-L immersion. A seat next to a large window allows one to project outward into the exterior realm while still feeling protected—for example, in the glass-enclosed atrium/courtyard at the literal heart the Maggie's Centre in Oldham, UK (see chapter 4). This type of NIC experience potentially helps ameliorate the deleterious aspects of the nature-degraded everyday world beyond. This can simultaneously promote positive social interactions if one so chooses. Provide safe, protected, semitransparent open spaces, ranging from small consulting rooms to large open-plan group activity rooms. Throughout, provide various alcoves and semiprivate *nodes*, places affording respite where one can sit quietly, read, or listen to music. Provide comfortable furnishings and equipment, with adaptable reconfiguration options, coordinated with the material finishes on the walls, floors, and ceilings.[14] Provide viewing stations overlooking N-L courtyards and, in winter, indoor gardens and greenhouses. These amenities can help re-establish N-L prospect-refuge behavioral patterns and can help restore positive cognitive attentional abilities in the patient (see chapter 4). Partially viewable nodes

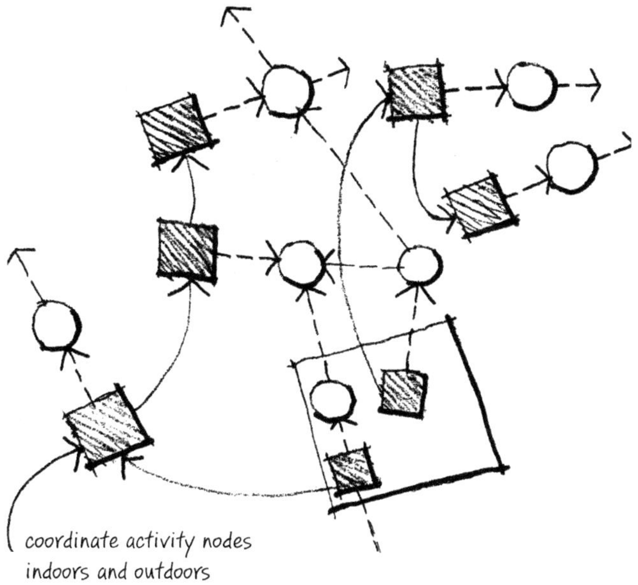

Figure A9. Prospect-refuge affordances. Drawing by Stephen Verderber.

and landmarks along pathways have proven beneficial in promoting the sense of perceptual mystery (prospect), prompting further inquiry if and when pursued further, especially if refuge-respite is rewarded through this type of exploration. A recent evidence-based research investigation examined self-rated attention restoration theory (ART) levels, first by following a group of respondents who walked through an actual outdoor wooded setting.[15] Next, in a controlled laboratory setting, a second (control) group of respondents only viewed a video of this same wooded nature walk. Exposure to the real natural setting, with its "high prospect" and relatively "low refuge," was found to be significantly restorative, by the first group of respondents (fig. A9).

4. BIOPHILIA AND ECOLOGICAL CONNECTIVITY

4a. Equitable Site Reclamation

Landscapes are destroyed everywhere by complex natural ecological processes combined with planned and unplanned adverse human actions. The unforeseen consequences are often catastrophic. One of the most egregious worst practices is the obsessive paving over of greenfield sites worldwide, adversely destroying countless natural ecosystems and bio-species' habitats. And, too often, the damage caused is irreversible. In the Anthropocene, posthumanist-inspired managed growth and site reclamation strategies are essential, in order to attempt to reinstate the ecological vitalization of these ruined habitats, ecosystems, and natural landscapes.[16] This will require removing the human species from its traditional pedestal at the apex of all other species and things and reconceptualizing our flawed species firmly *in* (not above) the ecological fray in its totality, in an attempt to function in synchronicity with nature in its full dimensions. The revitalization of damaged, degraded, abandoned parcels of land, sites previously paved/built over and subsequently suffocating, is a best practice in regenerative environmental design and in enhancing the health of all on an imperiled planet. Posthumanist public health and built-environment policies will help guide the equitable reclamation of these degraded and obliterated sites.

With the human predilection for real immersive contact with nature so deep rooted, the trend in urban waterfront redevelopment in North America and elsewhere over the past thirty years has been no accident. In Wilmington, North Carolina, its extensive boardwalk along the Cape Fear River represents the city's proactive reclamation of former industrial sites for new recreational and nature immersion uses. Rescue these sites, possibly for the construction of the NIC. Reclaim the massive abandoned parking lot of a former K-Mart or an abandoned indoor shopping mall parking lot, places where seagulls once congregated when it was a wetland, and now deserted. Reinstate the ecological *agency* of these and other degraded and lost sites by removing all significant traces of their ecological defacement, then build completely anew, from the dirt up, in ways that are unharmful from a health equity standpoint and without redestroying the best attributes of what was reclaimed (fig. A10).[17]

4b. Compositional Lightness

The progressive design principle of *causing no ecological harm* is gaining acceptance in the interdisciplinary field of posthumanist ethics; it is a precept adapted from the Hippocratic Oath. It involves regaining a site's intrinsic or naturalistic *agency*. This applies to reclaiming a brownfield in a medically underserved community, where a high percentage of the population has experienced chronic health inequities for generations. And it

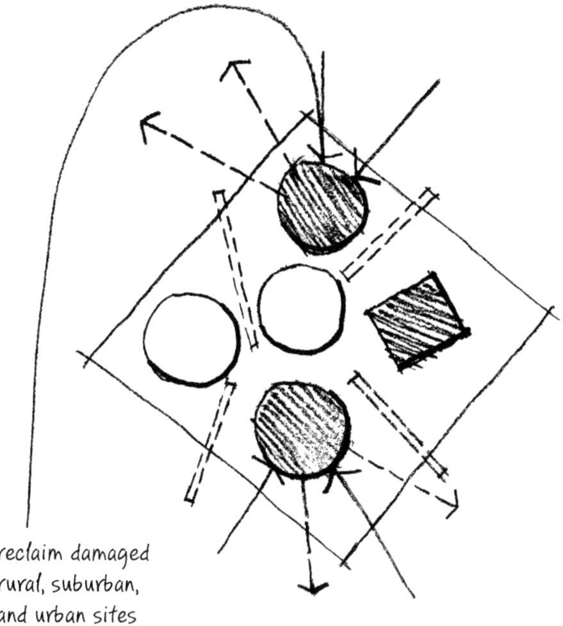

Figure A10. Equitable reclamation of lost sites. Drawing by Stephen Verderber.

equally applies at the other extreme, to a rural site with an unbuilt green-field. On sloping and irregularly shaped sites, urban or otherwise, seam-lessly embed part of the structure *into its site*, if practicable. This notion applies to residential architecture and, in particular, to private residences that cantilever (project outward) above and outward from their sites—such as structures that straddle two higher sides of a site or otherwise are ele-vated on piers or columns above the ground plane. Strive to inventively create the appearance of a building that floats.[18] This architectural strat-egy lifts the structure upward, allowing it to occupy perhaps an otherwise formerly uninhabitable site, perhaps even straddling a stream or creek, or on a hillside slope, drawing the building's inhabitants closer to nature while treading lightly on the reclaimed natural environment and respecting its intrinsic agency. The most daring of the Maggie's Centres built to date occupy previously dismissed or, at the very least, challenging sites, accord-ing to conventional health care facility site-planning best practices. These include Maggie's sites whose agency was reclaimed/restored from formerly paved-over parking lots (Manchester); or by demolishing an obsolete main-tenance building on a hundred-year-old hospital campus (Oldham); or by building on narrow, sloping, otherwise unredeemable land (Oxford). The latter was constructed directly across a main access road from its affiliated mothership institution. These three examples had all previously been rejected for other land uses, considered unsuitable for the construction of a health care facility (see chapter 4).[19]

4c. Virtual and Augmented Reality Therapy

Nature immersion simulation technologies have been demonstrated to be effective in psychiatric and substance abuse treatments. While severe disorders typically require pharmacological intervention, cognitive behavioral therapy is an effective treatment for anxiety and panic disorders, phobias, and obsessive-compulsive disorders. Anxiety disorders alone are estimated to currently afflict more than 40 million people in the US alone, and treatment fiscal expenditures total approximately $42 billion (USD) annually. Virtual reality (VR) technology has been applied in exposure therapy (VRET) and, in military contexts, has shown promise in the treatment of ADHD, depression, and numerous related mental health disorders. In this type of immersion therapy, simulated scenes are displayed on a large flat-screen monitor or experienced with the patient wearing headsets with viewfinders. This technique has proved successful in preparing soldiers for combat missions, in conducting difficult hostage negotiations on the battlefield, and in the treatment of PTSD among veterans returning from the Iraq War. This type of simulation treatment based on VRET does not, as a rule, require pharmaceuticals. Additional therapeutic examples include the use of nonhuman (surrogate) AI-bot "therapists."[20] Commercial providers of this type of software or hardware include CleVR (The Netherlands), Psious (Spain), and Mimerse (Sweden), VirtualRet, and Zen Zone. At the NIC, sound-sculpting software tools that psychologists and therapists use to treat phobias are techniques with potential therapeutic benefits in treating NDD, SAD, and related sensory deprivation diagnoses.[21] Treatments are administered in multisensory nature immersion rooms. These interior spaces support reasonably accurate multisensorial simulation modalities and are capable of "imitating" diverse exposure levels to both built and natural environments (fig. A11).[22]

4d. Horticultural Therapy

Many people who experience episodic or chronic health inequities are subject to anxiety and depression yet refrain from seeking clinical medical

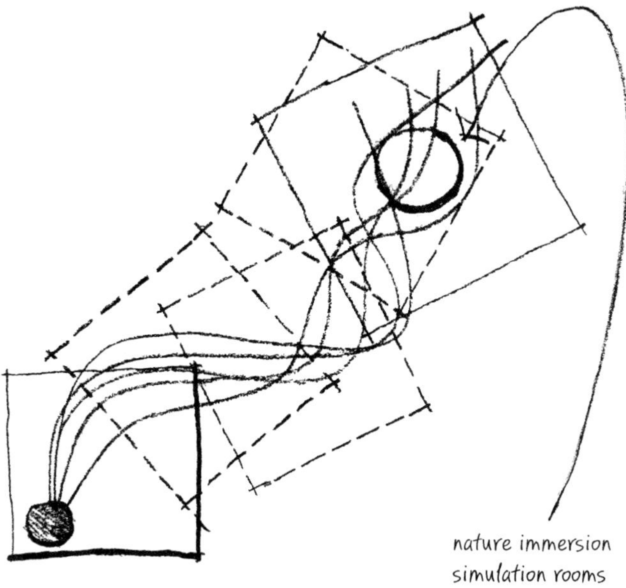

Figure A11. Virtual and augmented reality. Drawing by Stephen Verderber.

treatment. When they do look for professional help, they find that for one reason or another it is unavailable to them in their community. A low-cost alternative—nonpharmacologic horticultural therapy (NHT)—is receiving increased attention from health professionals and also from public health policy specialists. NHT encourages psychologically restorative human/ nature/plant interactions and is cited increasingly in discussion of the therapeutic role of biophilia in the built environment (see chapter 4). It consists of systematically and prescriptively employing plants, gardening, and landscaping in an effort to ameliorate diagnosed symptoms of depression and anxiety. Nature immersion therapies using NHT are potentially of effective use in the NIC to treat these particular mental health disorders in patients from diverse age, gender, cultural, and socioeconomic backgrounds, including the aforementioned populations who suffer from episodic or chronic health inequities. NHT is recommended as a baseline therapy treatment especially for elderly patients in both clinical and nonclinical settings.[23] And with respect to younger cohorts, in a recent study in Denmark with returning combat veterans, NHT activities, such as tree planting and the scheduled watering of plants, increased respondents' capacity for and interest in a heightened level of self-achievement while concomitantly reducing symptoms of PTSD.[24] One year after stage one of this laboratory investigation, the majority of the study's cohort were found to continue to be actively engaged in self-guided outdoor nature immersion activities, with NHT cited specifically as having improved their memory and thought processes by stimulating a desire for outdoor physical exercise and nature appreciation (fig. A12).

4e. Net-Zero Strategies / Stewardship

As is well known, the wealthiest countries in the world are its worst and most chronic polluters, while the poorest countries tend to always suffer the most adverse consequences. Not coincidentally, the poorest countries account for the largest percentage of persons who suffer from chronic health inequities. Thus any call for a new health care building type (such as the NIC) places the burden on those who advocate for it to be committed environmental stewards, especially in the case of countries with a high percentage of medically underserved populations. Tellingly, at COP28 in 2023, the world's petrostates fought fiercely against a resolution from 130 other nations for a definitive full-scale fossil fuel phase-out deadline. The world's petrostates continue to engage instead in a colossal fossil fuel *phase up*, assiduously working to double the rate at which they extract highly toxic substances from the earth.

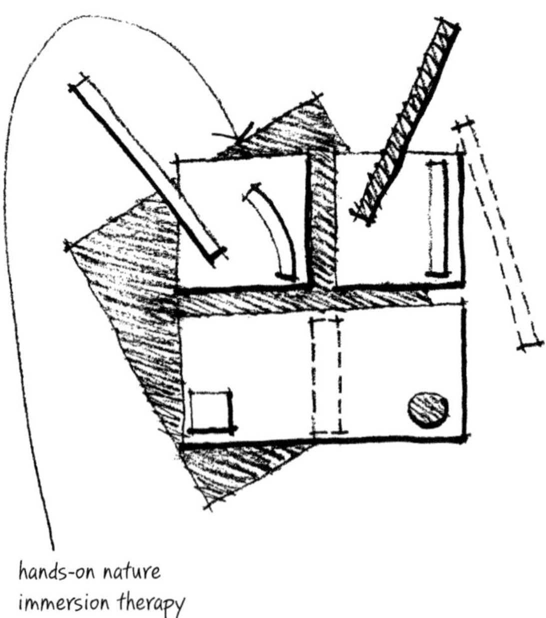

Figure A12. Horticultural therapy. Drawing by Stephen Verderber.

This is the root of the climate crisis: carbon emissions must plunge rapidly if we are to avoid complete climate breakdown, with catastrophic results. Meanwhile, the global fossil fuel industry continues to pour hundreds of billions into extracting more and more oil, gas, and coal, in a bet the world's nations will continue to be unsuccessful in their efforts to self-regulate carbon emissions.

Big Oil and natural gas cartels' trillion-dollar addiction to their profits trumps any real interest in transitioning their investments toward renewable energy sources. This is happening while their investor conglomerations largely remain silent, on the sidelines. But as Damian Carrington states, "This fight is existential for both the industry and the rest of civilization, although only one side can prosper in the long run. If this global mega-industry will not reform itself how will society end its hegemony?"[25] This is a question every public health, medical, and built-environment specialist must confront in the Anthropocene. As the adage goes, "Think global, act local." The NIC, as a building type, has the potential to symbolize a viable alternative in climate-responsive health care architecture (fig. A13).

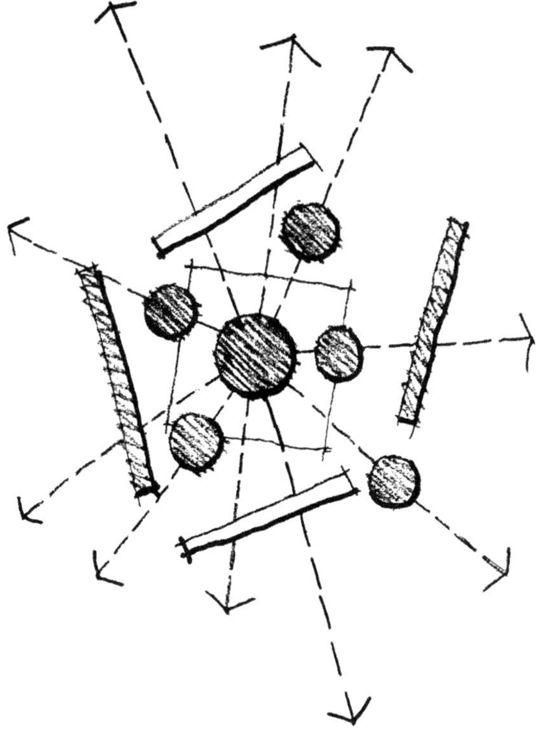

Figure A13. Net-zero strategies / stewardship. Drawing by Stephen Verderber.

Design Considerations for Equitable Eldercare Housing

Evidence-based environment and aging research has evolved significantly over the past fifty years, with this topic now recognized as a distinct subdiscipline. The evidence-based literature is multifaceted regarding the unique types of support older persons require to age successfully. And the case for according this research attention became even more urgent in the coronavirus pandemic, revealed in a recent comprehensive review of evidence-based environment and aging research conducted by a university-based team directed by this author. The period reviewed was from January 2005 to the end of 2022, examining the broad range of eldercare residential built environments, the caregivers who work in these settings, and the families of residents, focusing on semi-independent living options and 24/7 residential care settings.[1] It addressed two basic questions. First, what trends are discernable among older persons who reside in semi-independent noninstitutional residential settings, as well as individuals residing in 24/7 long-term care custodial institutions? Second, how, and to what extent did COVID-19 impact these residential settings and what are the implications for the future?[2]

An eight-part typology of this literature was identified. Fifty design considerations were distilled and are presented below for subsequent action, in the hope this compendium of design considerations will impact what actually gets built. These fifty considerations are presented here *both* for interpretation and application by public health specialists, medical professionals, architects who specialize in environment and aging, landscape architects, interior designers, planners, engineers, administrators, boards of directors, governmental agencies at all levels, private philanthropic foundations, and by grassroots eldercare advocacy organizations.

In light of current global aging demographic trends, action-based *timeliness* must be of priority. Demographic factors, together with the climate crisis, are intensifying the pressure to design and build more resiliently and intelligently for older persons than ever—and to design and build for this demographic cohort *faster*. In light of this urgency, each design consideration is essentially a *hypothesis* intended for further field testing, refinement, and amendment in the field. An underlying intent is for this compendium to enter the mainstream of public policy and professional practice discourses and become a part of ever evolving best practices in LTC facility renovations, additions, adaptive uses of existing eldercare architecture, and new construction. Each is written in cognizance of the ever-changing nature of local- and national-standard building codes and minimum standards regarding what gets built—or doesn't get built—and its architectural and landscape design quality. Regardless, the status quo in environment and aging built environments needs to be revamped. Many obsolete building codes and outdated assumptions are challenged in this compendium.

The compendium highlights emerging special off-site–built modular prefabricated design and construction. Modularity is a viable alternative to what are, by comparison, far more lengthy, redundant, finite resource–consumptive, and costly accepted design and construction practices. The compendium is structured as eight thematic categories, all of which directly or indirectly highlight the virtues of off-site–built modular prefabrication in design, construction, and administrative operations. The aim is to further propel forward design excellence in architecture for eldercare in 24/7 institutionally based care settings. These eight themes are listed below (and collectively illustrated in fig. B1):

1. site context and spatial organization,
2. private realm,
3. shared realms,
4. biophilia and nature connectivity,
5. circulation and navigation,
6. support amenities,
7. sensory and environmental supports, and
8. prefabricated housing for long-term care.

Note to readers: *At the end of each design consideration, related topics are listed and indicated in* **bold** *type. The intent is to aid the reader in seeking to cross-reference other individual design considerations within the compendium.*

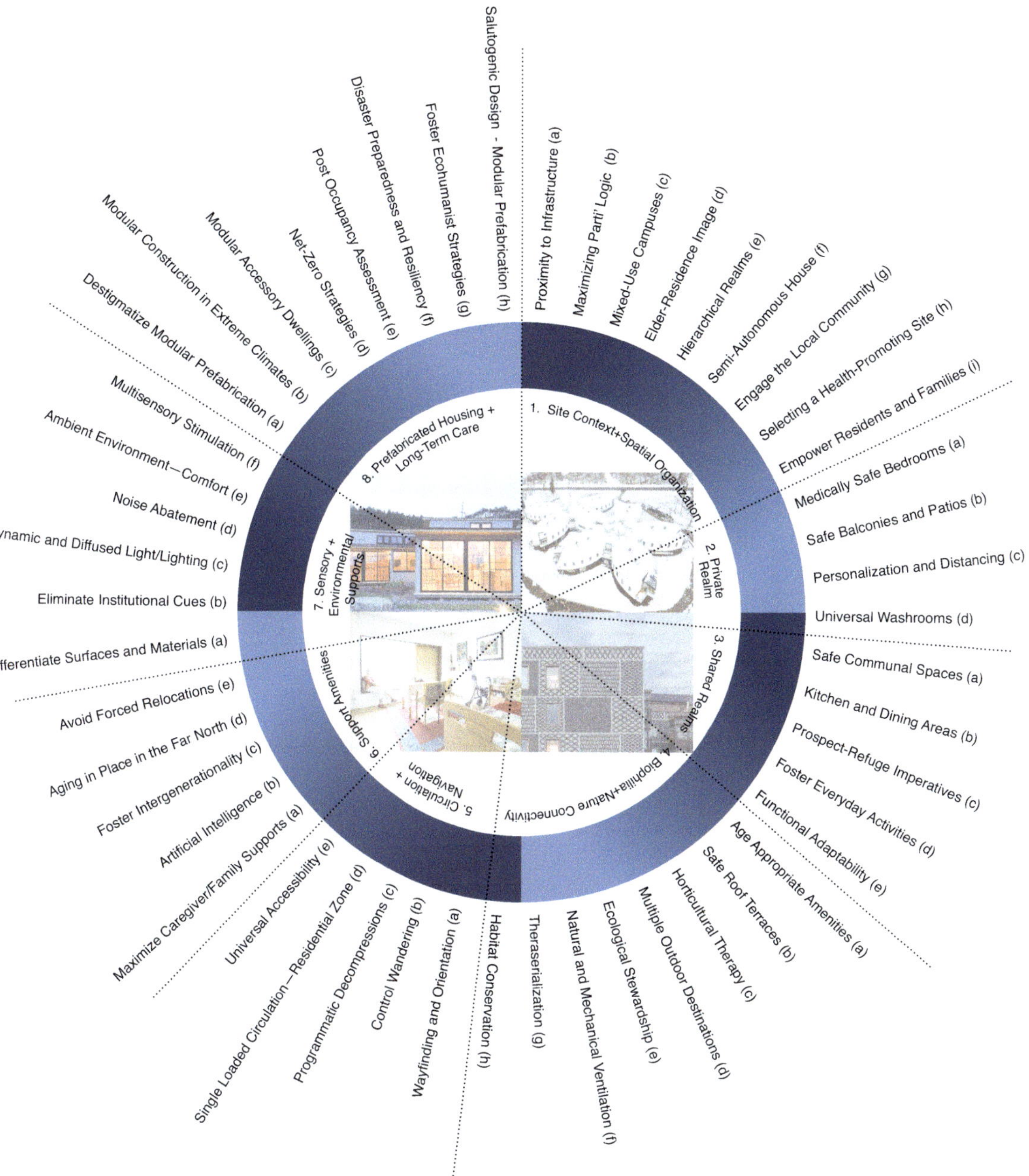

Figure B1. Equitable elder-residences for older persons: design considerations 1–50. Diagram by Stephen Verderber and Lucas Siemucha.

1. SITE CONTEXT AND SPATIAL ORGANIZATION

1a. Proximity to Infrastructure

In a recent research study a group of elderly residents were instructed to take photos of the most salient architectural and related features of their current long-term care residence. Features most closely reminding them of their longtime old neighborhood and their former home were self-photographed most frequently.[3] Living in a preferred residential setting is about somehow still feeling connected to the places, people, and things that trigger positive recollections from the past—places such as the local grocery store, bakery, pharmacy, hair salon, barber, and so on—even if these establishments may now no longer be within walking distance or independently accessible via public transit. A stream of related research in the interdisciplinary field of gerontology has shown residents often sorely miss their everyday routines from an earlier time in life, routines once taken for granted. The activities and the memories they trigger may prompt getting out and engaging in socialization. In light of this predilection, carefully plan to make their transition from their old neighborhood and former home to the long-term care (LTC) home as seamless as possible: psychologically, socially, and architecturally.[4] The importance of locating the LTC residence in close proximity to similar places (if not the actual places themselves) from the resident's past cannot be overestimated. The resident should feel a part of the rhythms of everyday life in the local community surrounding the LTC residence, versus socially and geographically autonomous.

First impressions warrant careful design consideration. Provide a porte cochere at the main entrance for protection from the elements and a sidewalk to enable walking to and from the parking area or possibly a nearby public transit stop, such as at the entrance of the Priory at Heritage Woods in Victoria, British Columbia. There, the residents of this model Green House® project (see section 1f) can also easily walk to the neighborhood public park (located just two blocks away), the commercial downtown area, and main public library. Close proximity to this town center establishes connectivity with the rhythms of everyday life. If and when walking becomes unfeasible for the resident, wheelchair-accessible vans are available on scheduled excursion days for transiting residents to local destination points, possibly including a nearby shopping mall, post office, movie theatre, and so on. Unfortunately, many normative activities of daily living (ADL) will likely become unattainable over time, due to a lack of physical proximity to these amenities, especially for those who reside in a rural area or a low-density, sprawling suburban community (fig. B2). **1c; 6c; 8a; 8b; 8d**

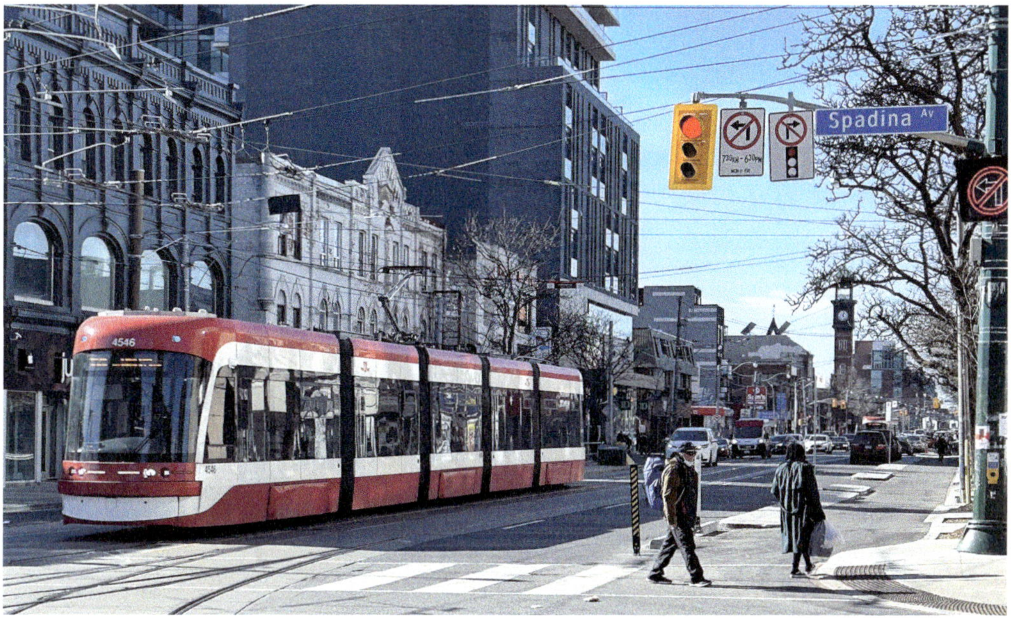

Figure B2. Transit and walkable amenities provide freedom of choice.
Photo by Stephen Verderber.

1b. Maximizing Parti Logic

Residential LTC facilities in North America too often inadvertently perpetuate preexisting health inequities. In many places the trend is to house as
many beds on a single site as is deemed economically "correct" by public
health policy specialists. Instead of designing for sixty beds, for example,
built facilities in the Toronto metropolitan area now house as many as
500–600 beds on a single site.[5] In terms of the quality of life for their
inhabitants, residents are thrust into a stultifying experience. These physical
environments can be psychologically and physically overwhelming—places
where any sense of individuality is evasive, if not impossible to attain. This
has profound ramifications for the architecture of massive LTC residences.
Bigger is by no means *better*. Internal navigation within these places is
difficult, because they are too large and confusing, adversely impacting
an already vulnerable population. For residents suffering from cognitive
impairments, excessively large, spatially complex physical settings pose
myriad challenges.[6] The individual may shut down—a state known as
learned helplessness— remaining cocooned in one's bedroom because
the built environment simply becomes too pressing to effectively comprehend. This constant balancing act between physical settings deemed
too physically challenging versus those which invite frequent daily usage

and sustained engagement as a function of the individual's personal level of physical and cognitive competency is known as *environmental press-competency theory*. More specifically, the effort required from the resident to obtain navigational mastery vis-à-vis their personal abilities, or competencies, is outstripped by the sheer resistance, or *press*, posed by that physical setting.[7] In many ways, the problem of mismatched press-competency levels among the residents in large LTC homes begins with the architectural functional brief. Instead of 300–400 beds, program these homes to house only 75–100 beds in semiautonomous buildings, with each building containing 12-15 beds maximum in a residential cluster. This one measure alone will foster a far more human-scaled, less pressing physical environment, because greater architectural legibility is tantamount to greater spatial comprehensibility.[8] From an environmental stress-reduction standpoint, seek to maximize occupants' executive cognitive functioning while avoiding excessive large and compositionally confusing (i.e., overly pressing) physical environments that can trigger cognitive disorientation, a condition that may force the resident to physically and socially withdraw (fig. B3). **1c; 1d; 1e; 1f; 4c; 4g; 8b**

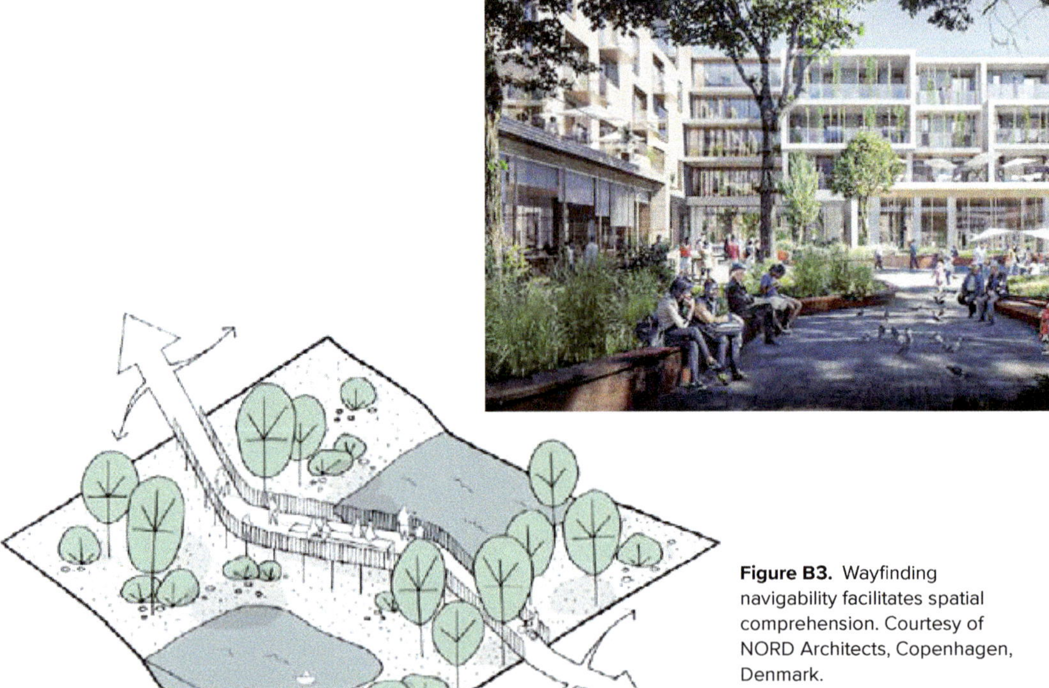

Figure B3. Wayfinding navigability facilitates spatial comprehension. Courtesy of NORD Architects, Copenhagen, Denmark.

referred to as the dwelling's *functional spillover syndrome*, such as when one's teenage son practices on his saxophone every afternoon from 4:00 to 6:00 p.m. virtually taking over the entire residence for the duration of his daily routine. The residential zones cited above have endured across time and space, manifesting cross-culturally, and have been given architectural expression in diverse socioeconomic contexts. For the older members of the household, these hierarchical spatial zones are relevant both in theory and in practical daily life. When applied to the LTC residence, they provide hierarchically clustered spaces designed to fluidly support diverse concurrent activities within one or two areas without overpowering all others. Examples include the provision of specific rooms/types for quiet time, socialization, personal hygiene, food preparation, dining, physical fitness, home office work, and space(s) for intimacy.[17] In an overcrowded LTC residence, on the other hand, individual rooms tend to become distorted and functionally convoluted, with their hierarchical adjacencies often being undiscernible and becoming dysfunctional.

Architectural dysfunction inhibits the use of hierarchical spaces for multiple functions—for example, a kitchen without countertop and stools for casual dining, a dining room unable to be used for non-dining functions, or lack of an exterior patio as a dining option. The absence of hierarchical spaces presents needless physical and psychological barriers from a *press-competency* perspective. A poorly designed wandering garden with too few places to sit and rest signifies excessive spatial compression, because it affords an insufficient hierarchical amenity—a condition frequently resulting from flawed facility programming (i.e., the brief) prior to the schematic architectural design phase.[18] Kitchens, communal dining areas, and outdoor spaces are all examples of the importance of spatial hierarchy in fostering fluid connectivity between adjoining spaces that afford opportunities for residents and visitors to obtain privacy and small group socialization. **1b; 1f; 3b; 4d; 4g; 7b**

1f. Semiautonomous Houses

Multi-site LTC residential care corporations are driven to maximize their return on capital investment, or ROI. But does this mean too many residents need to be forced into a single overcrowded building? This unfortunate and inequitable practice was first called out in the 1970s by vocal critics of the modern International Style machine-for-healing hospital.[19] In many places, still, health policies are complicit partners in the continuance of this false premise resulting in the continued erection of too-large LTC facilities. In the past, "bigger is better" may have made economic sense, but it represents inequitable health planning policy today and this warrants a thorough reappraisal. Architecturally, bigness per se is by no means a positive attribute, especially from the standpoint of creating a sustainably positive residential quality of life.[20] An overcrowded LTC residence with thirty or more beds per administrative unit represents a poor quality of life. Older LTC facilities from the 1960s to 1980s still remaining in operation are the worst offenders, continuing to subject their inhabitants to dehumanizing conditions, denying them an affirmative *residentialist* everyday reality. Instead, design and build interconnected, small-scale, semiautonomous clusters of residences—*houses*—in a shared campus-like setting using inventive design strategies, with each residence projecting an appropriate residentialist scale and image.

Semi-autonomous houses, with each comprising ten to fifteen residents, provide many opportunities to inventively plan and design deinstitutionalized, human-scale architecture within a campus context of interconnected yet semiautonomous buildings. For residents, the intrinsic virtues of these small-scale residential clusters, with their private and semiprivate realms, support the resident's activities of daily living—including opportunities for meaningful engagement with nature and landscape (N-L), improved nutritional health, and increased opportunities for socialization—without sacrificing privacy or engagement in prescribed daily therapeutic regimens and other activities.[21] As such, each semiautonomous house is organized around its residents' personal regimens: hygiene, dayrooms, dining, access to the outdoors. Design these houses so that residents, caregiver staff, and visitors can safely walk on a path or cross a lawn to visit any of the other houses on the campus, with adequate personal distancing and without having to pass through the most public spaces, such as the main lobby.[22] The Green House® model of long-term care is premised on this concept, a concept similarly applicable in horizontally configured midrise structures of four to seven levels (fig. B4).[23] **1b; 1d; 1e; 2c; 3b; 4d; 5c**

1g. Engage the Local Community

In 2022, more than 79,000 qualifying individuals in the Province of Ontario, Canada, were on waiting lists for home-based eldercare services. Nearly 38,000 of these applicants, all meeting the criteria for placement in a 24/7 LTC residence, would have to endure an especially

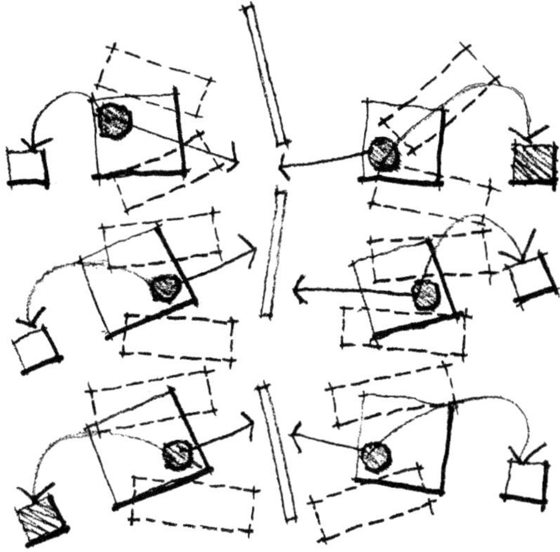

Figure B4. Semiautonomous houses. Drawing by Stephen Verderber.

lengthy wait of many years. This is how the supply-and-demand problem begins—a community's worsening shortage of services for seniors, due to a lack of public policy foresight, proper upfront planning, and vision.

The professional architectural community province—the Ontario Association of Architects (OAA)—has tried to break free from this supply-and-demand bottleneck by focusing its advocacy efforts on improving the quality of appropriately scaled architecture for qualifying older persons, doing so in response to a public health and medical crisis only worsening with each passing year. Through its committee structure, the OAA engages elected officials, advocating for improving the supply and quality of housing for the province's seniors. Sadly, the case for constructing facilities able to house tens of thousands of additional LTC beds was well documented before COVID-19, yet this growing crisis continues to be underprioritized politically. The architectural community has been primed to address this unmet housing need, although its hands remain tied, due to governmental bureaucracy—largely attributable to a procurement process bogged down in excessive political maneuvering, excessive red tape, the constant threat of NIMBYism erupting wherever a new LTC residence is proposed, and seemingly endless public consultations that can last years. Regardless, effective political support from the host local community is crucial, hinging on political and administrative leadership, buttressed by viable public health policies. Little can be accomplished unless the agency of the local *community* is carefully listened to and equitably respected, with higher-up decision makers then appropriately acting on what they learned through the community consultation process. It continues to be critical for decision makers at all levels to genuinely *hear* and comprehend what local advocacy groups and others most care about when it comes to 24/7 long-term custodial care places that perhaps their own parents and grandparents—now or in the future—will reside in. Formulate evidence-based architectural design strategies to address these medically underserved communities.[24] 4e; 4h; 6c; 8a–8h

1h. Select a Health-Promoting Site

Noncommunicable diseases are at epidemic levels among the aged in poor and wealthy nations alike, according to the World Health Organization.[25] Sedentary lifestyles and unhealthful consequences—with increasing numbers of medically underserved people reside in sprawling, auto-dependent urban centers globally—are well documented by epidemiologists internationally. The international public health community is in agreement on the importance of non–age discriminatory, equitable, health-promoting polices in combating current and future unhealthful built environments and the sedentary lifestyles they foster.[26] Comorbidities are on the rise among older persons: eating disorders, obesity, hypertension, type 2 diabetes, and depression. In North America, it is now widely accepted that post–World War II suburban sprawl had a major role in fostering these unhealthy lifestyles, in large part due to an overdependence on the automobile. Being obliged to drive everywhere all the time resulted in sitting still in traffic for long periods, when one could have been outdoors walking or bicycling between destination points. For older persons, endeavor to select an appropriate site for construction within a reasonable distance to neighborhood parks, nearby commercial establishments, and accessible health care resources—resources reachable on foot or via public transit, such as the excellent community infrastructure framework that surrounds the Priory at Heritage Woods in Victoria, BC. For active and semi-active older persons, the architecture should encourage their venturing out into the local community. The cumulative health benefits are manifold, because in the depths of suburbia, unsafe sidewalks (or their absence entirely) and excessive distances between destination points for trips render it nearly impossible to go anywhere without a car. This is why it remains so challenging to get older people to stop using their vehicles.[27] In short, advocate for resources close

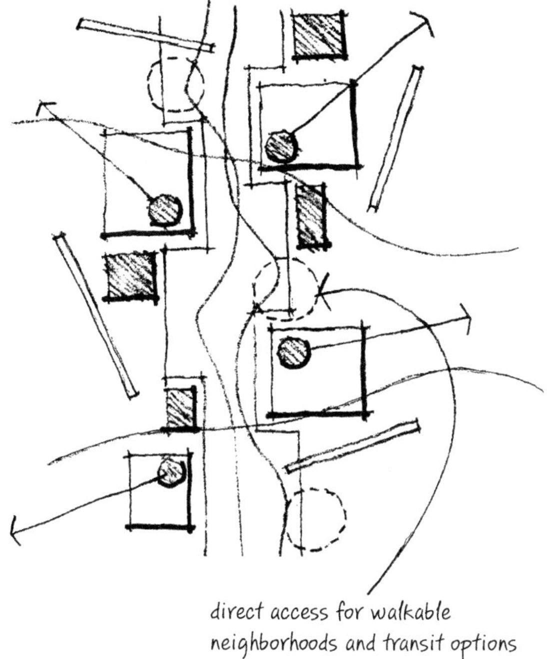

Figure B5. Equitable selection of health-promoting sites. Drawing by Stephen Verderber.

to the newly built LTC residence. Building new 24/7 eldercare residences too far from local supporting infrastructural resources. such as a transit stop, only exacerbates this isolating syndrome. All stakeholders working toward a common goal will be able to seek out, for example, reclaimed brownfield and greenfield sites near transit connections and a local park, increasing the probability of a higher usage rate by residents, as well as by family members and friends who, in rural contexts, need not travel fifty or a hundred miles or more by car (fig. B5).[28] **1a; 4e; 4h; 5e; 6d; 8a–8h**

1i. Empower Residents and Families

Older persons frequently lack personal or collective agency, which translates into scant political lobbying influence and limited effectiveness.[29] With many older individuals already suffering from societal non-agency and isolation—due to shunning, bullying, stigmas, and other discriminatory manifestations of ageism—an ideal place for heightened self-empowerment for both residents and families begins with confronting this lack of agency. For the inhabitants of an LTC residence, this entails reclaiming their sense of worth, expanding personal competency levels to cope with environmentally press-ing physical barriers, and, thereby, attaining a greater sense of personal control and predictability. This will release a hidden power, harnessing it in positive, mutually supportive, life-affirming ways. A supportive LTC residence respects the elderly persons' Bill of Rights, which affirms, in part, their right to information and to associated technical resources, to enable them to make the right decisions to enhance their well-being.[30] For this to occur in the everyday milieu means respecting the right to eldercare-centric health ser-vices, the right to medically safe 24/7 residential care options, and the right to public consultation at all times, especially when a new capital improve-ment project is proposed that requires the forced relocation of a current in-place residential population to an unfamiliar facility somewhere else.[31]

Encourage transparency in these public discourses, with meetings scheduled at convenient times for those who have busy schedules, and foster a forum to genuinely listen—without the baggage of hidden political agendas or merely giving lip service to decision makers—so they can genu-inely say "We heard the people out" following public consultation meetings. Prerequisite conditions also require respecting the agency of residents and their families in site selection and the architectural and landscape design of a proposed local LTC facility, including information on transit connections (a priority), future facility expansion options, and any local environmental impacts.[32] In the UK, in 2017 the Bradford City Clinical Commissioning Group initiated its Grass Roots Programme—a process drawing local stake-holders together to carefully review and comment on local planned health care projects—to assess proposed new therapy and counseling resources and establish effective political communications throughout this public con-sultation process.[33] In the first phase, more than 1,949 online posts related to patient and family feedback were received from 3,987 individuals, with 209 coming directly from elderly mental health patients and their families. **2c; 3c; 4a; 6a; 6c; 8a–8h**

2. PRIVATE REALM

2a. Medically Safe Bedrooms

From an infection control standpoint, even prior to the global onset of COVID-19, infectious disease specialists regarded shared (communal) bed-rooms, bathrooms, and showers as prime transmitters of communicable disease.[34] This became abundantly clear early on in the pandemic, due to the disproportionately high mortality rates linked with these conditions in long-term institutional care facilities. A deadly pattern emerged, beginning early in 2020, due to thousands of persistently overcrowded facilities that provided insufficient or no physical space for adequate personal distancing.[35] These obsolete conditions were a holdover from the 1960s and 1970s International Style, first-generation modern nursing home's four- to six- or even eight-bed open wards, with their communal hygiene spaces.[36] COVID-19 once and for all exposed the folly of overcrowdedness. Evidence-based research has clearly shown that communal sleeping and hygiene spaces are hazardous for both residents and the caregiver staff. During the pandemic, caregivers globally were themselves subjected to substandard conditions and viral outbreaks, often aided and abetted by the facilities' antiquated HVAC systems. Now coming under intense media scrutiny, thousands of health care provider organizations were suddenly thrust into the spotlight, seemingly overnight, and put under pressure to retrofit their facility *yesterday*.[37] Such a magnitude of retrofitting was often impossible to accomplish quickly, due to supply chain disruptions, labor shortages, high construction costs, and often mind-bending facility policies and spatial limitations, such as inoperable windows and excessive distance ratios from the unit's outer walls to its double-loaded central corridors. This left few to no good options for relocating residents within their present facility.[38]

Moreover, does completely vacating the facility, if even temporarily (for, say, a month), yield positive outcomes for the residents? No evidence-based data yet exists on this. Best evidence-based practices, however, now call for smaller-scale, semiautonomous *houses*, consisting of *private bedrooms* with *private bathrooms* provided for each resident, with a maximum of ten to fifteen beds per semiautonomous "house" (see section 1f). In summary, the evidence-based medical and architectural literature both support a thorough policy reappraisal—constituting a political and health policy reawakening long overdue. The prior seventy-year period (1955–2025) of overcrowded, unsafe LTC residences is over (fig. B6). **1f; 2c; 3b; 4f; 5e; 7e; 8c**

2b. Safe Balconies and Patios

Well-designed outdoor spaces immediately adjacent to the semiautonomous house are getaways—whether a balcony overlooking a courtyard, a ground-level patio with seating, or a quiet spot within a wandering garden with ample space to stroll around.[39] Attention restoration theory (ART, see chapter 4) posits that humans periodically need to get away psychologically, if only briefly, to restore their psychological attentional (coping) capabilities in the context of environmental press-competency, built-environment challenges. Balconies and patios function as viewing stations, allowing residents opportunities to satisfy these involuntary attentional needs by

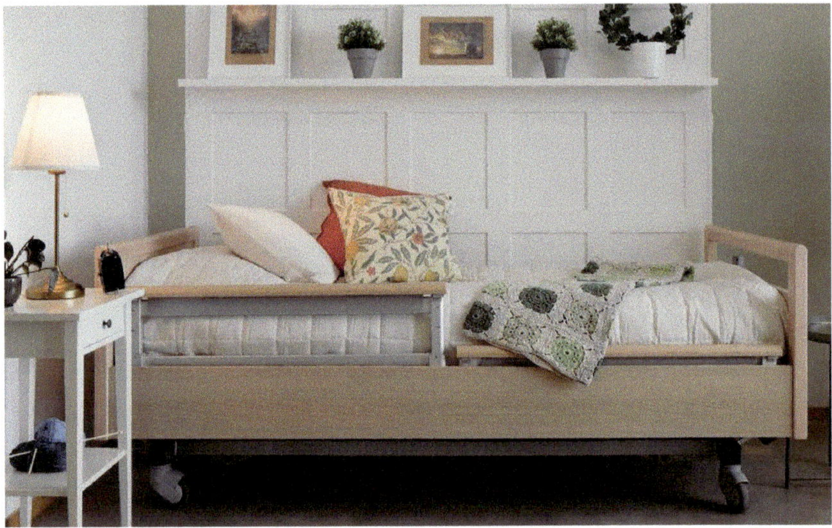

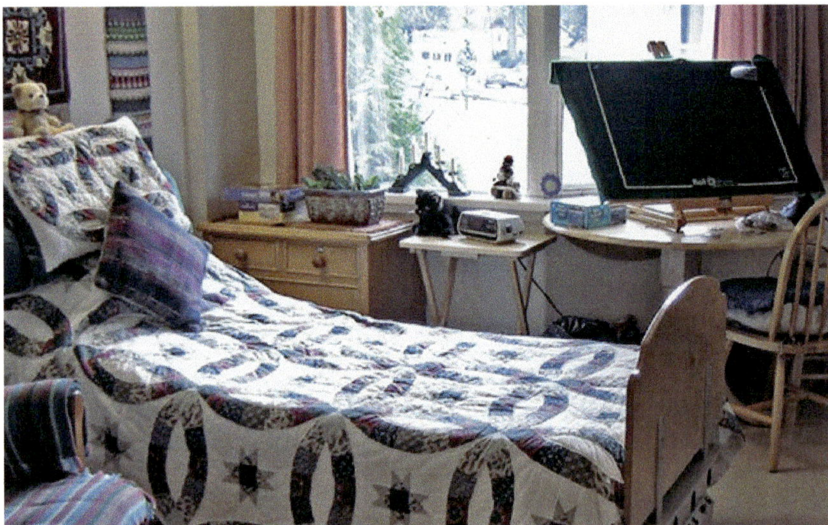

Figure B6. Medically safe bedrooms, personal distancing, and personalization. Courtesy of Max Plunger.

providing a new experience, if only for a few minutes. A balcony adjacent to a bedroom, an exterior terrace, or a sequestered patio next to a social activity room become adjunctive extensions to the bedroom and, by extension, to one's *domestic space*. They offer a break from overcrowded, over-stimulating conditions indoors, such as a too small and confining bedroom. Equally important, doors and windows looking onto these exterior spaces can transmit daylight and natural ventilation into the interior.[40] Provide a small table and a few chairs—such as in the recessed private balconies at the Wilder Kaiser nursing home (2017) in Austria—simultaneously protecting residents from excessive sunlight and inclement weather, shielding them from direct observation, and offering places for obtaining non-indoor respite. Provide space for plants. Design these areas and their volumes as outdoor extensions of the interior realm. Otherwise, if undersized and lacking in prospect-refuge opportunities, they will not be used. Above all, do not design these outdoor rooms to make the resident or visitor feel unsafe or in any way unprotected. If a private balcony adjacent to a bedroom cantilevers (projects) outward from the building's main envelope, create a microclimate effect with a roof canopy and provide between-balcony screens or partitions.[41] Balance microclimate conditions with residents' prospect-refuge predilections, supporting both quiet contemplation and socialization. In ground-level and lower-floor exterior spaces, provide visual screening with landscaping, trellises, and perimeter walls (fig. B7). **1d; 1f; 4f; 6a; 7b; 7c; 8a–8d**

2c. Personalization and Distancing

Building codes and minimum facility standards for nursing homes during the 1946–1985 period were basically modeled on the identical aesthetic and functional standards that governed the design and construction of the post–World War II International Style hospital. The dehumanizing atmosphere of the hospital-based geriatric units of the 1940s and 1950s, often housed in the back wards of acute care hospitals, were exported into the postwar nursing home. These places were confining, uninspiring, and, to their critics, symbols of society's scant regard for their inhabitants' dignity, privacy needs, or quality of life.

Establish policies to encourage the resident and family to personalize the *private bedroom*—something once virtually impossible in the aforementioned communal bedroom scenarios. For both the resident and family, room personalization opportunities and improved personal distancing options in eldercare residences has been empirically demonstrated to result in higher satisfaction levels and medically safer physical settings.

In light of the recent global reawakening to disease transmissibility issues among medically frail older persons post–COVID-19, administrative policies actively encourage resident/family personalizations of private bedrooms.[42] This best-practice policy supports promoting the resident's (and

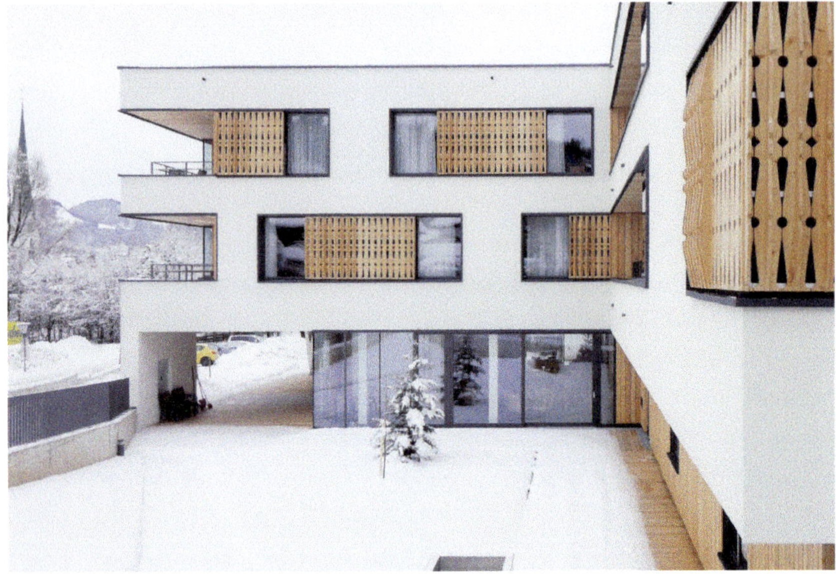

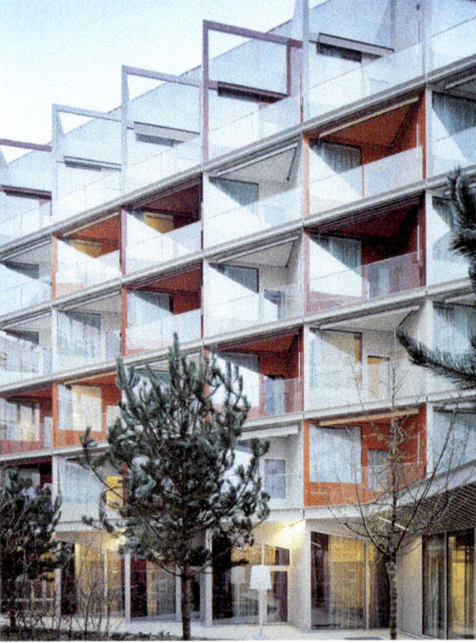

Figure B7. Outdoor spaces close by, for respite without compromising security. Courtesy of Óscar Miguel Ares Álvarez; courtesy of SRAP (Sedlak Rissland Architektur Partnerhaft), Nuremburg, Germany.

family's) personal and political agency, self-dignity, personal autonomy, and overall quality of life.

Effective ways to do this include the provision of individualized, recessed, doorway entry thresholds off the main corridor and wall-inset glass cases in recesses, with bedrooms sufficiently large for a proper display of meaningful mementos and photos featuring a collection of people and important events from earlier stages in life, together with miscellaneous artifacts and even furnishings brought in from the former longtime home. All these provide opportunities to share something about oneself with other residents and one's caregiver team, because then a resident becomes more than just a one-dimensional "old person."[43] These types of personalization measures were first pioneered in the architecture of Scandinavian eldercare residences, in order to make them feel more like home. They have since proven effective in diverse cultural contexts, ameliorating otherwise harsh, one-dimensional institutional conditions.[44] **1e; 4d; 5b; 5c; 5e**

2d. Private Washrooms

Semiprivate bedrooms with communal washroom and shower rooms are high-probability transmitters of infectious disease. Instead, provide both a private bedroom and a *private washroom/shower unit* for each resident. This design consideration will yield a lower disease transmission rate while also providing greater personal privacy and autonomy. This aspect of the residential unit may, in some situations, require some additional staffing, as the caregiver team frequently must attend to one resident at a time. Despite the staffing ramifications and equipment needed for this level of personalized care, it will elevate the resident's medical safety, privacy, self-dignity, and sense of personal control, as well as being commensurate with infection control and personal-distancing best practices.[45] Universal design standards are now widely accepted in the health care industry and are premised on the principles of nondiscrimination and equity in facility planning, architectural design, and construction.[46] Assistive technologies can help the resident more fully participate in activities of daily living, and in many ways this begins with a private bath/shower unit. From a health equity perspective, no resident should be prohibited or discouraged from using the private bathroom/shower unit, although this may be difficult to negotiate for some residents—a situation worsened by poor quality lighting, undifferentiated floor and wall surfaces, and badly designed fixtures such as grab bars and pull cords. In these eldercare residences, equitably design and equip the private bathroom/shower units to support a wide range of physical mobility, sensory, and cognitive abilities—for example, provide equivalent physical transference space on both sides of the commode to accommodate multiple transfer methods; position the commode in a direct sightline from the bed; and identifiably differentiate wall and floor surfaces with color-accented, multisensorial visual cues. Windows (perhaps specifying obscured glass, if the window has a low sill height) will further enhance and functionally activate these personal hygiene spaces, thus rendering them more homelike—residentialist.[47] **1f; 2a; 2c; 3b; 5e; 7a**

3. SHARED REALMS

3a. Safe Communal Spaces

COVID-19 disturbingly demonstrated how the built environment functions as a prime host for transmitting infectious disease. But disease transmission rates are but one metric in evaluating an LTC home's overall safety. According to the Centers for Disease Control and Prevention, each year an estimated 648,000 people in the US develop hospital-acquired infections, and nearly 75,000 victims die.[48] Many such illnesses and deaths are traceable to the use of pathogenic antibiotics, the very drugs whose purpose is to fight and eradicate infection. Residents with dementia often misconstrue what is needed and therefore are uncooperative regarding proper personal hygiene or in taking their prescribed medications. The resident may suffer from comorbidities, as well as longstanding health inequities, chronic infections from (but not limited to) substance abuse, a mental health disorder, a human immunodeficiency virus (HIV) infection, hepatitis B or C, or tuberculosis. Psychological and immunocompromising conditions pose risks to other residents' health, as well as that of caregiver staff, unless proper personal distancing occurs and PPEs are provided.[49] Besides the need for better infection control protocols, a number of recent advancements in facility security and surveillance technologies make it possible to establish layered, overlapping security zones, starting at the campus's perimeter and extending throughout, with concentric security rings culminating at the heart of the multiperson residence. Providing secure buffer zones at access points (doors) and extending these layers to semiprivate spaces indoors and outdoors can help ensure safe, secure communal spaces with infrared lasers, CCTV, and card-reader access devices. Balance campus-

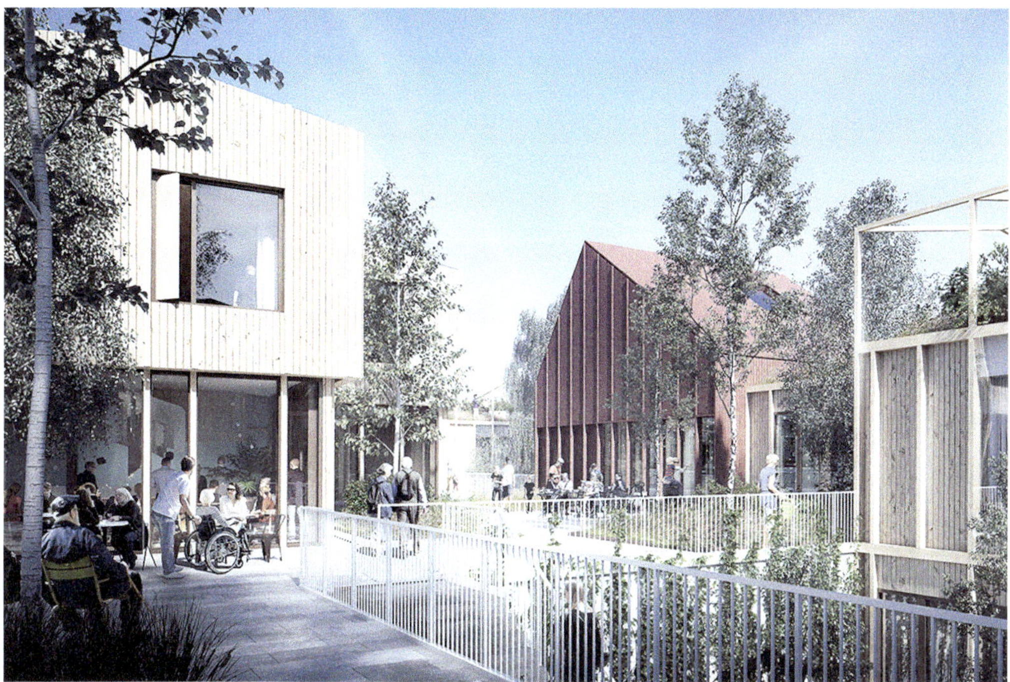

Figure B8. Protected courtyards promote nature immersion. Courtesy of NORD Architects, Copenhagen, Denmark.

wide security measures with the organizational medical care philosophy of distinguishing between passive and active security systems. These systems should be unobtrusively woven into the architectural fabric of the physical setting. This aspect will avoid costly retrofits down the road (fig. B8).[50] **2a; 2d; 5b; 5e; 6a; 8a–8h**

3b. Kitchen and Dining Areas

Stories abound of older persons with dementia who, for too long, continued to reside in their longtime dwelling too independently. For instance, one afternoon my own 92-year-old mother turned on her kitchen oven and then forgot about it, wandering off elsewhere within her home. The fire department, luckily, quickly arrived, because her daytime in-home caregiver thankfully arrived in time to call for help before a full-scale fire broke out in her kitchen. At this stage in life, an individual may become unable to perform basic activities of daily living—including maintaining proper personal hygiene, purchasing and preparing food, doing laundry, maintaining a clean home, and keeping abreast of personal finances, to name but a few essential ADLs. This is when living independently can be both a personal risk and a risk to others.[51] In an LTC residence, the central kitchen and dining area(s) provide safe, secure places in support of nutritional health while ideally offering freedom of choice for an individual to select where to eat, when, and with whom (as deemed feasible by the caregiver team).[52] Design these places to allow visiting family members to prepare a meal, perhaps together with the resident. Provide a sufficiently large, universally designed countertop eating area (with wheelchair under-table access), one to two refrigerators, a double-compartment sink next to a window (contributing to a homelike aesthetic), a microwave oven, a dishwasher, an adequate number of cabinets, and a full pantry. Locate these decentralized kitchen/dining areas at the heart of each ten- to fifteen-bed residential unit, and include an adjacent outdoor shaded terrace or patio for dining. Decentralized kitchen/dining areas will be most effective if designed to be residentialist, contributing to a universally designed, normative atmosphere. Provide enough space in these dining areas to accommodate everyone who resides in the semiautonomous house at once, including room for four dining tables, so multiple families can dine separately if they so choose. The incorporation of artwork, murals, and sufficiently large windows providing interesting views of N-L, enhance these dining spaces (fig. B9).[53] **1e; 3b; 3c; 5a; 6a; 7b**

3c. Prospect-Refuge

Prospect-refuge (P-R) behavioral accommodations contribute to greater overall well-being among older persons who continue to seek out engagement with the world around them but wish to do so without developing stress, due to overly pressing conditions. The provision of adequate personal space is a prerequisite for the resident being actively involved in this type of behavioral activity.[54] Overcrowded LTC residences are frequently too loud and lack respite areas, subverting or negating the resident's ability to successfully engage in psychological restoration activities. Getaway areas—a garden, pathways to destinations, balconies, window seats, semiobscured outdoor spaces, and terraces—allow a person to look outward beyond their immediate surroundings and view another scene or place safely (a *prospect*), without being observed (from a *refuge*), or to be with others in a somewhat less private setting.[55] Caregiver staff also need opportunities to get away from their routines and obtain respite. Breakrooms and indoor and outdoor spaces can be designed to accommodate P-R behaviors and N-L immersion. For a resident with a cognitive disorder,

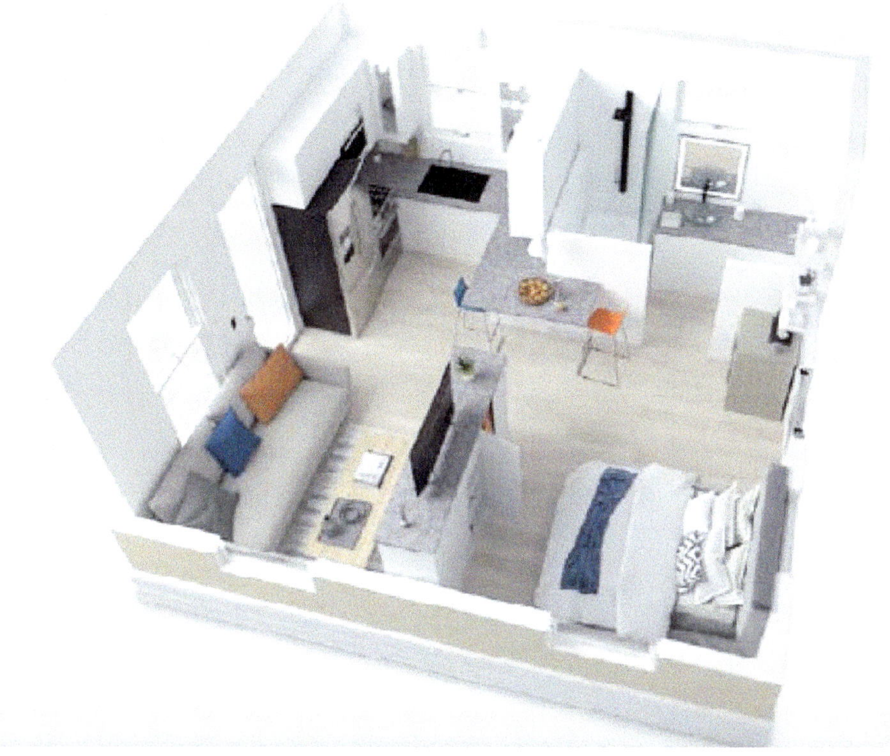

Figure B9. Adaptable kitchen and dining areas support informal uses. Courtesy of BOXABEL, Inc., Las Vegas, Nevada.

the wandering garden is a place to engage in P-R behaviors and N-L immersion.[56] Early on, select a site that allows for adequate exterior space for a campus plan of interconnected, semiautonomous residential units. Terraces, patios, walkways, and connecting footbridges can help facilitate residents' freedom of choice to circulate within and between these places and allow them to explore their surroundings. A network of interior and exterior paths and destination points will help prompt exploration and psycho-emotionally positive P-R behaviors within a safe and protected physical setting. Foster high congruence between these therapeutic physical settings and their potential for social activity by providing indoor and outdoor places to stop and sit, rest, and converse with others, either along the various paths or at destination points. Coordinate these P-R amenities to not inadvertently impinge on private or semiprivate zones or create conditions tantamount to overcrowding, with its unintended, pressing, functional spillover effects. Memory care residents in particular will benefit physically and cognitively from well-designed prospect-refuge options that draw them outward—both indoors and outdoors—beyond the safe personal zone of their private bedroom or semiautonomous house.[57] **1e; 4d; 5a; 5e; 6a; 7b**

3d. Foster Everyday Activities

A poorly planned and designed LTC residence can inadvertently foster acts of elder abuse. While these harmful actions can and do occur in all types of LTC homes, harsh lessons were painfully learned in the early months of the COVID-19 pandemic in 2020. Then, overcrowded and understaffed facilities were revealed to have relatively few and weakly enforced caring policies to encourage residents to participate in the normative activities of everyday life, because the medical risk was simply staggering, as personal distancing was often next to impossible.[58] From a personal-distancing viewpoint, a health-promoting facility is one where residents meaningfully engage in therapeutic treatments, physical activities, and social activities (e.g., watching a film with others). Biophilic possibilities include spending time outdoors on a nice day; attending a physical therapy session; dining; being in the wandering garden; or traveling off-site for an excursion into the community, such as a trip to the local public library or a live music event in the nearby park.[59] A well-designed LTC residence can dignify and empower. These settings are salutogenically designed with built-in positive distractions and, as such, actively help combat feelings of loneliness and isolation.[60] Ask the residents, "What are your favorite everyday activities?" Then design the campus and its positive distraction amenities accordingly. After the facility is open and fully occupied, adapt and further modify the physical environment by asking such questions as, "What activities of daily living do you consider to be of particular interest, now that you have lived here for three months?" The responses will probably not include a very challenging physical therapy session that required intensive voluntary attention. Instead, preferred positive distraction activities likely to be cited might include art therapy, a hair appointment, horticultural therapy, pet therapy, recreational therapy, time spent in the multisensory room (MSR), and trips taken off campus (fig. B10). Above all, spaces that allow a resident to be unduly out of sight can become a stage for elder abuse in facilities that already cause stress, due to overcrowded conditions. **1a; 1c; 3d; 4a; 4c; 5a; 5e**

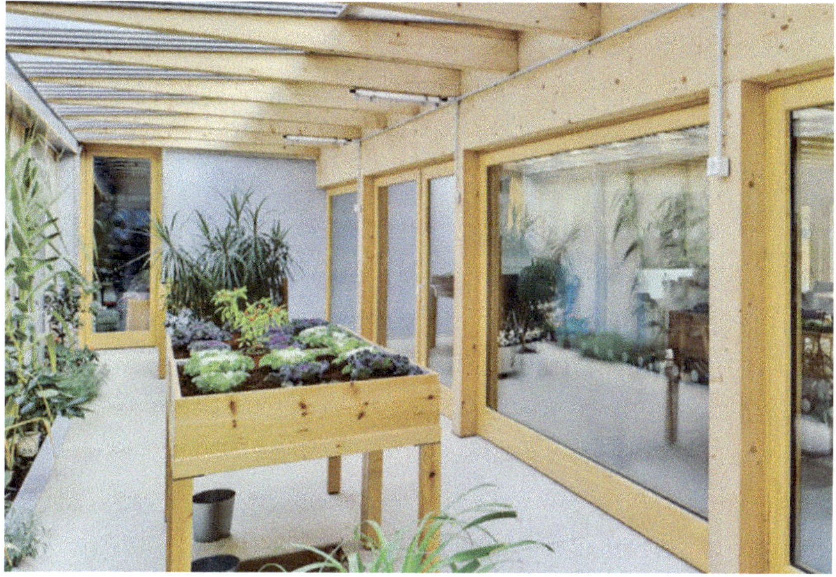

Figure B10. Design for a range of sensorily engaging activities indoors and outdoors. Courtesy of David Frutos via CSO Arquitectura, Mura, Spain.

3e. Functional Adaptability

Is it reasonable to expect a dayroom, in a single day, to equitably support activities as diverse as a group session, semiprivate weekend visits with family and friends, a birthday party, and so on?[61] Its dysfunctionality is likely due to having been undersized in the first place, and from then on it is subject to overprogramming—a problem in large part attributable to the anachronistic International Style nursing homes of the post–World War II era. Then, dayrooms (sadly, usually a single dayroom in a nursing unit with perhaps thirty or more beds), were sparsely furnished and located at the end of a long, drab, double-loaded corridor. By contrast, the space-planning and architectural design strategy in Scandinavia since the 1960s has been to provide multiple, adaptable activity rooms in support of a broad range of therapeutic, social, cultural, and recreational activities. Diverse events are prescheduled by staff or can occur simultaneously, with other scheduled activities by and for the local community arranged by affiliated civic groups.[62] This strategy is preferable from both quality-of-life and ADL standpoints. Provide interconnected, flexible, multipurpose rooms—some with higher ceilings, some with greater horizontal widths, and others comparatively smaller in size and more intimate—with most areas able to be partitioned into smaller spaces via moveable fold-away panels. Adaptable multipurpose rooms give residents options to get out of the comfort zone of their bedroom. These flexible spaces also host concerts, meetings, weekly events, holiday celebrations, concerts, and other activities. An on-site art gallery, winter garden, and greenhouse should be considered as multifunctional spaces.[63] Provide adaptable, rearrangeable furnishings; perhaps include a fireplace in the main multipurpose room; specify inviting colors throughout; employ natural materials and finishes for floors, ceilings, and wall surfaces; establish visual connections with N-L through large windows, portals, and other apertures, such as clerestories and skylights; and make use of varied geometries to avoid spatial repetitiveness (fig. B11). **2c; 3a; 3b; 3c; 4a; 6a; 6c**

4. BIOPHILIA AND NATURE CONNECTIVITY

4a. Age-Appropriate Amenities

Warehousing is a term used to describe a society's premeditated offloading and act of *uncaring* for its older citizens. The COVID-19 pandemic brought this "worst practice" to the forefront of public consciousness and was fueled by occurrences of unacceptably high mortality rates in LTC insti-

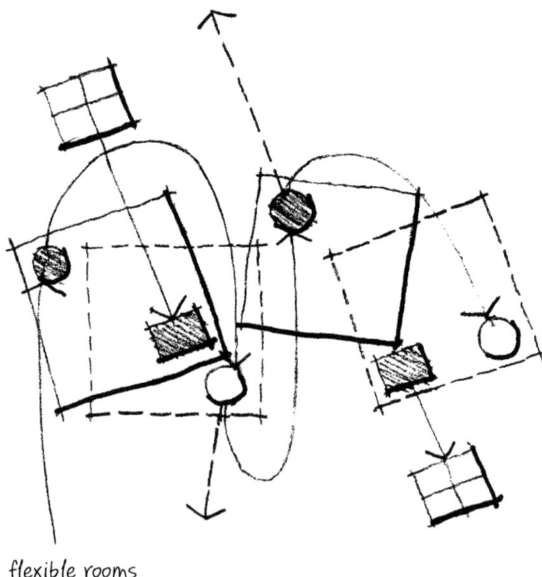

Figure B11. Explore the virtues of functional adaptability. Drawing by Stephen Verderber.

tutions throughout the coronavirus pandemic. In the 1960s and 1970s, a nursing home's physical environment was not primarily viewed through a therapeutic lens. Whether a particular nursing home's aesthetic vocabulary was particularly "liked" or not was not first and foremost in pre-architectural design, architect-client considerations, or so it seemed. A nursing facility's administrators were used to running and their architects to designing *hospitals* and therefore thought and acted as if a nursing home was a mini-hospital. As a lingering remnant of International Style minimalism, relatively little attention was accorded in providing non-stereotypical or above and beyond physical environment amenities for the inhabitants.[64] This was a main reason why these places appeared so threatening to younger people (this author included), who thought, "I don't ever want to end up THERE!"

Much evidence-based research published over the past thirty years points to the therapeutic value of providing life affirming N-L biophilic experiences geared specifically for the LTC resident. The operative assumption is that age appropriate biophilic activities will help keep older persons more actively stimulated and, hence, healthier longer.[65] Don't settle for the excuse, "We had no choice but to max out the building's ground floor footprint, even through this meant eliminating the landscaped courtyard and garden." From the outset, all stakeholders in the built outcome can advocate for activity-stimulating, biophilic N-L amenities, with their timeless intrinsic appeal, and this will outweigh shopworn stereotypes of what "slowing down" older persons might like or dislike.[66] Memory care gardens and wandering paths can be enlivening places—fully age appropriate—while allowing adequate social distancing best practices. Include comfortable seating and tables, where individuals can sit, simply contemplate alone, or converse with others. **3c; 5e; 6a; 6c; 8c; 8a–8h**

4b. Safe Roof Terraces

Alvar Aalto's (1898–1976) iconic rooftop terraces at his Paimio Sanitorium (1929–1933) near Helsinki, Finland, featured extensive natural plantings, as did the terraces located on the lower levels. Aalto's inventive incorporation of N-L in the treatment of tuberculosis was exceptional and extraordinary at the time, although its architectural precursors dated from the 1890s in the TB hospitals built in Switzerland and Austria. The N-L connectivity of Paimio and other progressively designed hospitals would be dismissed outright in the age of the high-tech megahospitals constructed post–World War II and throughout the 1960–1980 period in North America and elsewhere. Few nursing homes built during this period featured anything on a par with Aalto's heroic achievement at Paimio many decades earlier. The modern nursing home was taking its architectural cues from the acute care hospital of the era. There were no balconies, terraces, or related amenities to draw N-L into the 24/7 health care experience. *Patients* (as they were referred to then) in nursing homes had little measurable, therapeutically sustainable contact with nature, save for the view from a small window if their bed happened to be near one in a four- to six-bed ward—or from the dayroom or dining room on the unit. Even then, the view was likely of a parking lot, nearby building, or dimly lit lightwell—all poor substitutes for the real thing. Instead, inventively incorporate genuinely salutogenic architectural and landscape design strategies, creating safe, well-protected areas on the upper levels of the LTC home to celebrate and satisfy the biophilic human predilection for N-L immersion.[67] Undulating stepped-roof terraces, recesses in the building's envelope, balconies, exterior furnishings, greenhouses, and winter gardens with sliding and retractable walls/roofs and perhaps roll-up garage doors are feasible amenities in this regard. Provide shaded spaces with canopies, trellises, extended roof eaves, and deciduous trees and ground plantings without sacrificing residents' P-R behavioral predilections, personal safety, or security requirements. Provide rooftop terraces in the upper levels in midrise structures with four to seven levels (figs. B12 and B13). **1e; 2b; 4c; 4d; 5e; 6c; 7f**

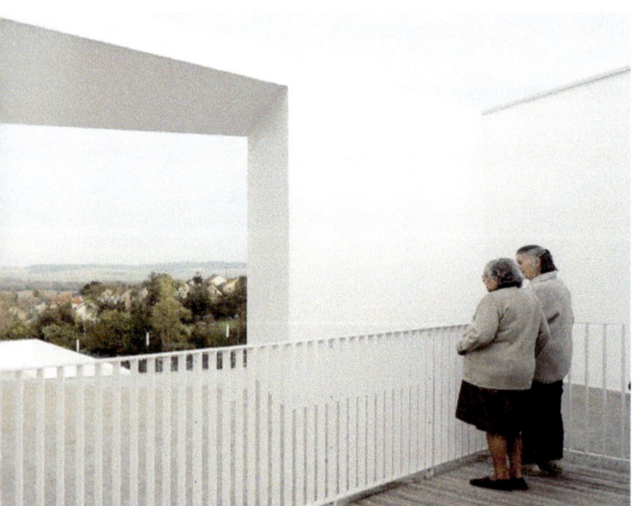

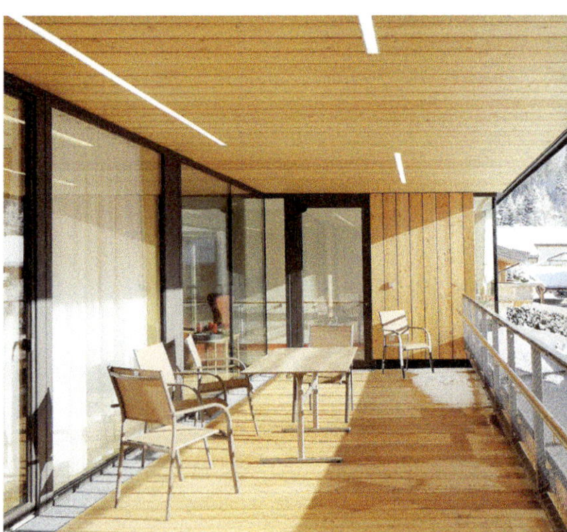

Figure B12. Encourage transactional indoor and outdoor connections. Courtesy of Atelier Zündel Cristea, Paris, France; courtesy of René Rissland.

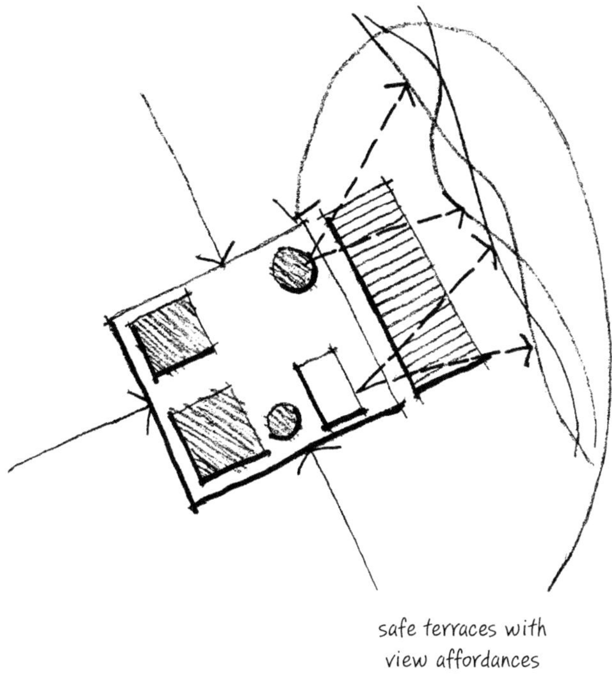

Figure B13. Provide safe, protected roof terraces. Drawing by Stephen Verderber.

4c. Horticultural Therapy

Eighteenth- and nineteenth-century convents, orphanages, and alms-houses often featured gardens maintained by a full-time groundskeeper who often resided on-site.[68] This was the case at the motherhouse of the Grey Nuns, in Montreal, Quebec, built in 1869. Gardening on the grounds of LTC residences is now referred to as *horticultural therapy* (HT). Timeless benefits of HT include providing respite, witnessing vegetation grow and flourish, and offering a locus for social interaction. And P-R behaviors (see section 3c) are an equally integral aspect of this type of indoor/outdoor therapy. Gardening also provides food to consume on-site or sell in the local market, or simply is a means to draw people together in a daily, seasonal, or year-round activities. Since opportunities for intergenerational participation are few and far between in most of today's eldercare facilities, HT allows friends and family opportunities to feel like real stakeholders in the larger LTC experience. Platform gardens and vegetable gardens are usually preferred for a unit housing ten to fifteen residents. For the relatively ambulatory and able bodied, standing and kneeling may still be possible without difficulty, although the physical range of movement for the wheelchair bound may be quite limited. For them, raised or platform gardening, whether in a greenhouse or an open-air garden, provides excellent access to N-L and allows the individual to self- plant, self-water, and self-weed plants from a stationary seated position. Platform garden plots, with equipment storage space in close proximity, are therapeutically similar in many ways to art therapy or occupational therapy. Provide seating nearby for periodic rests and socialization, allowing effective press-competency rebalancing. Design a hierarchy of HT opportunities with a main centralized garden supplemented by additional rooftop garden plots, perhaps one per semiautonomous residence. This decentralized network of microgardens can begin at grade level and extend to the uppermost roof terrace level. A rooftop (or ground-level) winter garden / greenhouse can function as the centerpiece of this lattice of spaces. These amenities have been identified in the evidence-based literature as fostering intergenerationality, allowing residents' children and grandchildren to partake on-site in gardening.[69] **2b; 3b; 4d; 4e; 5b; 5e; 6c; 7f**

4d. Multiple Outdoor Destinations

The COVID-19 pandemic brought to the forefront one particularly glaring shortcoming of many LTC facilities. The residents' confinement indoors throughout the height of the pandemic became a form of acute sensory deprivation. Without any opportunity to walk or be moved via wheelchair to outdoor destination points on-site or beyond, the adverse outcome was often environmental stress. Outdoor destination points provide multiple opportunities for attention restoration, greater cognitive clarity, lower rates of depression, and reduced rates of loneliness and isolation.[70] They can also have a positive influence on indicators of residents' physiologic stress levels: pulse rates, diastolic pressure, and degree of physical stamina.[71] It makes little sense to provide these amenities, however, unless physically accessible and visible from the interior, so residents can be aware of the existence of multiple outdoor exit options. A safe, protected garden can be but one of numerous outdoor destination points designed to be relatively easily accessible via a network of paths and ramps. Other destination points might include a fountain or a small pond, protected by railings with seating nearby; a gazebo; outdoor works of art; and multiple small-scale *landmarks* inviting residents to seek them out. Of course, the individual must be physically able to move about from points A to B to C and beyond without having to negotiate an excessively difficult set of obstacles, such

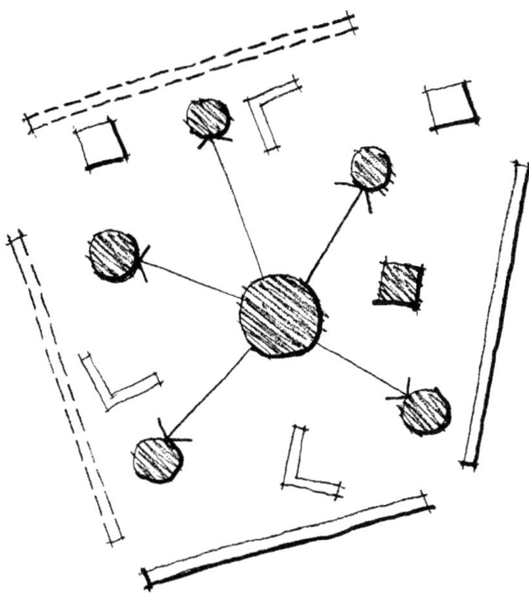

Figure B14. Provide coordinated outdoor destination points. Drawing by Stephen Verderber.

as a staircase or overly sloped ramp. Position these multiple destination nodes and landmarks in close proximity to one another and not too distant from the main building, with residents having the option to experience just one node without necessarily having to encounter all the others along the same path. Buffer these nodes from extraneous noise and visual distractions. Illuminate them—like an important civic landmark, such as a fountain, only on a smaller scale—especially within the wandering garden. Perimeter walls and fences should have *soft* boundaries, so individuals can safely remain within a strictly prescribed surveillance area, with their behaviorally warranted movements observable on CCTV monitors (fig. B14).[72] **1e; 2b; 3b; 3c; 4c; 5a; 5b; 5e**

4e. Ecological Stewardship

Long-term care residences are environmental polluters, with their toxic wastes typically ending up in the local landfill. It no longer suffices to hide behind elaborate public relations pronouncements while still eschewing ecological best practices. Many opportunities exist to do better—heritage buildings retrofitted for use as LTC facilities; pilot projects for total campus waste recycling programs; and sustainable land use best practices, such as on-site water retention (cisterns) and microgardening. Organizational and public policy leadership in environmental stewardship can help eradicate toxic chemicals from a local community's water supply and biological food chain. In North America, the LEED (Leadership through Energy Efficient Environmental Design)-affiliated "Green Guide for Health Care" began in 2002 as a joint effort between Health Care without Harm and the Center for Maximum Potential Building Systems.[73] It is a point-based metrics system for rating ecological performance, closely paralleling the mainstream LEED-certification rating program. In the UK, some years ago the National Health Service initiated an assessment tool called NEAT (National Emergency Access Target) for all its new construction and renovation projects and actively works to foster ecologically sustainable best practices. Similar equitably distributed ecological stewardship efforts are needed in medically underserved communities in North America and elsewhere. In the US, Catawba Hospital, a state-run psychiatric facility in Virginia, recently completed an extensive retrofitting of its large rural campus. All twenty-one buildings were retrofitted, including the buildings' HVAC systems, and the campus's central chilled water plant was replaced with a new, highly energy-efficient unit. This yielded significant energy savings by reducing the campus's total electrical power consumption, resulting in a corresponding decrease in the overall physical plant's annual operating costs.[74] This is but one recent example of the value of corresponding public- and private-sector partnering for greater ecological stewardship and responsibility. 3c; 4h; 6d; 8a–8h

4f. Natural and Mechanical Ventilation

The coronavirus pandemic underlined the medical importance of maintaining 24/7, proper natural and mechanical ventilation in LTC homes. The disproportionately high number of fatalities in improperly ventilated facilities reached a crisis level, although the seeds for this disaster were planted decades ago. Why was this facility-based oversight allowed to persist? Without adequate personal distancing measures, it became impossible to control the person-to-person transmission of COVID-19 in these eldercare residences. The myriad problems associated with overcrowded bedrooms, personal hygiene rooms, and social activity areas (such as dayrooms and dining rooms) became stressors for everyone, causing discomfort and, in the extreme, acute levels of residents' agitation. These built-environment shortcomings still manifest daily in many hundreds of older LTC homes, especially in eldercare residences built prior to 1990.[75] Eldercare residences with inoperable or poor-condition windows, inadequate HVAC systems, no mechanical air conditioning whatsoever, and insufficient numbers of negative pressure rooms constitute a serious ongoing health threat. Negative pressure rooms have been proven to help in combating infectious disease transmission, as the air pressure distributed within these rooms is lower than the air pressure outside.[76] When the door is opened, potentially contaminated air or allied toxic particulates will not flow outside the room into adjacent uncontaminated spatial zones. Instead, uncontaminated air will flow into the negatively pressurized room. Contaminated air is removed and filtrated (for purification) before being expelled to the outside the building envelope. Continuously monitor ambient temperatures and humidity levels, since excessive airflow rates can create drafts, causing discomfort and agitation among residents and, especially, persons with dementia.[77] There are four types of isolation rooms: class 5 (air pressure level), class P (positive air pressure), class N (negative air pressure), and class Q (quarantine). This typology should be comparatively assessed with respect to the planning and architectural design of an LTC residence. **1f; 2a; 2b; 4g; 5c; 5d; 7e**

4g. Theraserialization

The modernist architect Richard Neutra's (1892–1970) professional practice spanned five decades. Neutra's private residential commissions in Southern California pioneered the concept of rational transparency by means of meticulously composed indoor/outdoor spatial relationships—full-height windows, ample natural ventilation and daylight, inventive use of natural building materials, and unobstructed views. His unbuilt proposal in the 1930s for a hospital in Los Angeles expressed this same therapeutic amenity by providing patients with direct exposure to nature, as every inpatient room would be equipped with its own private outdoor balcony. Similarly, design strategies are available to provide direct exposure to and immersion in N-L in the contemporary LTC residence, and this can give the resident greater N-L agency. The evidence-based health-design literature points to the therapeutic value of architectural and landscape design strategies maximizing two-way visual and sensory/spatial transparency.[78] By contrast, psychologically and physically windowless spaces have empirically been associated with occupants' sensory deprivation and their corresponding decline in health status. And such suboptimal conditions are of particular concern with respect to the cognitively impaired. Health policies and design strategies that establish a multisensory interior space, connected with nature, draw natural light and fresh air into the building envelope. Theraserialization (see chapter 4 for a more in-depth discussion) is achievable both horizontally and vertically without restricting it to the ground level of a residence. Terraces, setbacks, cutouts, extended eaves, recesses, light wells, atria, skylights, clerestories, and splayed axes collectively allow the building to *therapeutically breathe*. Natural daylight, windows with views to the world beyond, and well-thought-out axial sightlines promote heightened navigational wayfinding behaviors, simultaneously reducing occurrences of agitation, especially among residents with dementia and related cognitive deficits.[79] Inventive applications of this strategy of theraserialization in architecture for health care also holds promise in countering sensory deprivation in midrise LTC facilities necessarily limited by their restrictive sites. In general, theraserialized design strategies emphasize single-loaded corridors affording full visibility of perhaps an adjacent exterior courtyard and ancillary outdoor spaces, allowing unobstructed views beyond, providing the resident with heightened personal agency. **1b; 2b; 3a; 3d; 4f; 5d; 5e; 7c**

4h. Habitat Conservation

A recent report by the World Wildlife Fund documents the dramatically declining status of the world's biospecies in the Anthropocene. The 2024 iteration of the biennial *Living Planet Report* noted a 73 percent decline in vertebrate populations from 1972 to 2020, warning that if current trends persist, the world will permanently lose tens of thousands of species.[80] The clear-cutting of Amazon rainforests (which, in 2020, set a record for total destruction), massive oceanic overfishing, and other destructive worst practices have made it imperative to rebalance habitat/species conservation with ecological best building practices, including land development priorities, ecological conservation, and reclaimed-site restoration priorities. This rebalancing must be compassionate and health equitable, supporting the demographic realities of aging populations around the world. *How* and *what* we build for older persons is equally as important as *where* we build. Whenever possible, in the process of selecting a building site, explore multiple configuration footprints and comparatively ascertain the merits and shortcomings of each. In the earliest phase of the LTC facility procurement process, examine circular, biaxial, rectangular, pointillistic, raised platform, and linear footprints for these 24/7 residential care buildings. Make a reasonable effort to reclaim a previously paved-over, formerly abandoned site and work to restore its intrinsic natural, ecological agency.[81] Work to conserve and preserve. When tree cutting is unavoidable, replant soon thereafter and continue to add further complimentary landscaping elements, thus contributing to the critical function of natural vegetation in absorbing carbon dioxide. The release of oxygen through photosynthesis acts as a natural air filter, stores carbon, and helps in mitigating global warming while improving air quality. **6d; 8b; 8a–8h**

5. CIRCULATION AND NAVIGATION

5a. Wayfinding

Over 5 million persons in the US suffer from some stage of dementia, and in Canada more than 747,000 live with Alzheimer's disease or a related cognitive disorder.[82] Worldwide, at least 55.2 million persons over age 60 live with dementia—a disease that is now a global health concern.[83] With so many people now living longer, the need for comprehendible architectural environments has never been more urgent. In North America alone, thousands of *memory care units* are expected to be established by renovated existing LTC homes, together with hundreds of newly built, 100 percent specialized *memory care–only residences*. In either scenario, these individuals will experience considerable difficulty in navigating their everyday physical environment. Currently, many LTC homes are deficient in the degree of wayfinding support they provide, because they are sensorily monotonous; physically unsafe, due to unnecessary barriers; and difficult to decipher, due to poor or nonexistent directional signage. Their internal circulation is confusing, with low overall spatial legibility. Redundant cueing has been an applied design strategy for more than forty years in these physical settings, to improve occupants' spatial wayfinding and ameliorate otherwise difficult-to-navigate architectural conditions.[84] This strategy consists of encoding the built environment with clearly legible, interpretable landmarks, indoor and exterior circulation paths, destination points, clearly marked edges, and safe vantage points. Differentiated materials and varied surface colors and textures have been proven to ease internal and external site navigation—for example, a floor surface patterned with color-coded materials demarcating the various internal circulation zones; recessed bedroom door thresholds along corridors in residential units; legible numerical room identification, whether during the day or at night; safe staircases; ramps; and color-differentiated floor, wall, and ceiling surfaces.[85]

An effective wayfinding measure is to create single-loaded corridors (versus the windowless double-loaded corridors in nursing homes of the past), thereby allowing the residents to more easily orient/reorient (cognitively reset) relative to spatial navigation. Single-loaded corridors are now supplemented with audio sounds and messages—triggered, for instance, by moving through a door threshold movement sensor. Multisensory assistive measures such as this help counter memory loss by allowing residents to retain a degree of mastery over their immediate physical environment.[86] And this palette of tech-assists is growing: AI and smart-house technologies now anticipatorily communicate with residents through triggered robotic functions, audio prompts, and face-recognition technology, potentially providing further assistive navigational support. Nonetheless, assistive spatial navigational technologies are currently not anticipated to ever fully replace human-to-human contact in 24/7 custodial care settings. **1b; 1e; 1f; 4d; 5b; 5c; 5d; 5e**

5b. Controlled Wandering

Stories abound of dementia wanderers who became lost and disoriented after having absconded from their home or institutional care residence, and subsequently die from an automobile accident or other adverse event. Even within the LTC residence and its grounds, wandering behavior can be a stressful responsibility for the caregiver staff.[87] Wandering poses a high risk for an individual who may inadvertently stroll away from the facility unchaperoned, perhaps seeking return to a locale remembered from the past, such as a workplace, a former home and neighborhood, or some other destination. Serial wanderers engage in this behavior to relieve their restlessness and agitation. While it is important to support self-dignity, freedom of choice, and freedom of movement, this must be tempered, channeled in a safe manner by means of protected wandering gardens and paths, spaces that have become widely incorporated into LTC residences in recent years.[88] This consist of at least one controlled outdoor wandering path with clearly demarcated and secure interior and exterior physical boundaries—locked doors, gates, and security systems for 24/7 visual monitoring. These spaces are designed with safe surfaces and features and often include protection from the elements vis-à-vis projecting roof eaves, ample indoor

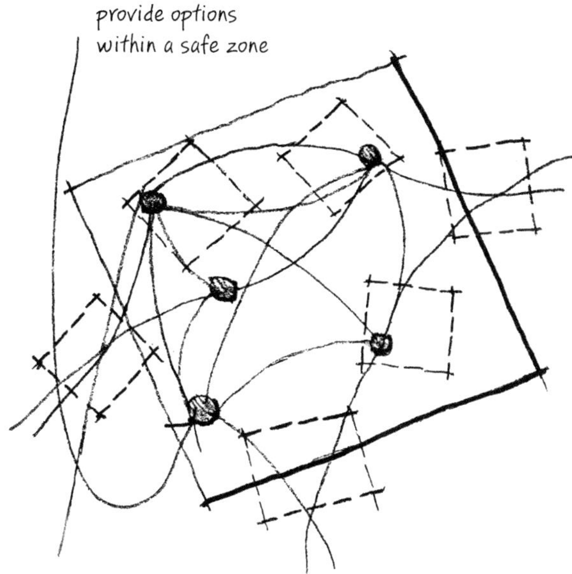

Figure B15. Design effective controls to prevent unsupervised wandering. Drawing by Stephen Verderber.

and outdoor lighting, and assistive technology, such as movement monitors. These amenities can encourage physical activity outdoors, allowing the residents to self-select their level of N-L immersion, which is further reinforced through horticultural therapy activities in or adjacent to the wandering garden, such as in a year-round winter garden or greenhouse. Unsanctioned physical movements can be unobtrusively monitored with assistive technology (see section 5a). Long staircases and irregular, steeply sloping surfaces and paths are a potential source of stress and agitation and only discourage prospect-refuge-seeking behaviors during controlled wandering sessions outdoors.[89] In sum, effective multisensory design strategies revolve around encouraging independence and personal autonomy outdoors in a safe, protected space, in a manner that fosters attention restoration (see chapter 4). Inventive redundant cueing and related navigational measures facilitates more adroit cognitive spatial orientation in interior and exterior wandering (fig. B15).[90] **4b; 4c; 4d; 5e; 7a; 7b; 7c**

5c. Programmatic Decompression

The modernist dictum "form follows function" drove the machine-for-healing hospital and the architecture of skilled nursing institutions in North America between 1946 and 1980. Spartan surroundings were predominant during this period—overwhelmingly minimalist, both aesthetically and function-ally. Quality of life dimensions of 24/7 custodial care in post-war nursing homes were frequently reduced to a prescriptive set of behavioral activities and rituals—work, sleep, eat, hygiene, rest, and so on—reductive behav-iors whose twentieth-century origins were traceable to the Staatliches Bauhaus (1919–1933) post-secondary design school in Dessau, Germany, commonly known as the Bauhaus. Many faculty and students in residence at the Bauhaus prior to Hitler's forced shutdown would rise to international prominence overseas as architects, industrial designers, and artists in the postwar decades. The reductive nature of the Bauhaus's educational ped-agogy yielded functional briefs that were translated and adopted in the planning and design of post-war custodial care nursing.

The essential elements of day-to-day life in these nursing homes became strictly utilitarian: monochromacy in interior circulation arteries; spatial restrictiveness, with not one square foot wasted; and pervasive aesthetic and functional indistinctiveness. These institutions often looked like they were designed and built as place to put society's *warehoused invalids*. By contrast, today a compassionate, therapeutically designed LTC residence and its N-L environs is free to express a homelike residential atmosphere.[91] Its architecture extends freely beyond a set of reductive, pro-grammatically and spatially compressed functional requirements. The rejec-tion of this institutionality is what guided the Maggie Keswick Foundation in developing the mission statement for its network of Maggie's Centres in the UK and elsewhere (see chapter 4 and appendix A). This document is a philosophical and pragmatic guide, extoling the virtues of *programmatic decompression* where the therapeutic amenity of informal, *in-between* inte-rior and exterior spaces is celebrated architecturally and viewed as equally important to other programmatically required rooms.

Informal as well as more formal (conventional) room types and their appointments are discussed in the Maggie's Centres functional brief. The high priority placed on the provision of in-between spaces resonates through the lens of prospect-refuge theory. This same thinking needs to be applied to LTC residences by designing numerous programmati-cally decompressed informal nodes and pockets throughout—including recessed, semisequestered seating alcoves, dining areas, and places to read or just chill that are aesthetically interesting yet universally accessible and navigable by persons with cognitive impairments (fig. B16).[92] **1b; 1e; 1f; 4g; 5d; 6a**

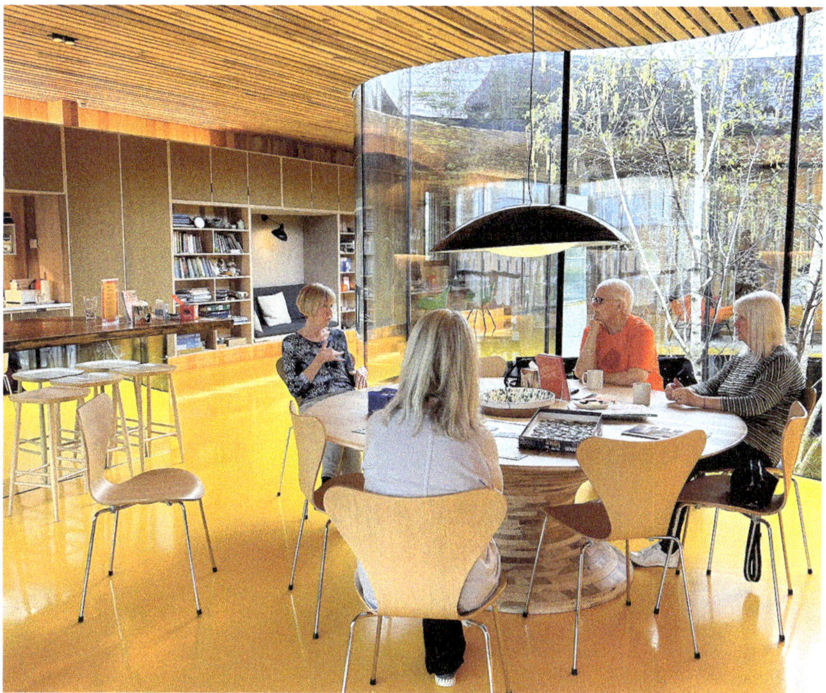

Figure B16. In-between spaces that *breathe* support cognitive respite. Photo by Stephen Verderber.

5d. Single-Loaded Circulation in the Residential Unit

Throughout the history of film, Hollywood has crafted and solidified negative stereotypes of hospitals, psychiatric asylums, and nursing homes, dramatizing their architecturally dehumanizing, restrictive conditions in film.[93] Scenes in *The Lost Weekend* (1945), *Shock Corridor* (1963), *The Godfather* (1972), *One Flew Over the Cuckoo's Nest* (1975), *Flatliners* (1999), *Girl Interrupted* (1999), *Lost in Translation* (2003), *Outbreak* (2004), *The Immigrant* (2015), and many other films featured archetypal, forbidding double-loaded corridors, symbolizing the utter inhumanity of institutionalization.[94] Where does the term *double-loaded* come from? It likely originated as a metaphorical reference to an unbroken row of rooms flanking either side of a common circulation path, or perhaps the double barrels of a shotgun. To this day, the long, narrow rowhouses in New Orleans are described as single- or double-loaded building types—a shot could pass through the entire house front to back, without hitting a wall because the bullet could pass through all doorways unimpeded. The process of programmatically decoupling the two rows of rooms flanking a common corridor in health care architecture began in earnest in the late 1990s in psychiatric treatment centers, hospices, and progressively designed LTC residences in Scandinavia and Asia. This alternative approach to achieving greater spatial openness to N-L content was not really new, because the thirty-two public Kirkbride insane asylums built in the US throughout the late nineteenth century (and much-copied elsewhere) featured single-loaded inpatient units that drew natural daylight and fresh air directly into every corridor and patient bedroom. These Kirkbride asylums have long since been thoroughly debunked as a building type for myriad reasons, although the practice of designing single-loaded LTC residential units has returned, for much the same reason: the ability to expose occupants to N-L affordances, including natural ventilation and daylight. Moreover, these environmental attributes are similar to theraserialization (see chapter 4 and above). The process of decoupling—eliminating one side of a corridor—yields more open visual and spatial N-L interior/exterior relationships.[95] An early contemporary example of this once-lost and now rediscovered design strategy was the Corinne Dolan Alzheimer Center (1988) in Ohio, with its pair of triangulated residential wings and a dayroom at the center (fig. B17). **1b; 1d; 1e; 1f; 5a; 7b; 7c; 7e**

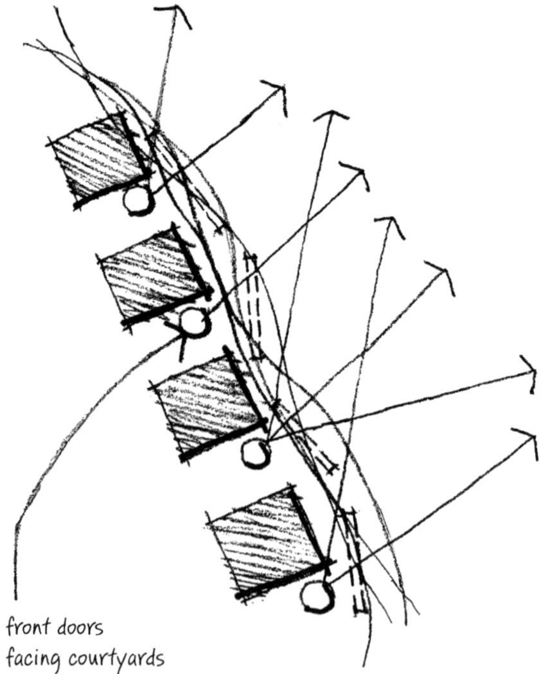

Figure B17. Single-loaded circulation arteries in residential units. Drawing by Stephen Verderber.

5e. Universal Accessibility

Universality denotes having the freedom of choice to participate in everyday activities of daily living without fear of stigmas or age discrimination. The strategy of universal design (UD) seeks to seamlessly and unobtrusively support this larger purpose.[96] Currently, there are three types of UD accommodations. *Accessible supports* are separate functional amenities, such as directly visible and usable wheelchair ramps for persons with physical limitations, thus fulfilling minimum building code requirements at the local, state, and federal levels. *Adaptable supports* are physical amenities that remain concealed or otherwise hidden (until needed) with adjustable or portable assistive technology amenities in response to an individual's specific physical and cognitive abilities. *Transgenerational design* is when a built environment is constructed from the outset to fully support a broad range of anticipated physical and sensory deficits commonly experienced across the life/aging spectrum, including associated losses of sensory and physical abilities. Support amenities include power-assisted doors, windows, and window treatments; chair lifts; lighting options; and fiber optics.[97]

Provide accessible and operable fixed and electronically or manually adjustable personal hygiene amenities—smart grab bars, adaptable fixtures, roll-in showers, and redundant cued audio alerts. With respect to physical ambulation amenities, UD calls for no uneven edges or steps, consistent riser and tread dimensions on stairs, and landings midway between the different stories in a building. Food preparation areas include adjustable-height kitchen counters, color-contrasted surfaces and material textures for the visually impaired, audio-tactile sensors, accessible ovens, and microwaves with adjacent countertops. Think of UD design strategies as a seamless continuum of physical environment affordances beginning with the resident's bedroom, extending throughout the entire building and campus, into the neighborhood, and beyond into the broader community (fig. B18). **2a; 2b; 2c; 2d; 3c; 3d; 4c; 5a; 5b**

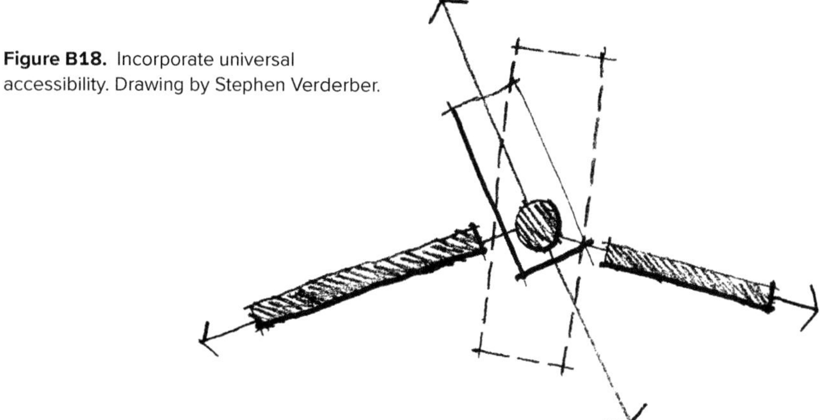

Figure B18. Incorporate universal accessibility. Drawing by Stephen Verderber.

6. SUPPORT AMENITIES

6a. Maximize Caregiver and Family Supports

During COVID-19, the administrators of many LTC homes were chastised for the substandard conditions their staff and residents endured. These facilities lacked the adequate physical space required for PPE storage and minimum personal distancing requirements (at least 6 feet of physical separation) and were unable to simultaneously provide sufficient space for the residents' and staff's prospect-refuge behaviors, with their role in minimizing infection transmission rates. With so little physical space available for built-environment support amenities to relieve the stresses caused by the coronavirus pandemic, unforeseen challenges arose. Prolonged lockdowns, lasting months (if not years), combined with high infection rates, made it difficult, if not impossible, for family members and friends to visit. As the pandemic wore on, with facility lockdowns frequently extended for indefinite periods, residents began to feel ever more disconnected and isolated. They were cut off from contact with the outside world, except for their direct caregivers who were able to come and go. This resulted in heightened social withdrawal, agitation behaviors, loneliness, and depression, in addition to the pandemic's increased mortality rates.[98] Spatial compression caused by too little caregiver and family support space, combined with effects of the lockdowns on them and on residents made it difficult for overworked caregivers and, especially, family members to feel connected.

Overcrowding is mentally unhealthy, and especially when the presence of caregivers and families is restrained or cut off entirely.[99] Space provided to obtain respite and social interactions, if equitably available to both caregivers and families, can close this gap. Alcoves, window seats, terraces, balconies, patios, multipurpose rooms, breakout meeting and consult rooms, breakrooms, kitchens, and storerooms for equipment and supplies provide assistive support for staff and family members.[100] In Australia, family-sized communal sleepover rooms are provided on-site in recently built hospitals for the families of Indigenous patients, if they elect to spend multiple days there, because the daily travel distances back home can be extreme (fig. B19). **3c; 3d; 4a; 5e; 6c**

6b. Artificial Intelligence and Long-Term Care

Machine learning–based artificial intelligence is evolving haphazardly, and its quick ascendance is raising vexing questions. There is room for

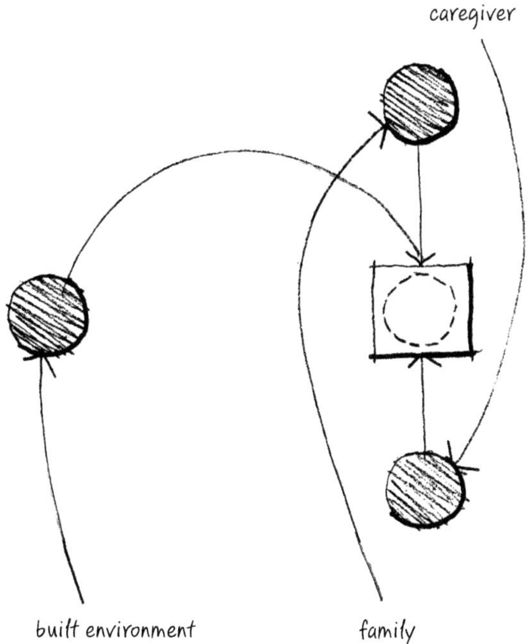

Figure B19. Equitably provide caregiver and family support amenities. Drawing by Stephen Verderber.

deep skepticism. Machine-learning technologies harvest vast quantities of existing information using highly complex algorithms. It is yielding major advances in computation and impacting our everyday lives—for better or worse.[101] Barriers to its further adoption in the everyday lives of older persons, whether in institutional care settings or otherwise, include data-source access restrictions associated with patient confidentiality laws, which disallow data harvesting. Other restrictions include limitations from industry-wide investment regulatory laws, private investor groups' mistrust of AI, and misaligned incentives between the public and private sectors. Perhaps most threatening is the fear that AI will destroy the livelihoods of health care professionals in key specialties, minimizing their degree of agency. It is already casting radiologists, among other specialists, out of work.

Without guardrails, AI's adverse impacts threaten current procedural, ethical, and legal norms. Regarding its architectural ramifications, it will undoubtedly have an impact on older persons' daily lives. Prosthetic technologies and universally designed smart houses already track navigational movements and incorporate informational triggers that allow a building, room, or outdoor space to be encoded to "speak" to the occupant/user (see section 5a). AI-assisted redundant cueing triggers provide assistance to a person approaching a staircase, door threshold, or other potentially pressing (challenging) condition. They can alert the individual to, say, an excessively bright room or one too dark to navigate safely. AI algorithms are comparatively assessing structural deformation probabilities; the deformational properties of complex, environmentally friendly materials and construction; and solar radiation penetration levels into any building envelope. They also predictably assess the building occupants' spatial movements. *Assistive design modeling* involves machine-learned systems that, within milliseconds, routinely comparatively assess dozens (if not hundreds) of architectural and site landscaping design solutions virtually simultaneously.[102] **3c; 5a; 5b; 5e; 7f; 8a–8h**

6c. Intergenerationality

Equitably designed intergenerational housing heightens older persons' well-being and health status by reinforcing their personal and collective agency.[103] In Canada, the British Columbia–based Happipad company successfully connects seniors, living independently in their longtime homes independently, seek more social contact and additional income with younger tenants looking for more-affordable housing options in the community.[104] This is just one adaptive housing strategy with intergenerational promise. Purpose-built intergenerational housing already exists in Calgary, Canada, where assisted, long-term, and palliative care housing is integrated within a single multigenerational setting. Similar cooperative living arrangements currently being built across Canada point to the many benefits of older persons living with and generally being closer to family members and others who may previously have been strangers, as well as being able care for grandchildren in a shared dwelling. These best practices promote normative domestic lifestyles, functioning as protective buffers against the adverse physical and emotional impacts of aging—loneliness, depression, physical ailments with inadequate social or medical support networks, the onset of frailty, and death.[105] Given the reality of the housing unaffordability crisis in much of North America, a complete rethinking is overdue regarding housing innovations for older persons and how these new options can best support the growing interest in intergenerational living arrangements—including scenarios where older persons reside in the LTC residence as part of shared-site multigenerational housing complexes. Until the current housing crisis can be rectified, elderhousing options are expected to only

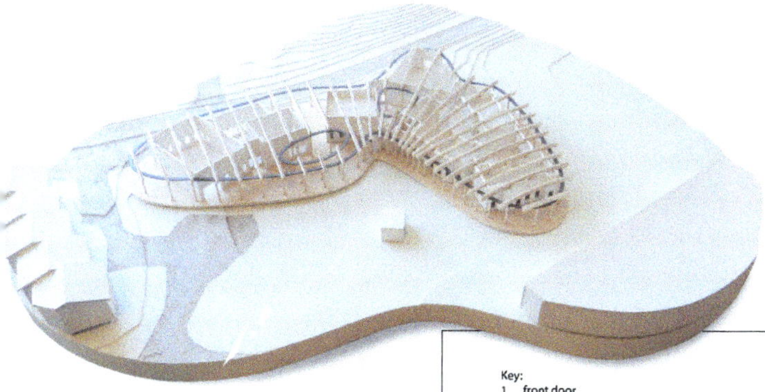

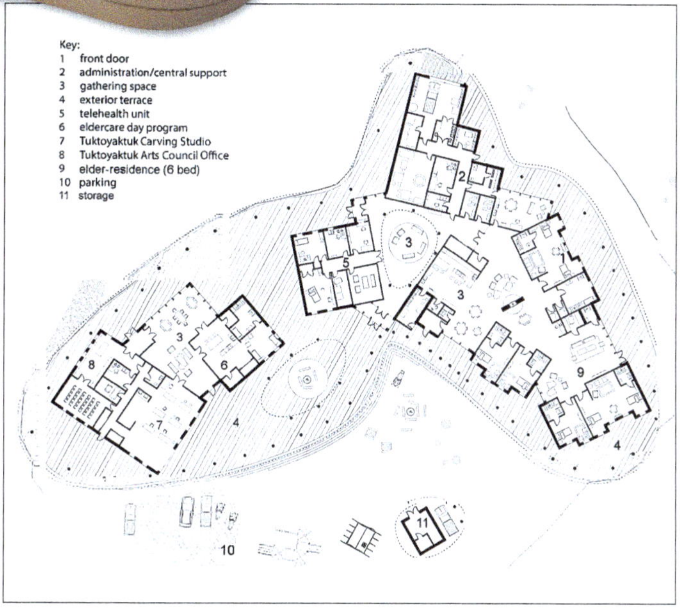

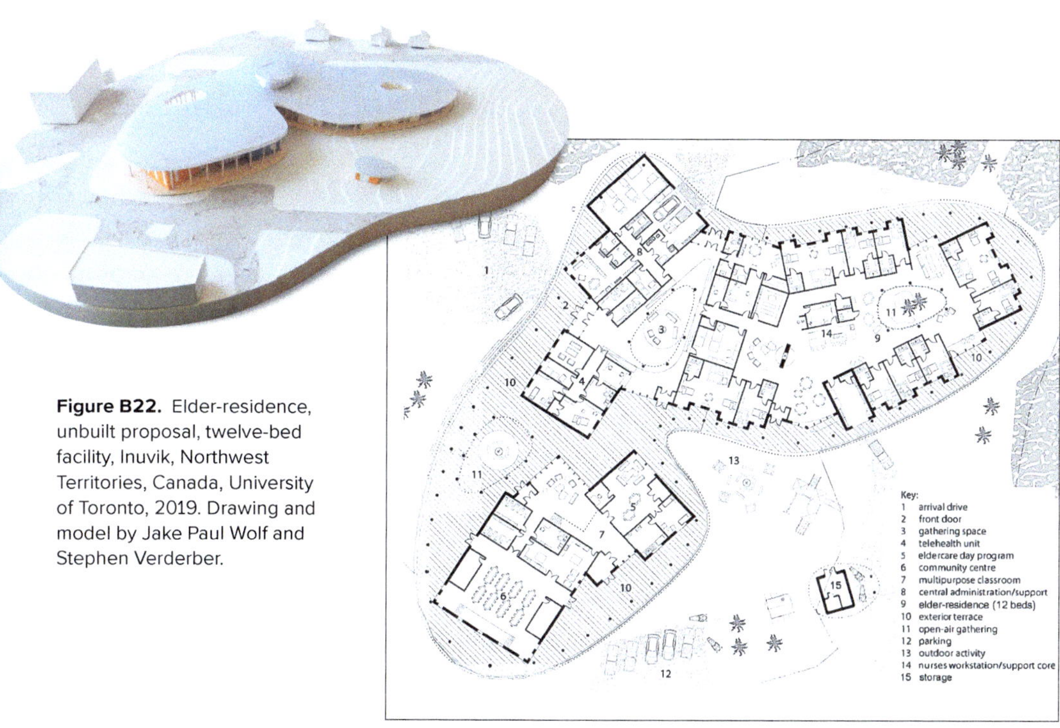

Figure B21. Elder-residence, unbuilt proposal, six-bed facility, Tuktoyaktuk and Aklavik, Northwest Territories, Canada, University of Toronto, 2019. Drawing and model by Jake Paul Wolf and Stephen Verderber.

Figure B22. Elder-residence, unbuilt proposal, twelve-bed facility, Inuvik, Northwest Territories, Canada, University of Toronto, 2019. Drawing and model by Jake Paul Wolf and Stephen Verderber.

6e. Avoid Forced Relocation

Is it ethical to force more than one hundred residents of an LTC home to relocate if there is nowhere for them to move? This is exactly what happened in the case of the Cedarvale Terrace LTC home in Toronto, Canada in 2025. This residence, licensed for 150 beds, was built in the days when they were still called nursing homes. It opened in 1973 in the Forest Hill section of Toronto. In 2022 a clever developer bought the land and building, intending to demolish this 1970s nursing home and construct a nineteen-level luxury condo tower.[111] A local architect hired by the developer conducted a "feasibility study" proclaiming the facility to be obsolete and wholly unworthy of renovation. Meanwhile, Toronto's City Planning Office appeared to be indifferent to the plight of Cedarvale's residents, claiming the developer possessed the full legal right to demolish the building and squash its provincially granted LTC bed licenses. One problem, however, was the Province of Ontario's wait list at the time, with more than 39,000 people who needed placement in an LTC home ASAP within the province. How could the community afford to lose 150 licensed beds when the provincial Ministry of Long-Term Care was urgently trying to build 30,000 new beds by 2030? Expectedly, the residents and their families were completely shut out of any serious consultation discussions on the possibility of saving Cedarvale Terrace. The adverse impacts of the forced relocation of these

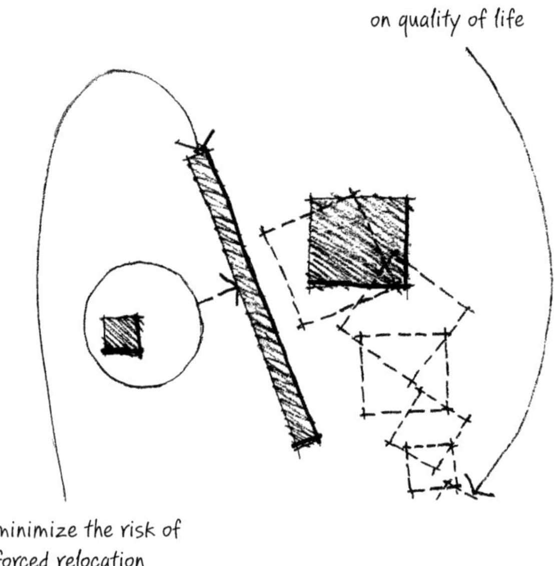

Figure B23. Advocate for non-forced relocation policies. Drawing by Stephen Verderber.

and other nursing home residents has been well known since the 1960s, when geriatric patients were forcibly moved from the back wards of old hospitals into newly built modernist nursing homes, without any family input whatsoever. This resulted in higher mortality rates among the relocated, a practice that unfortunately still continues.[112] But need it be this way? Public health policymakers in some locales are taking steps to rectify this potentially deadly "worst practice."[113] Alternatively, hold a series of pre-planning-stage consultations that involve *all* of the key stakeholders. Lend credence to their collective agency, carefully listening to and, where possible, accommodating/balancing this input. Genuinely address the concerns and priorities of local planning boards, developers, grassroots eldercare community advocates, LTC home operators, impacted residents and families, and the to-be-impacted (post-move) local community, because NIMBYism remains alive and well when it comes to institutionally based housing for older persons (fig. B23).[114] **6a; 8a–8h**

7. SENSORY AND ENVIRONMENTAL SUPPORTS

7a. Differentiated Surfaces and Materials

Injurious falls are a continuing major health risk among older persons. In the US, one in three people aged 65 or older falls at least once per year, and many of these falls occur at home. Fall frequency increases to one in two persons per year for those over 80 years of age. Worldwide, adults over 70, particularly females, have a significantly higher fall-induced mortality rate than younger people.[115] The severity of fall-related adverse outcomes increases with age. The most common are head injuries, severe fractures, and the onset post-fall anxiety disorders. Most fall victims experience multiple physical and sensory deficits over time—impaired eyesight, physical immobility, hearing loss, tactile insensitivity, olfactory-sense loss, and complicating comorbidities—with a high risk of the onset of additional frailty, and even death. This compounded adverse health status results in considerable difficulty in deciphering and navigating architecturally pressing physical features in the everyday physical environment. Panic sets in about venturing beyond one's immediate home turf into the outside world, for fear of falling again. This causes additional debilitating, compounded consequences for the individual, resulting in isolation, depression, social withdrawal, and further physical inactivity. The importance of nonpressing, redundant-cued architectural forms and spaces cannot be overemphasized. These support measures include the presence of signage at the bedroom door threshold (reinforcing who and where one is) and carefully synchronized colors schemes, together with distinctive surface materials, lighting switches on walls, emergency pull cords, and carefully transitioned floor surfaces, thereby making it easier to navigate a rapid transition from tile to carpet in a poorly lit corridor. More specifically, avoid abrupt transitions from carpet to wood or to a tiled floor. This helps to reinforce sensory/ambulatory orientation. Other design measures include multicued directional graphics, with room identification; varied colors and compositional forms; stairs with color-highlighted treads and risers; and adequate lighting levels to illuminate all interior surfaces day and night. Avoid overly stimulating, potentially confusing design strategies—where too much is happening, requiring many rapid decisions—as this can be off-putting, causing cognitive disequilibrium. Avoid "blind" staircases, sudden level changes, and confusing indoor and outdoor corridors. Place a high priority on the design of interior walls, provide varied ceiling heights, as well as color-coded flooring at bedroom door thresholds and entrances to other highly used rooms. Install motion sensors that trigger audio cues as one approach potentially dangerous spaces, such as a staircase, the edge of a balcony, and other architectural conditions that may otherwise pose undue physical and psychological risk. For example, provide extendable grab bars and related assistive devices in bathroom/shower units, and emergency pull cords located on the walls next to the commode, shower, and sink fixtures (fig. B24).[116] **2a; 3a; 4d; 5a; 5d; 5e; 7b; 7c; 7e**

7b. Eliminate Institutional Cues

Project a positive first impression.[117] A carefully designed front door to a private residence symbolically extends a welcoming hand outward, inviting one in.[118] Similarly, inviting exterior spaces and features on the grounds convey a positive, noninstitutional image as one approaches the front door. When a prospective resident and one's family members first arrive, they should not be put off by any image-based semblance of institutionality. This may sound obvious, but the fiscal pressures are immense to make these places too large by cramming too many beds into a single building. In stark contrast, recent evidence-based research on this issue strongly points to impersonally scaled facilities as far less preferred, compared with comparatively small-scaled LTC residential facilities. Unfortunately, entrenched

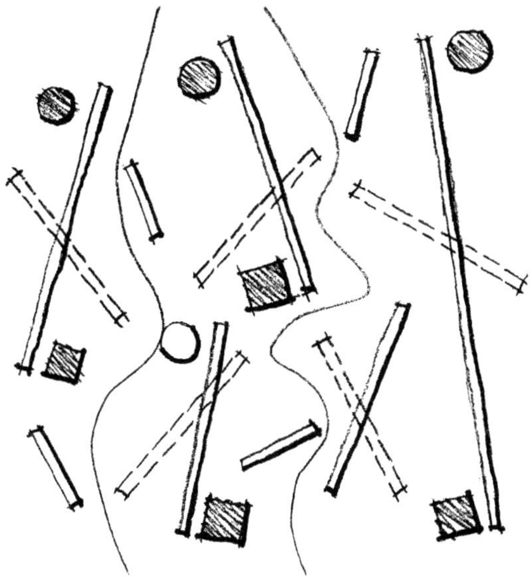

Figure B24. Design for differentiated interior surfaces, including ceilings. Drawing by Stephen Verderber.

governmental bureaucracies, competing financial interests, persistently outdated building codes, pressure to reduce construction costs, high land values, land scarcity, inflation, supply chain issues, and bed overdensification frequently result in architectural mistakes. With the architectural profession not at the table early on when health policies are set, this is when the original design intent can become obliterated amid a cornucopia of conflicting interests. Nonetheless—and this cannot be overemphasized—this *institutionalization syndrome* can be avoided if clients, when working closely with their architectural and landscape design team, respect the team's agency. Work with associated governmental oversight agencies from the outset, establishing clear protocols and performance metrics. *Otherwise, the architect's hands risk being tied before a project even begins*. This can easily happen during a project's earliest scoping phase, prior to the site planning, programming, and schematic design. And it can also happen during construction. The elimination of counterproductive facility institutionalization begins with a shared bold vision to reinvent this building type, starting with breaking down its massiveness and its excessive bed capacities.[119] Work towards adopting compassionate, equitable design strategies in creating a village-like atmosphere composed of residentially scaled compositional elements—semiautonomous *houses*—within a smaller-scaled microcampus setting that features effective navigational wayfinding and high levels of multisensory legibility and comprehensibility. A 24/7 custodial care setting that projects a poor architectural image on first impression faces an uphill challenge. (fig. B25). **1b; 2c; 3a; 4f; 5a; 5c; 7c; 7e**

7c. Dynamic and Diffused Light/Lighting

Our circadian rhythms (CRs) function on an approximately twenty-four-hour rhythmic cycle, controlled by the brain's suprachiasmatic nucleus, located in the hypothalamus of the brain. CRs are controlled/governed mainly by natural and artificial light.[120] The duration of one's exposure to these light sources, their intensity, and their spectral properties all bear on our patterns of daily living and well-being. CRs are most sensitive to short wavelength (blue) light, with a peak spectral sensitivity at around 460 nm, a spectral condition most prevalent during daylight hours. Myriad physiological changes occur with aging. These can affect the rhythm of our behaviors, internal temperature regulation, and hormone releases, causing sleep disturbances and increased daytime napping patterns. These outcomes are more pronounced in individuals with Alzheimer's and related cognitive impairments. Persons with impaired vision and mobility are prone to adverse CR impacts caused by insufficient illumination, whether from natural or artificial sources. Recent research indicates that significant exposure to bright light during the day and dim light at night is best suited to maintaining CRs among

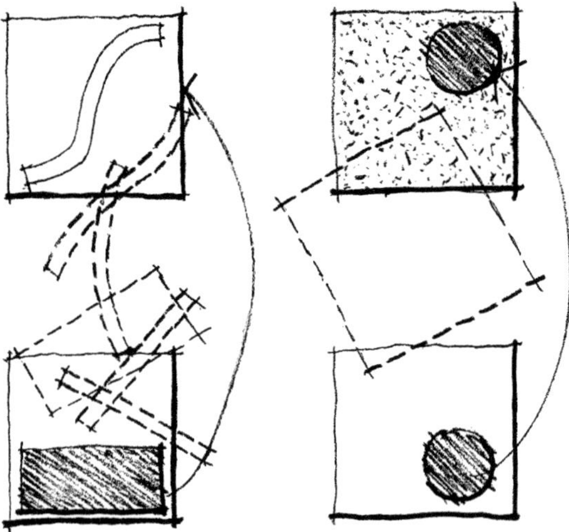

Figure B25. Eliminate anachronistic institutional cues. Drawing by Stephen Verderber.

older persons who reside in LTC settings.[121] It is therefore recommended to therapeutically incorporate an orchestrated blend of natural daylight with artificial illumination, including ultraviolet light sources. The interior lighting scheme should be based on cool, high lighting levels during the day and warm, low lighting types/levels in the evening, in order to reduce excessive circadian stimulation. A twenty-four-hour balanced exposure to multiple light sources is associated with increased sleep efficacy and lower rates of clinically diagnosed depression and agitation, as measured by standardized health status indicators.[122] The varied types of light fixtures (incandescent, LED, florescent) and different transmission apertures for natural daylight (skylights, clerestories, windows, doors) when carefully orchestrated, allow occupants to obtain maximum freedom of choice by having attained a proper balance of lighting during the day and through the evening hours.[123] Overexposure to artificial, bright light sources during the night suppresses melatonin secretion, which increases sleep disturbance patterns among older persons (fig. B26).[124] **2a; 2b; 4g; 5a; 5d; 8a–8h**

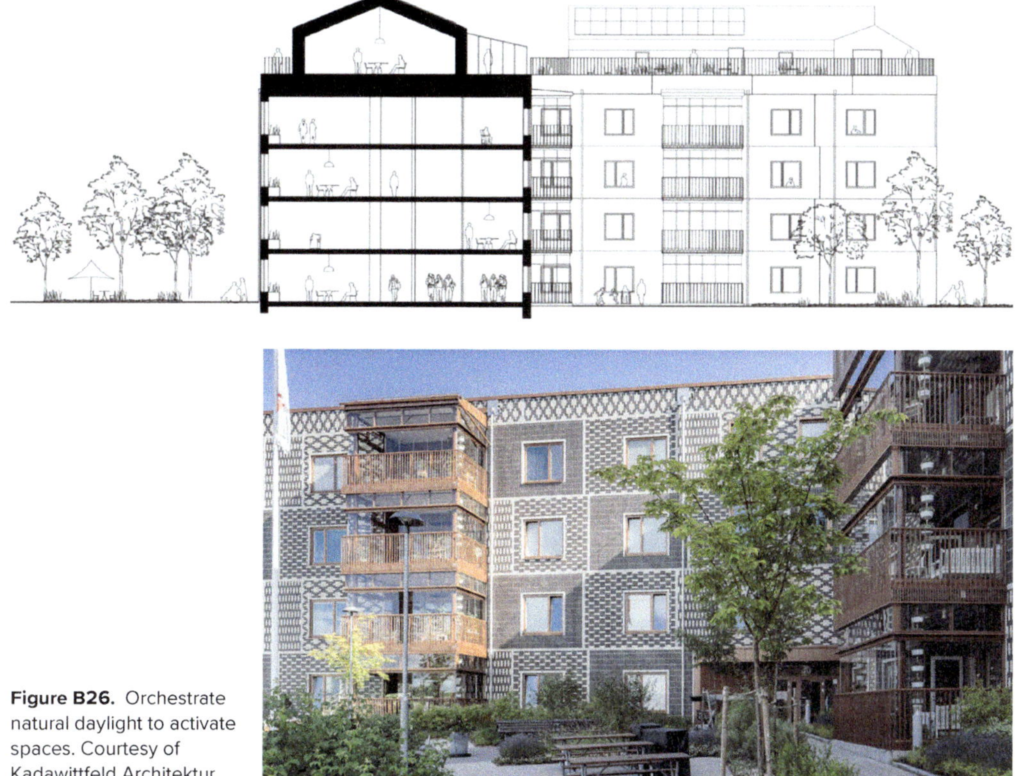

Figure B26. Orchestrate natural daylight to activate spaces. Courtesy of Kadawittfeld Architektur, Aachen, Germany.

7d. Noise Control

Noise is an ongoing concern in all health care facilities and is especially problematic in acute care medical centers, psychiatric institutions, and residential care settings for older persons.[125] Abrupt changes in ambient noise levels can cause agitation, possibly resulting in a violent outburst, especially at night, because sudden or repetitive noises disrupt circadian rhythms and sleep patterns.[126] The poor acoustical conditions caregiver staff often must cope with over months and years can contribute to increased worker burnout, absenteeism, and job dissatisfaction. In a recent empirical study, five LTC institutions in Belgium were examined before and after acoustic interventions were introduced.[127] Sound measurements were recorded in individual bedrooms, living rooms, and corridors to identify typical noise levels during the day. Acoustic intra-room (reverberation time) and inter-room (airborne and impact noise insulation levels) performance parameters were measured and compared. Noise levels in LTC homes triggered a stress response from measurements as low as 65 dB. Acoustical interventions—such as curtains, wall and ceiling panels, ventilation grills, and floating floors—were effective in reducing ambient noise. Staff caregivers also found that these interventions resulted in a quieter, more pleasant overall ambiance. Noise control is integral to well-being. Other recent research in these settings has employed phenomenological data collection methods to examine the noise quotient of music.[128] Certain types of ambient sounds have been found to normalize a setting, with their normative attributes even encouraging residents to draw closer socially, which can help ameliorate feelings of loneliness and social disconnection. Cross-cultural factors also greatly influence whether one person's perceived "noise" is another's tolerable or even desirable ambient sound. **1a; 1c; 3c; 3d; 6a; 7b; 8a–8h**

7e. Ambient Comfort

Residents with dementia are particularly unable to articulate what it is that is making them feel physically uncomfortable. And among all older persons, recent evidence-based research has found excessively hot and humid conditions to be a source of physical discomfort, and even death. Such conditions contribute to higher mortality rates, especially among persons living in unairconditioned private homes and apartments.[129] Comfortable ambient temperature and humidity conditions require defined metrics to assess optimal ambient thresholds suitable for this especially vulnerable population. Currently, however, there are no universally accepted models/metrics for application in LTC residences worldwide. The thermal comfort standards established by ASHRAE (an international society of heating, refrigerating, and air-conditioning professionals) attempt to address basic environmental and human-comfort minimum requirements for occupants' activities, recommended clothing types, and the most propitious kinds of building insulation.[130] It therefore continues to be difficult to apply standards equitably in all normative housing situations, largely due to residents' and their caregivers' transient nature, age and gender differences, diverse cultural backgrounds, and individual preferences. In general, due to their slower metabolic rates, older adults will prefer a *somewhat* warmer indoor ambient environment than younger individuals. An optimum temperature for sedentary older adults is above 77°F (25°C).[131] Radiant heat surfaces are preferable, with typically cold-to-the-touch surfaces (e.g., bathroom surfaces and fixtures) kept sufficiently warm. In general, systematically calibrate indoor heat/humidity levels on a 24/7 basis, balancing the residents' and the caregiver team's preferences and minimum thermal comfort requirements.[132] Provide operable windows, satisfactory natural air movement, low relative humidity, a suitable air exchange (ventilation) system with negative pressurization, appropriate weatherproofing, and energy-saving fixtures and appliances.[133] Thermal comfort levels are also mediated through effective daily use of manual or technology-assisted window blinds and screening devices. **2a; 2b; 2c; 3c; 4c; 4f**

7f. Multisensory Stimulation

In a multisensory room at the Coaldale Health Centre, Herman Stroeve loops strands of color-changing fiberoptic lights about his hand, not unlike a coil of rope. The strands glow in the darkened room. As he handles them, captivated, this long-term care resident softly reminisces about fixing a fence and mending a trough. "We'll see how that works," says Stroeve, who once ran a feedlot operation. He then sets down the lights, satisfied. Later, resident Evelyn Herter watches images of kittens and puppies projected onto the wall, as she snuggles a plush kitten placed in her lap by a recreation therapist. "Oh, they're so sweet," Herter exclaims. "So soft!"[134]

This recreation therapist, with eighteen years' experience, had wished for a special multisensory stimulation room (MSR) like this for years. This past summer it became a reality. Similar rooms have been created at Cardston and Crowsnest Pass Health Centres and the Geriatric Acute Rehabilitation Unit (GARU) at Chinook Regional Hospital in Alberta, Canada. Evidence-based research supports multisensory rooms in LTC residential environments, especially for the nonpharmaceutical behavioral treatment of individuals with dementia. This type of treatment space centers on music, massage therapy, aromatherapy, doll/animal/toy–assisted therapy, and Snoezelen technology. These interventions are proven effective in helping reduce agitation, depending on the diagnosed stage of dementia. For years Snoezelen rooms, proven popular for stimulating the senses, have been an integral part of the Sunrise Assisted Living Centers in the US and elsewhere. These rooms typically are centrally located within the LTC residence, although once-removed from the activity heart of public zones, because external noises and visual distractions should minimized.[135] A well-designed and equipped MSR is typically a windowless world unto itself, with comfortable furnishings—a place where full-immersion N-L therapy and related stimuli are electronically activated for varied lengths of time, depending on the prescribed treatment regimen for each individual. These rooms are therefore intentionally designed to be blank canvasses. Their nondescript aesthetic minimalism, however, is misleading to an untrained observer, because the blank surfaces are entirely activated in highly choreographed, digitally guided displays of multisensory information.[136] **4a; 4c; 4d; 7a; 7b; 7c; 7e**

8. PREFABRICATED HOUSING FOR LONG-TERM CARE

8a. Destigmatize Modular Prefabrication

The promise of modular construction in the housing industry remains unfulfilled. The hospital segment of the global health care industry, however, already makes considerable use of modular, off-site prefabrication methods, and in that sector of the industry, there is no longer any stigma attached to this method of design and construction. But the situation remains different in the arena of "conventional" modular housing for older persons. Historically, retiree trailer parks and mobile camper trailers have been the most well-known factory-built modular housing types for this demographic. But this elderhousing has long been viewed as impermanent, structurally insubstantial, socially stigmatized, and, at worst, outright dangerous, due to its so-called flimsy construction and total failure in light of extreme weather events, such as tornados. Despite stereotypes and the susceptibility to structural failure, overall the off-site–built prefabrication industry in North America has moved forward. In recent years it has attained an unprecedented level of sophistication through customization, overall better quality control, and proven advantages of labor- and material-cost optimization during fabrication and in transiting, as well as in the evolution of best practices in on-site installation protocols.[137] The five basic types of prefabricated structures for health care are: (1) portable tent-based and pneumatic structures; (2) vehicular nomadic (portable) units; (3) portable or fixed-site intermodal containerized systems; (4) portable or fixed-site flat-pack, lift-up, and pop-up systems; and (5) fixed-site or portable hybrid systems.[138] These modular typological variants provide architects and engineers with multiple options to design housing for applications around the globe. A careful and precise pre-design planning, manufacturing, and assembly specification phase/process for every component part is critical. First and foremost is the dictum "honor the match line"—that is, the connections between two or more modular components, which can range from the most minute coupling brackets, interlocking wall panels, to complete modular housing units placed alongside or stacked atop one another.[139] Key concerns include meticulous attention to site preparation; efficient transportation logistics; well-conceived sequenced production methods; reliable sources for materials and manufacturing; reliable HVAC, electrical, and plumbing systems; adaptability to occupants' evolving needs; the incorporation of salutogenic and biophilic design features; and occupant safety and security. Be aware of and use every means to eradicate potential adverse impacts from toxic building materials that may foster physical illnesses such as respiratory problems. In sum, if thoughtfully done, off-site–built prefab modularity offers a viable procurement strategy in the burgeoning arena of housing for older persons (fig. B27).[140] **1d; 1f; 2a; 2b; 2c; 2d; 3a; 4c; 5e**

8b. Modular Construction in Extreme Climates

Circumpolar nations will experience unprecedented public health challenges brought on by the warming climate. In Far North Canada, as elsewhere, First Nations communities are aging at a rapid rate. The vast physical distances between settlements in this region pose a logistical challenge when planning, designing, and constructing housing and health care facilities.[141] Indigenous communities have historically been medically underserved, with their health care facilities having been built over the twentieth century by colonialist governmental agencies that too frequently perpetuated inequitable, culturally incompatible medical care approaches.[142] These same problems have existed and continue to occur in extreme climate regions near the equator, where the living conditions of older persons and others are now hotter, wetter, and more humid. Standard facility procurement strategies commonplace elsewhere make little sense in extremely cold and extremely hot regions. Rapid responsiveness and cultural appropriateness, including due respect for local vernacular building traditions, are being recognized as more essential than ever. Many small-scale, village-like health care facilities are needed, built in close proximity to where older residents have lived for most (if not all) of their lives—as opposed to large-scale, impersonal institutions, especially those constructed on remote sites far from their ancestral village. For these, among other reasons, cultural appeasement governmental policies continue to be rejected by Indigenous communities in these regions. They are skeptically viewed as perfunctory, politically motivated gestures to end historically ingrained cultural dismissiveness.[143] Instead, awareness of Indigenous cultural behavioral and social traditions, cognizance of key health indicators within a local population, a genuine appreciation for the virtues of small-scale vernacular building types, and respect for the long-standing healing role of nature are of high priority.

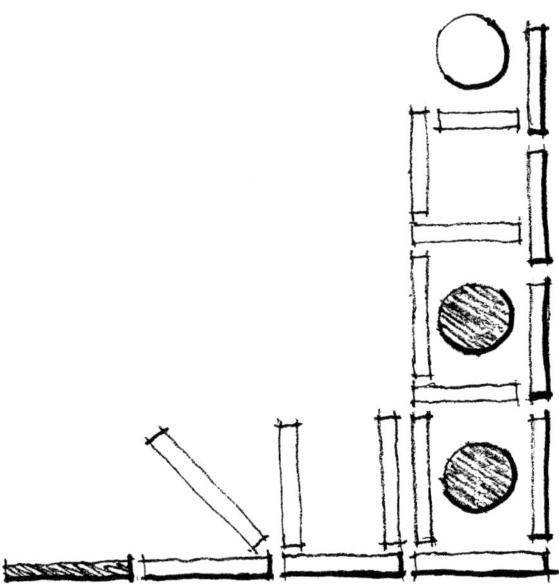

Figure B27. Explore the virtues of modular prefab elder-residences. Drawing by Stephen Verderber.

The elders who live in these communities are revered for their agency and are highly deserving of culturally appropriate, dignified, self-empowering housing. But beware, as local building sites may be seasonally limited, with the few local access roads perhaps being inaccessible at times, due to extreme weather events of long duration. Building materials may be scarce locally due to the weather, supply chain disruptions, and shortages of local skilled construction workers (fig. B28), **1a; 1b; 1c; 4e; 4h; 7b; 7c; 7e; 8a**

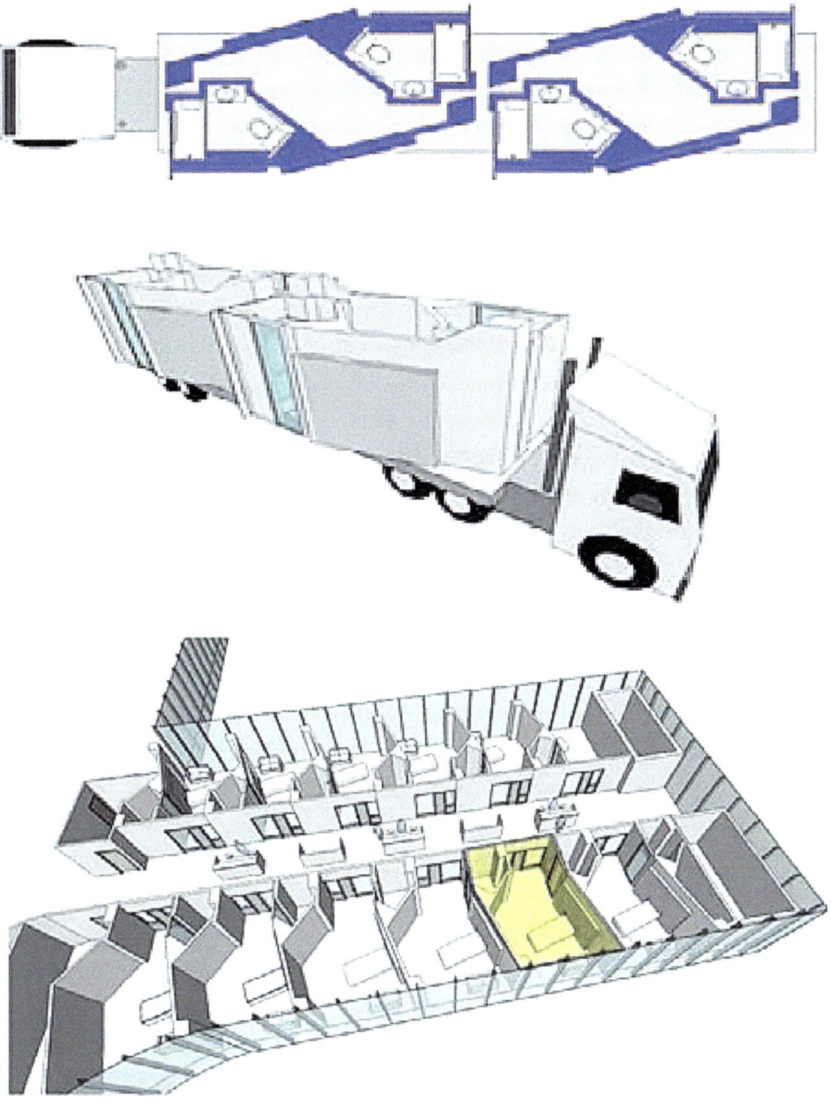

Figure B28. Prefab modular elder-residences. Courtesy of NBBJ Architects, Seattle.

8c. Modular Accessory Dwellings

The prospect of building prefabricated modular housing for a community's aging population can stir local resistance. This is due to the ongoing threat of NIMBYism, as much as anything else. Opponents will cite its "ugliness" and its threat to local property values. But, with increasingly unaffordable housing options and a growing percentage of families and individuals unable to purchase a home at any price point, what are the options? Those who wish to become homeowners must move ever farther from urban centers as part of the ever-worsening "drive until you qualify" (for a mortgage) syndrome.[144] From a zoning and building code perspective, an LTC residence is typically classified as a stand-alone, single-land-use building type. This needs to change.[145] It is far wiser to reclassify this type of housing. This allows other types of housing, such as ADUs and intergenerational housing options, to be built on shared sites. The well-established Scandinavian intergenerational housing model provides an excellent example of mixed-use/mixed-site accessory housing, a type widely known as *echo housing*. Accessory dwelling units—perhaps consisting of ten to fifteen homes/townhomes—are feasible, on shared sites, for occupancy by family members and visiting friends. These units can be owned or rented, with some set aside for individual day or short-term rentals by visiting friends and relatives. For families of older persons who presently live far from an elder-residence, this type of shared site housing allows them to be nearer to their aged relatives. Off-site–built modular elderhousing is especially well suited for this hybridic procurement strategy. Modular ADUs can be located on the ground level of a multilevel residence, in a different wing, or entirely separate from the LTC residence but still on a shared site. Provide each ADU with a full kitchen, a minimum of two bedrooms, two to three bathrooms, ample living and recreational space, a backyard or side yard, and access to parking close by.[146] Explore innovative ways to interweave these two distinct building types—LTC residences and ADUs—together. Creative cross-building–type thinking is needed and holds much promise in providing deinstitutionalized, equitable housing options for older persons who may otherwise feel warehoused and kept apart from the mainstream of society (fig. B29). **1d; 1f; 3b; 6c; 8a–8b; 8d–8h**

8d. Net-Zero Strategies

Life-cycle assessments, eco-balancing, and cradle-to-grave metrics are important tools in determining the energy performance rate of prefabri-

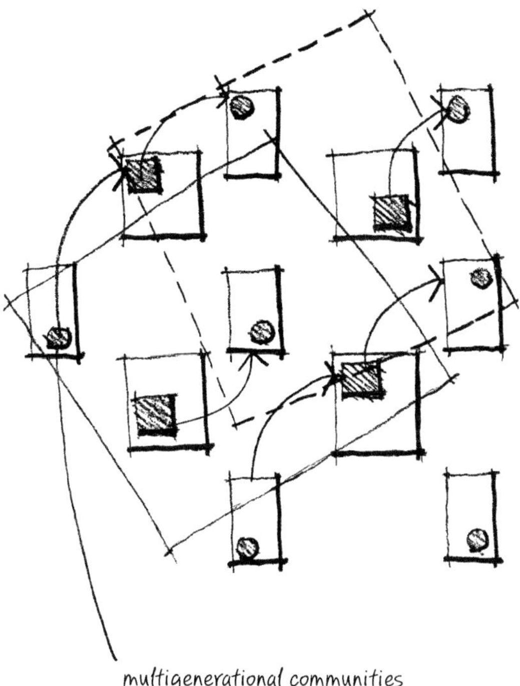

Figure B29. Modular accessory dwelling unit (ADU) elder-residences. Drawing by Stephen Verderber.

cated modular housing. The aim is to achieve *net-zero*, or carbon neutral, ecological sustainability through inventive health policy and design strategies, to reduce the adverse environmental impact of prefabricated modular architecture for older persons. Such measurable positive net gains are accruable in the form of *givebacks*. The aim of achieving carbon neutrality begins at the earliest stages of a capital improvement process, involving all key stakeholders.[147] The facility's expected occupancy lifespan/cycle is determined beforehand, be it 20 years, 30 years, or longer. Other determinants include environmental control systems, the type of modular construction (lift-pack, containerized, or hybrid), monthly and annual maintenance and upkeep costs, and relevant future adaptive expansion or retrofitting options. Anticipate projected occupant satisfaction as a function of these improvements, monitor the building envelope's functional performance, address biohazardous and solid waste disposal factors, and employ precise metrics to assess current and future resiliency.[148] Relevant metrics include atmospheric acidification, eutrophication, fossil fuel depletion rates, smog formation, ozone depletion rates, ecological toxicity, a comparative assessment of transiting pros and cons, and on-site water retention and recycling expectancies. Environmental programs for practical application to buildings include ISO14000—the most generally applicable and flexible program— developed by the International Standards Organization (ISO); the Building Research Establishment Environmental Assessment Methodology (BREEAM), launched in 1990; and BREEAM Canada and BREEAM/Green Leaf Canada's CSA Plus 1132 Standard. The US Green Building Council's Green Building Challenge is an international building assessment tool generally equivalent to the well-known LEED program in North America. In Australia, use of the National Australian Building Environmental Rating System (NABERS) is now widespread. Another assessment tool is the *embodied energy concept*, or the sum total of energy required to extract the necessary raw materials and then produce, transport, and assemble all modular componentry on the construction site.[149] **4e; 4h; 8a–8c; 8e–8h**

8e. Post-Occupancy Evaluation

More and more health care organizations are using post-occupancy evaluation (POE) metrics to measure the performance of their capital improvement projects.[150] In part it is an outgrowth of the US Institute of Medicine's 1999 landmark report, *To Err is Human*, which launched the patient/staff safety movement in North America. More recently, in a chapter on the supportive role of the physical environment, the widely cited 2022 report, *The National Imperative to Improve Nursing Home Quality*, discusses at some length the value of conducting systematic POEs of LTC residential facilities.[151] The report's use of evidence-based metrics is of foundational importance in drawing the public's attention to patient safety, especially in combating the high incidence of acquired infections and related adverse medical events that can occur during hospitalization, as well as in LTC facilities. Accordingly, it behooves the direct care provider organization to adopt a tailored POE methodology which will then help configure health policies to improve the habitability and quality of life for those in 24/7 custodial care. Top-down corporate initiatives are doomed to fail. This is especially so if they are initiated solely for marketing or other promotional purposes. It will accomplish little in the long run. Instead, establish thoughtful, grassroots-level, evidence-based POE facility assessment strategies. Then apply the results to design strategies grounded in measurable outcome metrics, acknowledging the full agency of all key stakeholders. Pay particular attention to the end users who live and work there.[152] This methodology was utilized to assess the performance of the first four Green House® case studies (fig. B30).[153] Many untapped opportunities await to apply POE methodologies to modular pre-fabricated residential facilities for older persons everywhere. **2a; 2c; 5e; 6a; 8a–8d; 8f–8h**

8f. Disaster Preparedness and Resiliency

Every health care organization needs an emergency preparedness plan, ready for immediate implementation. It is a strategic plan of potentially immense benefit in anticipating and responding to current and future adverse events, especially in medically underserved communities with persistent health inequities within the local population. Rising sea levels, intense rainstorms, hurricanes and typhoons, periods of drought and associ-ated water shortages, large-scale urban wildfires at the rural/urban interface (such as what occurred in Los Angeles in January 2005), and other disas-ters are predicted to trigger more frequent human and ecological catastro-phes in the future. In the case of St. Rita's Nursing Home in St. Bernard Parish in suburban New Orleans, the floodwaters from Hurricane Katrina in August 2005 filled this one-level facility nearly up to the ceiling within twenty minutes.[154] The owners of this nursing home were later put on trial for thirty-five counts of negligent homicide and twenty-four counts of cruelty to the elderly and infirm patients who drowned that night *in their beds and wheelchairs*.[155] In their defense, the owners maintained that keeping these frail patients in place was safer than subjecting them to the trauma of a forced evacuation. Eight long years later, the owners were acquitted of any guilt in the residents' deaths, yet this tragedy serves as a cautionary tale for the operators of LTC homes everywhere. The fact remains that every LTC organization should have a well-rehearsed emergency action plan in place, in the event that staff and patients must be rapidly evacuated off-site or to safe quarters elsewhere on the same site. LTC facilities, whether prefab modular or otherwise, now require emergency preparedness plans that address security measures to counter any acts of elder abuse while a facil-ity is in lockdown or in the process of being evacuated. Hold preparatory evacuation drills on a regular basis, perhaps once per month, since a rapid, adroit response could prove the difference between life and death. Draft the action plan from the outset of the capital improvement project, include built-in resiliency measures as part of equitable due diligence, including site selection and the type of modular prefab construction (containerized, lift-pack, or hybrid). Build and evaluate mock-up simulations prior to full scale construction (see chapter 3), and pretest a manifold of anticipated facility performance metrics in the face of possible calamity. **1a; 6c; 8a–8e; 8g; 8h**

8g. Ecohumanist Stewardship

Ten territories for *ecohumanist* engagement in architecture and health were defined by Terri Peters and Stephen Verderber in 2017:

1. minimization of the facility/campus's carbon footprint,
2. resilient and regenerative care settings,
3. the use of functional deconstruction strategies to reduce the sheer scale of health care institutions,
4. the role of landscape therapeutics and nature in treatment and healing,
5. the role of residentialism versus the anachronistic traditions of sheer institutionalism and custodialism,
6. special emphasis on stakeholder advocacy and social inclusiveness,
7. the value of therapeutic interior realms,
8. the incorporation of tectonic innovation,
9. the creative repurposing of existing resources to new uses versus their thoughtless demolition, and
10. the importance of interdisciplinary knowledge mobilization, so valuable new knowledge actually gets put to use.[156]

More specifically for modular prefabricated LTC architecture, carefully choose engineered prefab modular-building-material palettes and assembly systems to eliminate excess material waste. This can reduce the total project delivery cost, improve efficiencies, address ecological concerns, and decrease total energy expenditures. Applying building information modeling (BIM) in health care facility planning and design, combined with a controlled—versus controlling—use of LEAN in the building's design and delivery procurement strategies, can also reduce total project costs[157] BIM allows its users to monitor occupants' daily energy consumption, apply waste management best practices, and ensure building code compliance in existing, new, and renovated LTC facilities. Additional applications include geothermal-system modeling; comparative ratings of carbon neutral materials and building assemblies; off-site prefabrication options for modular components; lighting and natural ventilation choices; rainwater harvesting methods with respect to roofs, including green roofs; and site landscaping options, such as xeriscaping. The International Facility Management Association has a section that specifically addresses these aspects of ecologically responsive health care facilities.[158] **4e; 4h; 6d; 8a–8f; 8h**

8h. Salutogenic Design and Modular Prefabrication

The fact remains the vast majority of 24/7 long-term care custodial residences in North America and elsewhere do not really therapeutically/salutogenically support their inhabitants' quality of life. This is an urgent concern in the Anthropocene in the face of global resource depletion; the climate crisis; escalating land, labor, construction costs; and the unfortunate ramifications of unmitigated local grassroots NIMBYism. More and more, modular prefabricated long-term care housing is a therapeutic/salutogenic design, best-practice strategy for housing older persons in need of 24/7 care. A recent case study was funded by the government of Finland, in collaboration with Aalto University and the University of Helsinki.[159] This research team comparatively examined the efficacy of multiple anticipatory design methods in the planning and construction of modular health care facilities, concluding that such methods can be invaluable in this type of modular housing. Off-site options allow relocating manufacturing and assembly processes offsite, thus reducing competition between the industrial trades for space and time, and further expediting project schedules—all resulting in the more orderly staging of project deliverables to the job site. This also means fewer work-related injuries, because manufacturing and assembly processes normally occur in a more controllable shop environment (unaffected by weather, for example). Building componentry stays cleaner and is less vulnerable to sustaining damage on-site, while also reducing the amount of rework and punch list items requiring attention later on. Components and assemblies produced off-site can be made quicker, versus the longer time sequences required to manufacture them on-site. The these component systems can be transited and installed when the construction site is ready to accept them. Off-site prefabrication reduces the amount of pre-purchased materials and decreases environmental waste that would otherwise be sent to the local landfill. Excess labor, in terms of time spent walking around the construction site to find a particular tool or piece of equipment, is also reduced.[160] Building owners and their design/construction teams retain a greater degree of control and agency with respect to their legal financial liability, because with factory-made componentry, quality control can be maximized, resulting in fewer component failures and on-site accidents. This can also improve post-construction servicing and lifespan maintenance in the field. All this is achievable without sacrificing careful attention to therapeutic/salutogenic architectural and landscape-site design strategies (fig. B30).[161] **1a; 1c; 4a; 4c; 4f; 4g; 5c; 8a–8g**

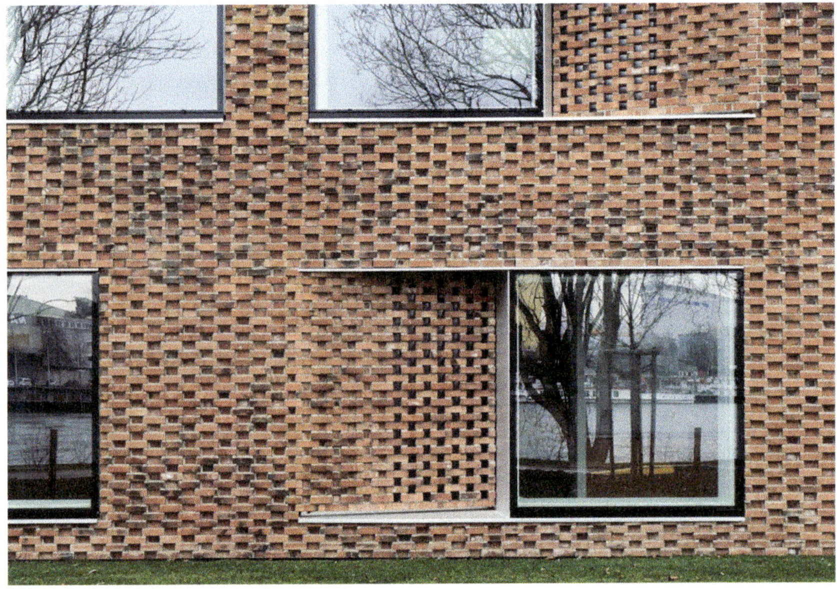

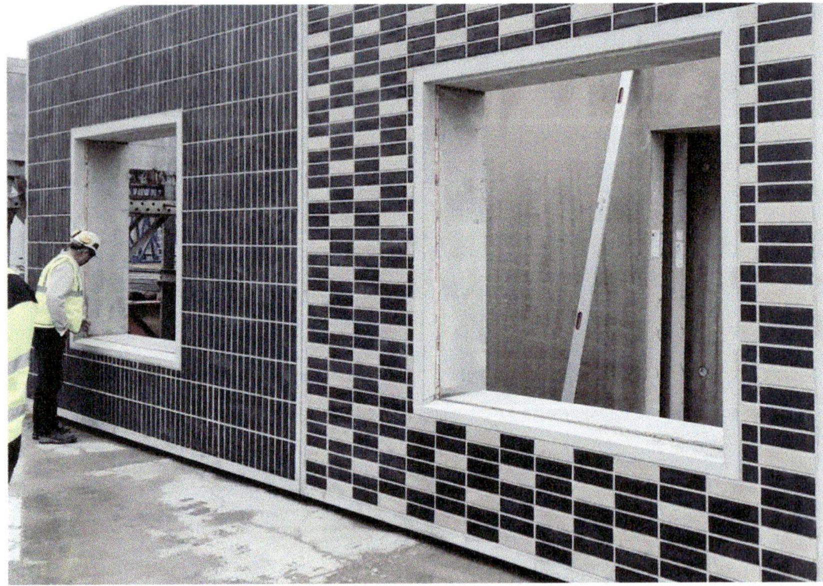

Figure B30. Incorporate salutogenic design concepts in prefab modular elder-residences. Courtesy of Kadawittfeld Architektur, Aachen, Germany.

Notes

Chapter 1

1. Rosner, D. (2010). "Spanish Flu, or whatever it is . . .": The paradox of public health in a time of crisis." *Public Health Reports*, 125(3): 37–47. https://doi.org/10.1177/00333549101250S307.
2. Yong, E. (2021). "How public health took part in its own downfall." *The Atlantic*, 23 October. https://www.theatlantic.com/health/archive/2021/10/how-public-health-took-part-its-own-downfall/620457/.
3. Hill, H. W. (1913). *The New Public Health*. London: Ulan Press.
4. Yong (2021).
5. Special September 2003 theme issue of the *American Journal of Public Health*, 93(9). Articles addressed historical advocacy in public health, nineteenth-century slum conditions in New York City and other industrialized American cities, the social and political history of zoning, and impacts of urban sprawl on unhealthful outcomes, including chronic disease in automobile-centric, post–World War II suburbia. One article directly addressed the role of public health inequities in the built environment.
6. Public Health Ontario (2022). *Health Equity*. Public Health Ontario, 9 May. https://www.publichealthontario.ca/en/health-topics/health-equity.
7. Braveman, P., and Gruskin, S. (2003). "Defining equity in health." *Journal of Epidemiology & Community Health*, 57(4): 254–258. https://jech.bmj.com/content/57/4/254.
8. Kawachi, I., Subramanian, S. V., and Almeida-Filho, N. (2002). "A glossary for health inequities." *Journal of Epidemiology & Community Health*, 56(9): 647–652. https://jech.bmj.com/content/56/9/647.
9. Fisher, T. (2022). *Space, Structures and Design in a Post-Pandemic World*. London and New York: Routledge.
10. United Nations (2023). "World population projected to reach 9.8 billion in 2050, and 11.2 billion in 2100." United Nations Department of Economic and Social Affairs. https://www.un.org/en/desa/world-population-projected-reach-98-billion-2050-and-112-billion-2100
11. Curtis, W. J. R. (1996). *LeCorbusier: Ideas and Forms*. New York: Phaidon Press.
12. Waters, C., and Zalasiewicz, M. (2018). "The Anthropocene and its Golden Spike." In Burtynsky, E., Baichwal, J. E., and de Pencier, N. (eds.), *Anthropocene*. Toronto and Ottawa: Art Gallery of Ontario / National Gallery of Canada.
13. Rosendale, S. (2002). *The Greening of Literary Scholarship: Literature, Theory and the Environment*. Iowa City: University of Iowa Press.
14. Buell, L. (2003). *Writing for an Endangered World: Literature, Culture, and Environment in the U.S. and Beyond*. Cambridge, MA: Belknap Press / Harvard University Press.
15. Stewart, F. (1994). *A Natural History of Nature Writing*. Washington, DC: Island Press.
16. Wohlleben, P. (2015). *The Hidden Life of Trees: How They Feel, How They Communicate*. Munich: Ludwig Verlag.
17. Andrews, G. J., and Duff, C. (2019). "Matter beginning to matter: On posthumanist understandings of the vital emergence of health." *Social Science & Medicine*, 226 (3): 123–134.
18. Burtynsky, E. (2018). "Life in the Anthropocene." In Burtynsky, E., Baichwal, J. E., and de Pencier, N., p. 189.

19. Pruss-Ustun, A., and Corvalán, C. (2006). *Preventing Disease Through Healthy Environments: Towards an Estimate of the Environmental Burden of Disease; Executive Summary.* Geneva: World Health Organization.

20. Guenther, R., and Vittori, G. (2013). *Sustainable Healthcare Architecture*, 2nd edition. New York: Wiley.

21. Steffen, W. B., Wendy, D., Owen, L. G., and Cornelia, L. (2015). "The trajectory of the Anthropocene: The great acceleration." *The Anthropocene Review*, 2(1): 81–98.

22. Whitmee, S., Andy, H., Frederick, C. B., Capon, A., and Dias, B. F. (2015). "Safeguarding human health in the Anthropocene epoch: Report of the Rockefeller Foundation *Lancet* Commission on Planetary Health." *The Lancet*, 386(10007): 1973–1928.

23. Darimont, C. T., Cooke, R. B., Bourbonnais, M. L., et al. (2023). "Humanity's diverse predatory niche and its ecological consequences." *Communications Biology*, 6(2): article number 609. https://www.nature.com/articles/s42003-023-04940-w. Also see Semeniuk, I. (2023). "Study lays out full extent of humans as global predators—and it's a big problem." *The Globe and Mail*, 30 June. https://www.theglobeandmail.com/canada/article-study-lays-out-full-extent-of-humans-as-global-predators-and-its-a-big/.

24. Trevor, H. (2016). "Healthcare in the Anthropocene: Challenges and opportunities." *Healthcare Quarterly*, 19(3): 17–22.

25. Colbert, C. (2021). "King tides are coming to parts of flood-prone South Florida." CNN, 11 September. https://www.cnn.com/2021/09/11/weather/king-tides-florida-flooding/index.

26. Lahiri, T., and Li, J. (2022). "Shanghai's perpetual lockdown is only getting worse." *Quartz*, 9 May. https://qz.com/2163159/shanghais-perpetual-lockdown-is-only-getting-worse.

27. Taleb, N. M. (2007). *The Black Swan: The Impact of the Highly Improbable.* New York: Random House.

28. Michelle, H. (2020). "216 homes flood in St. Charles Parish after storm drops 12 inches of rain in 2 hours." *Nola*, 15 May. https://www.nola.com/news/weather/article_11e8bbf0-96bd-11ea-adbd-7b20fd418991.html.

29. Mann, M. E. (2022). *The New Climate War: The Fight to Take Back Our Planet.* Washington, DC: PublicAffairs. If Plan A is to ameliorate or at least contain the most serious consequences, what will define any Plan B? In a Plan A world, architecture and planning unfortunately cannot get past obsessing over the idea of sustainable, resilient, or net-zero design as being sufficient in the climate crisis. Recent scientific reports predict that the earlier estimated projections of mass population displacements from rising sea levels have been too low. Instead of some 50 million people being forced to move to higher ground over the next thirty years, the oceans will likely rise higher than predicated, with a coastal diaspora at least three times larger. By 2100, the number of climate refugees could surpass 300 million.

30. Bingler, S., and Pedersen, M. C. (2020). "Planners talk about resilience in the face of climate change: We need to start using a different R word." *The Washington Post*, 17 February. https://www.washingtonpost.com/opinions/2020/02/17/climate-hope-best-prepare-worst/.

31. Hobbes, M. (2020). "America is not set up for this." *HuffPost*, 26 April. https://www.huffpost.com/entry/america-not-set-up-for-coronavirus-fema-disaster-preparedness_n_5ea491f3c5b6d37635909669.

32. Multihazard Mitigation Council (2019). *Natural Hazard Mitigation Saves: 2019 Report.* Washington, DC: National Institute of Building Sciences. https://www.nibs.org/projects/natural-hazard-mitigation-saves-2019-report.

33. El Akkad, O. (2021). "The climate refugees are coming: Countries and international law aren't ready for them." *The Globe and Mail*, 31 July. https://www.theglobeandmail

.com/opinion/article-the-climate-refugees-are-coming-countries-and-international
-law-arent/.

34. Lustgarten, A. (2020). "Climate change won't stop for the coronavirus pandemic."
ProPublica, 13 April. https://www.propublica.org/article/climate-change-wont-stop
-for-the-coronavirus-pandemic.

35. Gunn-Wright,   R. (2020). "Think this pandemic is bad? We have another crisis
coming." *The New York Times*, 15 April. https://www.nytimes.com/2020/04/15
/opinion/sunday/climate-change-covid-economy.html.

36. Kaplan, S., and Kaplan, R. (1982). *Cognition and Environment: Functioning in an
Uncertain World*. New York: Praeger. Also see Lawton, M. P. (1985). "The elderly
in context: Perspectives from environmental psychology and gerontology."
Environment and Behavior, 17(4): 501–519.

37. Ferguson, N. (2021) *Doom: The Politics of Catastrophe*. New York: Penguin Press,
chapter 3.

38. Festinger, L. (1957). *A Theory of Cognitive Dissonance*. Stanford, CA: Stanford
University Press.

39. Ferguson (2021), p. 102.

40. Morrow, A., and Alex, C. (2021). "Finger-pointing begins over collapse of Miami
condo amid search for survivors." *The Globe and Mail*, 28 June. https://www
.theglobeandmail.com/world/us-politics/article-finger-pointing-begins-amid
-continued-search-for-survivors-at-miami/.

41. Verderber, S. (2005). *Compassion in Architecture: Evidence-Based Design for
Health in Louisiana*. Lafayette: Center for Louisiana Studies. An earlier version of
these four constructs was included in that book, which received the Places Award
for 1986 from *Places* magazine and the Environmental Design Research Association.
Also see Moffat, D. (2006). "Compassion in architecture: Evidence-based design for
health." *Places*, 18(3): 23–27.

42. Teirstein, Z. (2022). "FEMA is giving homeowners money to prepare for floods—
or move away." *Grist*, 23 March. https://grist.org/politics/fema-is-giving-homeowners
-money-to-prepare-for-floods-or-move-away/. Also see Stein, M. I. (2018). "How to
save a town from rising waters." *Bloomberg*, 24 January. https://www.bloomberg
.com/news/articles/2018-01-24/moving-a-louisiana-town-out-of-the-path-of-climate
-change.

43. Myers, J. (2019). "This man is turning cities into giant sponges to save lives." World
Health Forum, 28 August. https://www.weforum.org/stories/2019/08/sponge-cities
-china-flood-protection-nature-wwf/. Also see Lubell, S. (2020). "Commentary:
Past pandemics changed the design of cities: Six ways COVID-19 could do the
same." *Los Angeles Times*, 22 April. https://www.latimes.com/entertainment-arts
/story/2020-04-22/coronavirus-pandemics-architecture-urban-design.

44. Heilmeyer, F. (2022). "Is this floating headquarters a model for waterfront workplaces?"
Metropolis, 7 March. https://metropolismag.com/projects/rotterdam-floating-office/.

45. *Oxford English Dictionary*, 3rd edition (2023), s.v. "Anthropocene, n. and adj."

Chapter 2

1. Herman, J. L. (2015) *Trauma and Recovery: The Aftermath of Violence—from
Domestic Abuse to Political Terror*. New York: Basic Books.

2. Verderber, S., and Fine, D. J. (2000). *Healthcare Architecture in an Era of Radical
Transformation*. New Haven, CT: Yale University Press. Also see Verderber, S.
(2003). "Architecture for health—2050: An international perspective." *The Journal
of Architecture*, 8(3): 281–302.

3. Kiple, K. F., ed. (1997). *Plague, Pox & Pestilence*. New York: Barnes and Noble.

4. Verderber (2003), p. 282. Also see Montague, J. (1982). "Hospitals in the Muslim Middle East: A historical overview." In Bradfer, F. (ed.), *Architecture Hospitalière: Part I, Islamic Hospitals*. Washington, DC: Center for Research in Architecture, Catholic University of America.

5. Montague (1982).

6. Ferguson, N. (2022). *Doom: The Politics of Catastrophe*. London: Penguin Books, pp. 121–129.

7. Thompson, J., and Goldin, G. (1975). *The Hospital: A Social and Architectural History*. New Haven. CT: Yale University Press.

8. Ferguson (2022), p. 126.

9. Dubos, R., and Dubos, J. (1952). *The White Plague: Tuberculosis, Man and Society*. New Brunswick and London: Rutgers University Press.

10. Verderber (2003), p. 288.

11. Kiple (1997), p. 27. It was called the "bubo plague" in Europe. Bubos are, as the name bubonic implies, the disease's telltale symptom. Once a person is infected with *Yersina pestis*, their lymphatic system attempts to collect the infection in the lymph nodes. These frequently swell to the size of an egg—or even a grapefruit—into what is called a *bubo*. Because fleas typically bite an exposed area of the human body, such as the limbs or face, these bubos are accessible targets. If the infection reaches the lungs, however, it manifests as pneumonia. In this mode the disease passes from human to human, bypassing rats and fleas.

12. Kiple (1997), p. 29.

13. Kiple (1997), p. 62.

14. Carmichael, A. G. (1997). "Leprosy: Larger than Life." In Kiple (ed.), pp. 50–57. By the twelfth century, the number of hospice institutions devoted to caring for lepers and other types of outcasts increased exponentially. Leprosaria, or specialized asylums, appeared across Western Europe. The incarceration and care of lepers was strictly enforced, while Catholic Church–ordered public decrees warned of the danger to the community's spiritual and public health, similar to published edicts on the presence of Jews and heretics. In 1179, the Third Lateran Council decreed that all lepers were to be permanently segregated. They were required to wear cowbells or hold hand-clappers, to announce their presence wherever they went; wear a yellow cross on their garb; and tap a long stick on the pavement whenever they appeared in public. Lepers were banished to remote hamlets, later known as leper colonies, usually far from medieval cities and towns.

15. Foucault, M. (1963). *The Birth of the Clinic: An Archeology of Medical Perception*. Translated by Sheridan Smith, A.M. (1994). New York: Vintage Books.

16. Ferguson (2022), p. 150.

17. Humphreys, M. (1997). "Typhoid and its Carriers." In Kiple (ed.), pp. 14–15.

18. Crosby, A. (1997). "Influenza: In the Grip of the Grippe." In Kiple (ed.), pp. 148–153.

19. Thompson and Goldin (1975), chapter 3.

20. Thompson and Goldin (1975), p. 52.

21. Debono, G. (2020). "When breaching quarantine was a matter of life and death." *Times of Malta*, 24 May. https://timesofmalta.com/articles/view/when-breaching-quarantine-was-a-matter-of-life-and-death.794096.

22. Thompson and Goldin (1975), p. 49.

23. Thompson and Goldin (1975), p. 51.

24. Thompson and Goldin (1975), p. 66.

25. Masson. G. (1957). "Lazzaretto in Ancona." *The Architectural Review*, 122(727): 116. Also see Camaioni, C., Di Prospero, L., D'Onofrio, R., Pierantoni, I., Renzi, A., and Sargolini, M. (2017). "The ideal Adriatic city." In Cocci G. R., D'Onofrio, R., and

Sargolini, M. (eds.), *Quality of Life in Urban Landscapes: In Search of a Decision Support System*. New York: Springer, pp. 245–281. https://doi.org/10.1007/978-3 -319-65581-9_23.

26. Ocaña, Q. L. (2007). "El lazaretto de Mahón." *Medicina y Seguridad del Trabajo*, 53(207): 63–69. Also see Bonastra, Q. (2017). "El lazaretto de Mahón." *Atlas Digital de los Espacios de Control*, 14(1): 32–42.

27. Silver, C. P. (1998). "Brunel's Crimean War hospital—Renkioi revisited." *Journal of Medical Biography*, 6(2): 234–239. Also see Merridew, C. G. (2014). "I. K. Brunel's Crimean War hospital." *Anesthesia and Intensive Care*, 42(3): 13–20.

28. Carmichael (1997), in Kiple (ed.), pp. 66–67.

29. Continuing a persistent pattern across hundreds of years, governments provided inadequate taxpayer funding for these public health enclaves. In Hawaii, the government emphasized the extreme contagiousness of the disease, and Molokai's leper colony was left to fend for itself. This was the case until Norwegian scientist Dr. Gerhard-Henrik Armauer Hansen (1841–1912) traveled there in 1873 to study this disfiguring disease firsthand. Robert Louis Stevenson (1850–1894) also visited Molokai in 1889 and spent twelve days there, shadowing the colony's leprosy-ridden director, Father Damian. Father Damian would die soon afterward.

30. Carmichael (1997), in Kiple (ed.), pp. 56–57.

31. Anderson, N. (2021). "The U.S. Columbia River Quarantine Station." Lewis and Clark National Historic Trail Experience. https://lewisandclark.travel/nomination/the-u-s -columbia-river-quarantine-station/. Also see Paulu, T. (2007). "Quarantine Station: Family transforms former medical center into museum to bring local history to light." *Longview Daily News*, 15 May. https://tdn.com/lifestyles/quarantine-station-family -transforms-former-medical-center-into-museum-to-bring-local-history-to-light/article _976b4daf-9496-5421-9d6a-be64de26e8d1.html.

32. Humphreys, M. (1997). "Malaria: 'Evil' Air and Mosquitos." In Kiple (ed.), pp. 98–101.

33. Weber, J. (1880). *Illustrated Europe, Davos*. London: Thames.

34. Weber (1880), pp. 75–79.

35. Colomina, B. (2019). *X-Ray Architecture*. Berlin: Lars Müller, pp. 35–36 and 72–74. Colomina cites Josef Hoffman's Purkersdorf (1903), outside Vienna; Otto Wagner's Steinhoff (1807) in Vienna; an unbuilt proposal (1914) for the Palmschoss heliotherapy center in the mountains near Brixen, Italy; Jan Duiker and Bernard Bijvoet's Zonnestraal (1928) in Hilversum, The Netherlands; Richard Docker's sanitorium (1928) in Waiblingen, Germany; Werner Hebebrand and Willi Kleinertz's Sonnenblick sanitorium (1931) in Marburg, Germany; Josep Lluis Sert's Dispensario Antituberculoso (1934) in Barcelona; and William Ganster and William Pereira's Lake County Tuberculosis Sanitorium (1939) in Waukegan, Illinois.

36. Dubos and Dubos (1952), pp. 144–145.

37. Verderber, S. (2010). *Innovations in Hospital Architecture*. London and New York: Routledge, chapter 2.

38. Dubos and Dubos (1952), p. 181.

39. Byerly, C. R. (2010). "The U.S. military and the influenza pandemic of 1918–1919." *Public Health Reports*, 3(125): 82–91. In the US alone, at least 550,000 died, ten times the number of those who were killed in combat in WW I. In India, the situation was far worse, with as many as 20 million dead. The pandemic caused the most harm per capita, however, in Western Samoa, where 7,542 out of a population of 38,302 died in an eight-week period in 1918.

40. Fisher, E. F., ed. (2012). *Envisioning Disease, Gender, and War*. New York: Palgrave Macmillan. Also see Winter, J. (2006). *Remembering War: The Great War between Memory and History in the Twentieth Century*. New Haven, CT, and London: Yale

University Press; Phillips, H., and Killingray, D. (2003). *The Spanish Influenza Pandemic of 1918–19: New Perspectives*. London: Routledge; and Blanchot, M. (1995). *Writing of the Disaster*, translated by Smock, A. Lincoln and London: University of Nebraska Press.

41. Sontag, S. (1978). *Illness as Metaphor*. New York: Farrar, Straus and Giroux. Also see Crosby, A. F. (1989). *America's Forgotten Pandemic: The Influenza of 1918*. Cambridge: Cambridge University Press; and Barry, J. M. (2004); and *The Great Influenza: The Epic Story of the Deadliest Plague in History*. New York: Viking. Other books on the 1918 pandemic include Hochling, A. A. (1961). *The Great Epidemic*. Boston: Little Brown; Collier, R. (1974). *The Plague of the Spanish Lady*. New York: Athenaeum; Pettit, D. A., and Baile, J. (2008). *A Cruel Wind: Pandemic Flu in America 1918–1920*. Murfreesboro, TN: Timberlane; and Honigsbaum, M. (2009). *Living with Enza: The Forgotten Story of Britain and the Great Flu Pandemic of 1918*. New York and London: Palgrave Macmillan.

42. Remarque, E. M. (2009 [1920]). *All Quiet on the Western Front*. New York and London: Palgrave Macmillan.

43. Crosby, A. F. (1997), in Kiple (ed.), p. 153.

44. Kolata, G. (1999). Flu. New York: Farrar, Straus and Giroux, pp. 38–40. It is noteworthy that few army physicians and commanders who experienced the Spanish flu pandemic firsthand wrote about it.

45. Howard, E. (1902) *Garden Cities of To-morrow*, 2nd edition. London: S. Sonnenschein, pp. 2–7.

46. Verderber, S. (2012). *Sprawling Cities and Our Endangered Public Health*. London and New York: Routledge, chapters 2–4.

47. Lindheim, R. (1979/80). "How modern hospitals got that way." *The Co-Evolution Quarterly*, Winter: 62–73.

48. Verderber and Fine (2000), chapters 2–5.

49. Tripp, A. R., Goad, P., and Logan, C. (2018). *Architecture and the Modern Hospital: Nosokomeion to Hygeia*. London and New York: Routledge. Also see Verderber, S., and Refuerzo, B. (2020). *Innovations in Hospice Architecture*, 2nd edition. London and New York: Routledge.

50. Kisacky, J. (2017). *Rise of the Modern Hospital: An Architectural History of Health and Healing, 1870–1940*. Pittsburgh: University of Pittsburgh Press, p. 152.

51. Kisacky, J. (2021). "Consequences of migrating U.S. contagious facilities into general hospitals, 1900–1950." *Health Environments Research & Design Journal*, 15(1): 45–61.

Chapter 3

1. Verderber, S. (2023). "Pandemical healthcare architecture, social responsibility, and health equity." In Tural, E., Ortega-Andeane, P., and Ruggeri, D. (eds.), *Environment and Health: Global/Local Challenges and Actions*. Proceedings of EDRA 54, Environmental Design Research Association, Mexico City, June 2023, pp. 219–231.

2. Worldometers (2024). "COVID-19 coronavirus pandemic." Worldometers. https://www.worldometers.info/coronavirus/?utm_campaign=homeAdvegas1 [no longer being updated].

3. Kurtz, A. (2020). "An Israeli hospital set up an emergency care ward in 72 hours." *The Algemeiner*, 22 March. https://www.algemeiner.com/2020/03/22/an-inraeli -hospital-set-up-a-covid-1.html.

4. Barcelona Convention Bureau (2020). "Vall d'Hebrón temporary hospital providing care for 132 COVID-19 patients." Barcelona International Welcome. https://www.barcelona.cat/internationalwelcome/en/noticia/first-temporary-hospital-for-covid -19-patients-now-operative_93404.htm [no longer available].

5. Otis, J. (2020). "COVID-19 numbers are bad in Ecuador: The president says the real story is even worse." National Public Radio, 20 April. https://www.npr.org/sections /goatsandsoda/2020/04/20/838746457/covid-19-numbers-are-bad-in-ecuador-the -president-says-the-real-story-is-even-worse.

6. Fisher, T. (2008). "Public interest architecture: a needed and inevitable change." In Bell, B., and Wakeford, K. (eds.), *Expanding Architecture: Design as Activism*. New York: Metropolis Books.

7. United Nations (2022). *World Population Prospects 2022*. New York: United Nations Department of Economic and Social Affairs, Population Division. https://www.un.org /development/desa/pd/content/World-Population-Prospects-2022.

8. Verderber, S. (2021). "Pandemical healthcare architecture and social responsibil- ity—COVID-19 and beyond." Centre for Design + Health Innovation White Paper, University of Toronto.

9. Kieran, S., and Timberlake, J. (2004). *Refabricating Architecture*. New York: McGraw-Hill

10. Verderber, S. (2016). *Innovations in Transportable Healthcare Architecture*. London and New York: Routledge, pp. 61–64. There are three broad types of off-site–built prefabricated buildings for health care. The first, redeployable health centers (RHCs), typically for use in nondisaster situations, are off-site–built vehicular mobile clinics—a portable but nonmotorized facility or a hybrid that combines elements of both. The second are redeployable trauma centers (RTCs), best suited to provide emergency and intensive care for victims of disaster. A prefabricated modular RTC is capable of being expanded from one unit to as many as twenty modules on a single site and is adaptable to diverse climate and site conditions in the field. The third—Permanent Modular Installations (PMIs)—are either complete turnkey pack- ages built off-site, or any constituent modular component assembly or individual part built off-site and then transported to a second site for permanent installation. Recent integrated design/build techniques, such as building information modeling (BIM), now enable the total automation of the building process in a manner that saves time, improves overall quality, and minimizes waste materials and the use of nonrenew- able resources.

11. M-RAD (2020). "COVID-19 mobile testing units featured in Designboom." M-RAD, 11 May. https://www.m-rad.com/covid-19-mobile-testing-units-featured-in-designboom/.

12. Ravenscroft, T. (2020) "Grimshaw designs range of shipping-container coronavirus testing centres." Dezeen, 3 June. https://www.dezeen.com/2020/06/03/grimshaw -shipping-container-coronavirus-testing-centres/.

13. MacLennan, R. (2020) "Citizen Care Pods provide mobile COVID-19 testing and screening." *Ontario Construction News*, 29 September. https://www.ontario constructionnews.com/citizen-care-pods.

14. Perkins & Will (2020). "A COVID-19 mobile testing solution." Perkins & Will, 21 April. https://perkinswill.com/news/a-covid-19-mobile-testing-solution/.

15. Designboom (2020). "Opposite Office proposes to turn Berlin's Brandenburg airport into COVID-19 'superhospital,'" Designboom, 31 March. https://www.designboom .com/architecture/opposite-office-berlin-brandenburg-airport-covid-19-superhospital -03-31-2020/.

16. Myers, S. L. (2021) "Facing new outbreaks, China places over 22 million on lockdown." *The New York Times*, 13 January. https://www.nytimes.com/2021/01/13/world/asia /china-covid-lockdown.html.

17. Verderber, S. (2021). Host structures chosen by the student teams included tem- porarily shuttered gyms in community recreational centers, retail commercial struc- tures, churches, a terminal at Pearson International Airport, a YMCA, and an art

museum. The program brief called for a lift-pack system, with an arrival, registration, and waiting area; five CNST rooms; five rooms for immunizations; workspace for staff personnel; a service entrance; and plug-in power generation for negative air pressurization. This lift-pack system must be able to be transported via truck. IT, HVAC, electrical, and plumbing systems run beneath a raised platform, with ramp and stair access. The modules feature lighting units suspended from an open grid, which also facilitates airflow. Internal circulation isolates nonsymptomatic from symptomatic individuals. Parking is provided on-site, as is space for individuals to queue outdoors, weather permitting.

18. NCKU [National Cheng Kung University] (2020). "NCKU, BAF co-design for COVID19 prototype of emergency quarantine hospital." NCKU, 29 April. https://web.ncku.edu .tw/p/406-1000-206984,r2845.php?Lang=en.

19. FuturArc (2020). "Modular design of mobile hospitals for the treatment of COVID-19." FuturArc, 16 April. https://www.futurarc.com/project/modular-design-of-mobile -hospitals-for-the-treatment-of-covid-19/.

20. Wang, J., Zhu, E., and Umlauf, T. (2020). "How China built two coronavirus hospitals in just over a week." *Wall Street Journal*, 6 February. https://www.wsj.com/articles /how-china-can-build-a-coronavirus-hospital-in-10-days-11580397751. A small army of earthmovers expediently prepared the site for the first facility. The hospital's foundation consisted of several layers of fibrous-matting insulation, with interspersed layers of concrete. Up to 7,000 people worked around the clock in three shifts.

21. Griffiths, J., Sidhu, S., and Gan, N. (2021). "WHO team in Wuhan begin long-delayed coronavirus investigation after clearing quarantine." CNN, updated January 28. https://www.cnn.com/2021/01/26/asia/who-coronavirus-team-wuhan-china-intl-hnk /index.html.

22. HAHA Architects Group (2020). "Rescue center." Prefab Modular Homes and Build-ings. https://blog.prefabium.com/2020/05/emergency-modular-hospitals-projects .html. The construction documents for this project are available online on the archi-tectural firm's website, as open access documents. Also see Archdaily (2020). "Alternative healthcare facilities: Architects mobilize their creativity in fight against COVID-19." Archdaily. https://www.archdaily.com/937840/alternative-healthcare -facilities-architects-mobilize-their-creativity-in-fight-against-covid-19/5e99c9a3b 357653cb1000102-alternative-healthcare-facilities-architects-mobilize-their -creativity-in-fight-against-covid-19-image.

23. Khan, Z. (2020). "CURA pods to help hospitals expand ICU capacity to treat COVID-19 patients." Stirworld, 27 March. https://www.stirworld.com/see-news-cura-pods-to -help-hospitals-expand-icu-capacity-to-treat-covid-19-patients. Also see Adlakha, N. (2020). "In Italy, two designers convert shipping containers into COVID-19 care pods." *The Hindu*, 21 April. https://www.thehindu.com/sci-tech/technology/designers -carlo-ratti-and-italo-rota-on-their-connected-units-for-respiratory-ailments-cura /article31394435.ece.

24. HGA (2020). "STAAT MOD™ critical care units address COVID-19 hospital bed shortage." *HGA News*, 3 April. https://hga.com/staat-mod-critical-care-units-address -covid-19-hospital-bed-shortage/.

25. Archdaily (2020). "Monash Health RESUS Facility / SPACECUBE." Archdaily, 20 July. https://www.archdaily.com/943908/monash-health-resus-facility-spacecube/.

26. Verderber, S., and Fine, D. J. (2000). *Healthcare Architecture in an Era of Radical Transformation*. New Haven, CT, and London: Yale University Press, chapter 3. In the case of the Crystal Hospital, a 100-bed configuration of this unbuilt proposal is hypothetically depicted as having been installed at the Hôtel Dieu in Lévis, Québec. Radial patient-care healing houses contain ten beds each, with privacy pull curtains

separating beds not positioned along an outer wall. The beds face a central staff work core, with a hand-sanitizing station and the nurse's station. These modules plug into a custom-built shipping container with staff and patient supports, including a washroom/shower, storage area, mechanical/HVAC/IT equipment, and a staff restroom/shower. Aggregate "crystals," consisting of five radial pods each (10 feet × 5 feet), are plugged into a common work zone, which itself is plugged into the facility's main arrival-intake module.

27. World Health Organization (2022). *INITIATE2 Infectious Disease Treatment Module. Technical Report.* Geneva: World Health Organization. The 2022–2024 WHO-IDTM project design team consisted of Michele DiMarco and Anna Silenzi (project director and o-director, respectively, WHO, Geneva, Switzerland), Kyle Basilius (Parkin Architects, Vancouver, British Columbia), Chantel Trudel (professor, Carleton University, Ottawa, Ontario), Nigra Marianna (PhD and postdoctoral fellow, Royal Polytechnic University of Turin, Italy), Meagan Webb (H. H. Angus & Associates, Ltd., Vancouver, British Columbia), Troy Savage (Mazzetti, New Haven, Connecticut), Cosci Massimiliano and Stefano Guagliardo (United Nations World Food Programme, Rome, Italy), Willy Schlein (LS3P Architects, Greenville, South Carolina), and Stephen Verderber (University of Toronto).

28. Antonovsky, A. (1979). *Health, Stress and Coping.* San Francisco: Jossey-Bass.

29. Golembiewski, J. (2012). "Psychiatric design: Using a salutogenic model for the development and management of mental health facilities." *World Health Design*, 5(2): 74–79.

30. Kellert, S. (1997). *The Value of Life.* Washington, DC: Island Press. Also see Kellert, S. (2008). "Dimensions, elements, and attributes of biophilic design." In Kellert, S., and Heerwagen, J. (eds.), *Biophilic Design: The Theory, Science and Practice of Bringing Buildings to Life.* Washington, DC: US Green Building Council. Also see Kellert, S. (2018). *Nature by Design: The Practice of Biophilic Design.* New Haven, CT: Yale University Press.

31. Wilson, E. O. (1984). *Biophilia.* Cambridge, MA, and London: Harvard University Press.

32. Peters, T., and Verderber, S. (2021). "Biophilic design strategies in long-term residential care environments for persons with dementia." *Journal of Aging and Environment*, 12(3): 11–29.

33. Verderber, S., and Peters, T. (2021). "Integrating LEED with biophilic design affordances—toward an inclusive rating system." In Battisto, D., and Wilhelm, J. J. (eds.), *Architecture and Health: Guiding Principles for Practice.* London: Routledge, pp. 311–327.

34. Browning, W. D., Ryan, C., and Clancy, J. O. (2014). *14 Patterns of Biophilic Design.* New York: Terrapin Bright Green. Also see Ryan, C. O., Browning, W. D., Clancy, J. O., Andrews, S. L., and Kallianpurkar, N. B. (2014). "Biophilic design patterns: Emerging nature-based parameters for health and well-being in the built environment." *Archnet—International Journal of Architectural Research*, 8(2): 62–76. https://earthwise .education/wp-content/uploads/2019/10/Biophilicdesign-patterns.pdf. There are three patterns. The first is *nature in physical space*—visual connectivity with nature, nonvisual connections with nature, nonrhythmic sensory stimuli, thermal and airflow variability, the presence of water, dynamic and diffuse light, and connections with natural ecological systems. The second is *nature analogies*—biomorphic forms and imagery (material connections from or inspired by nature) and the amelioration of discombobulation (overcomplexity versus patterned order). The third is the *nature of the physical space*—prospect-refuge behaviors, the function of mystery and intrigue, and the role of risk-reward behaviors.

35. Reed, P., and Lushniak. R. (2020). "Infectious diseases and public health in a field hospital." In Bar-On, E., Peleg, K., and Kreiss, Y. (eds.), *Field Hospitals: A Comprehensive Guide to Preparation and Operation*. London and New York: Cambridge University Press, pp. 245–255.

36. Lamontagne, F., Fowler, R. A., Adhikari, N. K., et al. (2017). "Evidence-based guidelines for supportive care of patients with Ebola virus disease." *The Lancet*, 391(10121): 700–708. Also see Wilson, D. (2015). "Inside an Ebola treatment unit: A nurse's report." *American Journal of Nursing*, 115(12): 28–38.

37. Verderber, S. (2016), chapters 5 and 6.

38. Verderber, S. (2016), p. 140.

39. Verderber, S. (2016), p. 141.

40. Gillis, K., and Gatersleben, B. (2015). "A review of psychological literature on the health and wellbeing benefits of biophilic design." *Buildings*, 5(3): 948–963. For a detailed overview of attention restoration theory, also see Kaplan, S., and Kaplan, R. (1989). *The Experience of Nature: A Psychological Perspective*. New York: Cambridge University Press; Kaplan, S. (1995). "The restorative benefits of nature: Toward an integrative framework." *Journal of Environmental Psychology*, 15(2): 169–182; Kaplan, S. (2001). "Meditation, restoration, and the management of mental fatigue." *Environment and Behavior*, 33(2): 480–506; Kaplan, S., and Berman, M. G. (2010). "Directed attention as a common resource for executive functioning and self-regulation." *Perspectives on Psychological Science*, 5(1): 43–57; and Ohly, H., White, M. P., Wheeler, B. W., et al. (2016). "Attention restoration theory: A systemic review of the attention restoration potential of exposure to natural environments." *Journal of Toxicology and Environmental Health, Part B*, 19(7): 305–343.

41. Verderber (2016), p. 141.

42. Djalali, A., Ingrassia, P. L., and Della Corte, F. (2014). "Identifying deficiencies in national and foreign medical team responses through expert opinion surveys: Implications for education and training." *Prehospital and Disaster Medicine*, 29(4): 364–368.

43. Norton, I., von Schreeb, J., Aitken, P., Herard, P., and Lajolo, C. (2013). *Classifications and Minimum Standards for Foreign Medical Teams in Sudden Onset Disasters*. Geneva: World Health Organization.

44. World Health Organization / Pan American Health Organization (2010). *Proceedings of the WHO/PAHO Technical Consultation on Foreign Medical Teams (FMTs) Post–Sudden Onset Disasters (SODs)*. Geneva: World Health Organization. The ethics component of the WHO standards is based on the World Medical Association's (WMA) *Medical Ethics Manual* and includes considerations in times of disasters (when resources are severely restricted), patient confidentiality, and the need for informed consent (wherever practicable). Besides WHO, the United Nations–based Inter-Agency Standing Committee (IASC) aims to provide a framework for coordinating multiple national health care systems seeking to provide disaster relief to achieve mutually agreed-upon goals and to minimize service gaps. Also see Lofti, T., Bou-Karroum, L., Darzi, A., et al. (2016). "Coordinating the provision of health services in humanitarian crises: A systematic review of suggested models." *PLOS Currents*, 8(2): 47–50.

45. Nerlander, M. P., and von Schreeb, J. (2020). "Definitions, needs, scenarios, functional concept, and modes of deployment." In Bar-On, E., Peleg, K., and Kriess, Y. (eds.).

46. Jobe, K. (2011). "Disaster relief in post-earthquake Haiti: Unintended consequences of humanitarian volunteerism." *Travel Medicine and Infectious Disease*, 9(1): 1–5.

47. Nerlander and van Schreeb (2020).

48. Nerlander and van Schreeb (2020), p. 20.

49. Lu, D., and Flavelle, C. (2019). "Rising seas will erase more cities by 2050, new research shows." *The New York Times*, 29 October. https://www.nytimes.com/interactive/2019/10/29/climate/coastal-cities-underwater.html.

50. Toole, M. J., and Waldman, R. J. (1990). "Prevention of excess mortality in refugee and displaced populations in developing countries." *Journal of the American Medical Association*, 263(24): 3296–3302. Also see Watson, J. T., Gayer, M., and Connonly, M. A. (2007). "Epidemics after natural disasters." *Emerging Infectious Diseases*, 13(1): 1–5.

51. Ligon, B. L. (2006). "Infectious diseases that pose specific challenges after natural disasters: A review." *Seminars in Pediatric Infectious Diseases*, 17(1): 36–45.

52. Sullivan, S. M., and McDonald, K. W. (2006). "Post–Hurricane Katrina infection control challenges and the public health role at a mobile field hospital." *American Journal of Infection Control*, 34(5): E11–E12. Also see Lichtenberger, P., Miskin, I. N., Dickinson, G., et al. (2010). "Infection control in field hospitals after a natural disaster: Lessons learned after the 2010 earthquake in Haiti." *Infection Control and Hospital Epidemiology*, 31(9): 951–957.

53. Hatch, C. R. (1984). *The Scope of Social Architecture*. New York: Van Nostrand Reinhold.

54. Dutton, T. (1996). "Cultural studies and critical pedagogy." In Dutton, T., and Mann, L. H. (eds.), *Reconstructing Architecture: Critical Discourses and Social Practices*. Minneapolis: University of Minnesota Press, pp. 158–201.

55. Verderber, S. (2003). "Compassionism in the design studio in the aftermath of 9/11." *Journal of Architectural Education*, 52(3): 48–62. Also see Verderber (2016).

56. Fife, R., and Chase, S. (2022). "Mobile hospitals that cost Ottawa $300 million sit in storage while Omicron strains Canada's health system." *The Globe and Mail*, 14 January. https://www.theglobeandmail.com/politics/article-federal-mobile-hospital-units-sitting-in-warehouses-as-omicron-surges/.

57. Fife and Chase (2022).

58. Le Corbusier (1923). *Towards a New Architecture*. Translated by Etchells, F. (1984). New York: Holt, Rinehart and Winston.

59. Kronenburg, R. (1995). *Houses in Motion: The Genesis, History and Development of the Portable Building*. London: Academy Editions.

60. Zolli, A., and Healy, A. M. (2012). *Resilience*. New York: Free Press, pp. 6–11.

61. Wallace-Wells, D. (2019). *The Uninhabitable Earth: Life after Warming*. New York: Tim Duggan Books. Also see Stiglitz, J. (2020). "Conquering the great divide." *International Monetary Fund Finance & Development Report*, September. https://www.imf.org/en/Publications/fandd/issues/2020/09/COVID19-and-global-inequality-joseph-stiglitz.

Chapter 4

1. Brown, H. (2023). "Sorry, honey, it's too hot for camp." *Radio Atlantic*, 6 July. https://www.theatlantic.com/podcasts/archive/2023/07/sorry-honey-its-too-hot-for-camp/674621/.

2. Cunsolo, A., and Ellis, N. A. (2018). "Ecological grief as a mental health response to climate change–related loss." *Nature Climate Change*, 8(2): 275–281.

3. Padhy, S. K., Sarkar, S., Panigrahi, M., and Paul, S. (2015). "Mental health effects of climate change." *Indian Journal of Occupational Environmental Medicine*, 19(3): 3–7.

4. Cianconi, P., Betrò, S., and Janiri, L. (2020). "The impact of climate change on mental health: A systematic descriptive review." *Frontiers in Psychiatry*, 11(2): 74. https://doi.org/10.3389/fpsyt.2020.00074.

5. Helm, S. V., Pollitt, A., Barnett, M. A., Curran, M. A., and Craig, Z. R. (2018). "Differentiating environmental concern in the context of psychological adaption to climate change." *Global Environmental Change*, 48(2): 158–167.

6. World Health Organization (1986). The Ottawa Charter for Health Promotion. Geneva: World Health Organization. https://www.who.int/publications/i/item/WH-1987.

6. Kahneman, D., Diener, E., and Schwarz, N. (1999). *Well-being: The Foundations of Hedonic Psychology*. New York: Russell Sage Foundation.

7. Barnosky, A. D., Matzke, N., Tomiya, S., et al. (2011). "Has the Earth's sixth mass extinction already arrived?" *Nature*, 471:51. https://doi.org/10.1038/nature09678.

8. Bittle, J. (2023). "The American climate migration has already begun." *The Guardian*, 23 February. https://www.theguardian.com/commentisfree/2023/feb/23/us-climate-crisis-housing-migration-natural-disasters.

9. Bathiany, S., Dakos, V., Scheffer, M., and Lenton, T. M. (2018). "Climate models predict increasing temperature variability in poor countries." *Science Advances*, 4(2): 1–10.

10. Strona, G., and Bradshaw, C. A. (2018). "Co-extinctions annihilate planetary life during extreme environmental change." *Scientific Reports*, 8(2): 1–12. https://doi.org/10.1038/s41598-018-35068-1.

11. Comtesse, H., Ertl, V., Hengst, S. M., Rosner, R., and Smid, G. E. (2021). "Ecological grief as a response to environmental change: A mental health risk or functional response?" *International Journal of Research in Public Health*, 18(2): 734–743.

12. UNHCR (2023). *Global Trends Report*. UNHCR, the UN Refugee Agency. https://www.unhcr.org/globaltrends.

13. USDA Forest Service (2023). "Loss of Open Space." Forest Service, US Department of Agriculture. https://www.fs.usda.gov/science-technology/loss-of-open-space.

14. Labbé, S. (2022). "How Canada's biggest cities are losing their green space." *Vancouver Is Awesome*, 20 November. https://www.vancouverisawesome.com/highlights/how-canadas-biggest-cities-are-losing-their-green-space-6121617.

15. Clemence, S. (2023). "The last place on earth any tourist should go." *The Atlantic*, 3 July. https://www.theatlantic.com/science/archive/2023/07/antarctica-tourism-overcrowding-environmental-threat/674600/.

16. Seligman, M. E. (1972). "Learned helplessness." *Annual Review of Medicine*, 23(1): 407–412. Also see Peterson, C., Marer, S. F., and Seligman, M. E. (1995). *Learned Helplessness: A Theory for the Age of Personal Control*. New York: Oxford University Press; and Maier, S. F., and Seligman, M. E. (2016). "Learned helplessness at fifty: Insights from neuroscience." *Psychological Review*, 123(4): 349–367.

17. Dodd, H. F., FitzGibbon, L., Watson, B. E., and Nesbit, R. J. (2021). "Children's play and independent mobility in 2020: Results from the British Children's Play Survey." *International Journal of Environmental Research*, 18(8): 4334. https://doi.org/10.3390/ijerph18084334. Also see Levs, J. (2017). "Whatever happened to go outside and play?'" CNN, 2 October. https://www.cnn.com/2013/03/22/living/let-children-play-outside/index.html.

18. Stephen, K., and Kaplan, R. (1983). *Cognition and Environment: Functioning in an Uncertain World*. New York: Praeger.

19. Daniel, T. C. (2001). "Whither scenic beauty? Visual landscape quality assessment in the 21st century." *Landscape and Urban Planning*, 54(2): 267–281. Further discussion is available in Wohlwill, J. F. (1983). "The concept of nature: A psychologist's view." In Altman, I., and Wohlwill, J. (eds.), *Behavior and the Natural Environment*. New York: Plenum Press, pp. 5–37. Also see Eder, K., and Ritter, M. (1996). *The Social Construction of Nature: A Sociology of Ecological Enlightenment*. London: Sage; and Evernden, N. (1992). *The Social Creation of Nature*. Baltimore: Johns Hopkins University Press.

20. Fromm, E. (1964). *The Heart of Man*. New York: Harper and Row.

21. Wilson, E. O. (1984). *Biophilia: The Human Bond with Other Species*. Cambridge, MA: Harvard University Press.

22. Kellert, S. R. (2008). "Dimensions, elements, and attributes of biophilic design." In Kellert, S. R., Heerwagen, J. H., and Mador, M. L. (eds.), *Biophilic Design: The Theory, Science and Practice of Bringing Buildings to Life*. New York: John Wiley & Sons.

23. Browning, W. D., Ryan, C. O., and Clancy, J. O. (2014). *14 Patterns of Biophilic Design*. New York: Terrapin Bright Green.

24. Peters. T., and Verderber, S. (2022). "Biophilic design strategies in long-term care residential environments for persons with dementia." *Journal of Aging and Environment*, 36(3): 227–255. https://doi.org/10.1080/26892618.2021.1918815.

25. Appleton, J. (1996). *The Experience of Landscape*, revised edition. London: Wiley.

26. Hartig, T. (2021). "Restoration in nature: Beyond the conventional narrative." In Schutte, A., Torquati, J. C., and Stevens, J. R. (eds.), *Nature and Psychology*. New York: Springer, pp. 89–151.

27. Hildebrand, G. (1991). *The Wright Space: Pattern and Meaning in Frank Lloyd Wright's Houses*. Seattle: University of Washington Press. Also see Hildebrand, G. (1999). *Origins of Architectural Pleasure*. Berkeley: University of California Press. In distilling thirteen characteristics of the prospect pattern, Hildebrand acknowledged that Wright did not use all of them in all his houses, although most of his major houses had at least ten of the following elements:

    1. major interior spaces elevated above the ground level,
    2. fireplaces withdrawn from the perimeter envelope,
    3. low ceilings,
    4. built-in seating and cabinets,
    5. upward-sweeping ceilings,
    6. interior views into contiguous interior spaces,
    7. ample glazed windows and doors,
    8. generous elevated terraces,
    9. deep overhanging eaves,
    10. an externally prominent central chimney,
    11. horizontal bands of windows,
    12. conspicuous balconies or terraces, and
    13. a strong connection between interior and exterior realms.

Nevertheless, there is no way to know with certainty if this was what Wright was specifically seeking to achieve. In 1985, a well-known theorist in architecture, Christian Norberg-Schulz, stated that Wright was instead "destroying the traditional 'box' by creating a new interaction between the inside and outside, an inner world of protection and comfort." Also see Norberg-Schulz, C. (1985). *The Concept of Dwelling*. New York: Rizzoli.

28. Dosen, A. S., and Ostwald, M. J. (2016). "Evidence for prospect-refuge theory: A meta-analysis of the findings of environmental preference research." *City, Territory and Architecture*, 3: article 4. https://doi.org/10.1186/s40410-016-0033-1.

29. James, W. (1892). *Psychology: The Briefer Course*. New York: Holt.

30. Kaplan, S., and Kaplan, R. (1989). *The Experience of Nature: A Psychological Perspective*. New York: Cambridge University Press.

31. Kaplan, S. (1995). "The restorative benefits of nature: Towards an integrative framework." *Journal of Environmental Psychology*, 15(2): 169–182. Also see Kaplan, S. (2001). "Meditation, restoration, and the management of mental fatigue." *Environment and Behavior*, 33(2): 480–506. This theory has also been applied to the study of attention deficit hyperactivity disorder (ADHA), postcancer treatments, treatments

for postcombat-acquired PTSD, and related post-traumatic disorders. Also see Kuo, F., and Taylor, A. F. (2001). "A potential natural treatment for attention-deficit hyper-activity disorder: Evidence from a national study." *American Journal of Public Health*, 94(9): 1104–1109.

32. Louv, R. (2005). *Last Child in the Woods: Saving Our Children from Nature-Deficit Disorder*. Chapel Hill, NC: Algonquin.

33. Louv, R. (2009). "No More 'Nature Deficit Disorder,'" *Psychology Today*, 29 January. https://www.psychologytoday.com/intl/blog/people-in-nature/200901/no-more-nature-deficit-disorder.

34. Kuo, F. (2013). "Nature-deficit disorder: Dosage, and treatment." *Journal of Policy Research in Tourism, Leisure, and Events*, 5(2): 172–186. Also see Van den Berg, A. E., Maas, J., Verheij, R. A., and Groenewegen, P. P. (2010). "Green space as a buffer between stressful life events and health." *Social Science & Medicine*, 70(6): 1203–1210.

35. Pergams, O., and Zardiac, P. (2006). "Is love of nature in the U.S. becoming love of electronic media? 16-year downward trend away from national parks visits explained by watching movies, playing video games, internet use, and oil prices." *Journal of Environmental Management*, 80(1): 387–393. Also see Wells, N., and Lekies, K. (2006). "Nature and the life course: Pathways from childhood nature experiences to adult environmentalism." *Children, Youth and Environments*, 16(2): 1–24.

36. Karieva, P. (2008). "Ominous trends in nature recreation." *Proceedings of the National Academy of Science*, 106: 2757–2758.

37. Fletcher, R. (2017). "Connection with nature is an oxymoron: A political ecology of nature-deficit disorder." *The Journal of Environmental Education*, 48(4): 226–233.

38. Hartig, T. (2008). "Greenspace, psychological restoration, and health inequality." *The Lancet*, 372: 1614–1615.

39. Thompson, J. D., and Goldin, G. (1975). *The Hospital: A Social and Architectural History*. New Haven, CT: Yale University Press, pp. 3–6.

40. Garraty, J. A., and Gay, P. (1972). *Columbia History of the World*. New York: Harper & Row.

41. Irvine, K. N., and Warber, S. L. (2002). "Greening healthcare: Practicing as if the natural environment really mattered." *Alternative Therapies in Health and Medicine*, 8(1): 76–83.

42. Marcus, C., and Barnes, M., eds. (1999). *Healing Gardens: Therapeutic Benefits and Design Recommendations*. New York: Wiley.

43. Nightingale, F. (1859). *Notes on Hospitals*. London: Parker and Son, pp. 95–96. Also see Anon (2004). "*Notes on Hospitals*, third edition and enlarged." *Journal of Mental Science* 10(2): 403–416. Inpatient pavilions, in her view, were to be no more than two levels in height, with landscaped open-air exterior side courts between the patients' housing pavilions, featuring gardens for use by patients. Windows were tall, reaching to 1 foot from the ceiling "so as not to trap foul air," with sills no higher than 30–36 inches above the floor. For Nightingale, it was better for a ward to be too light than too dark. The importance of engaging nature and outdoor views were strictly prescribed in *Notes on Hospitals*. St. Thomas Hospital (1868-1871) in London, on the Lambeth Palace Road directly across the Thames from Parliament, was the first hospital to incorporate Nightingale's ideas. She implored the architect, Henry Currey (1820–1900), to add as many large windows as possible to the neo-Gothic facades of the patient wards, to the point where Currey frustratingly exclaimed, "If I add any more, Miss Nightingale, the entire thing will come crashing down!" At her insistence, her architect specified a continuous open-air terrace for patients along the River Thames, running the entire length of this hospital.

44. Howard, E. (1902). *Garden Cities of To-morrow*. London: Swan Sonnenschein. Howard advocated for greenbelts, ample parkland, and expansive gardens in the Victorian Age. Town and country life were to be melded. Miasma theory attributed epidemic diseases, like cholera, to bad air emanating from contaminated ecological sources, such as foul pools of stagnant water. Far-reaching public health reforms ensued.

45. Hewitt, R. (2006). "The influence of somatic and psychiatric medical theory on the design of nineteenth century American cities." *History of Medicine Online*. https://www.priory.com/ital/influence.htm.

46. Brooks, H. A. (1966). "Frank Lloyd Wright and the Wasmuth Drawings." *The Art Bulletin*, 48(6): 193–202. Wright referred to the American prairie as the archetypal symbol of endless landscape, whereas Schindler favored horizontal functionalism, making extensive use of visual transparency in his private residential commissions in Los Angeles from the 1920s through the 1950s, beginning with the Translucent House (1927).

47. Neutra, R. (1954). *Survival through Design*. Oxford: Oxford University Press. Also see Lamprecht, B. (2016). *Neutra*. Cologne: Taschen. John Lautner, Hugh Jacobson, and other architects made extensive use of visual transparency in their International Style residential architecture.

48. Leatherbarrow, D. (2002). "Sitting in the city, or the body in the world." In Dodds, G., and Travenor, R. (eds.), *Body and Building: Essays on the Changing Relation of Body and Architecture*. Cambridge and London: MIT Press, pp. 47–59.

49. Hartig, T., van den Berg, A., Hagerhall, C. M., et al. (2011). "Health benefits of nature experience: Psychological, social and cultural processes." In Nilsson, K., Sangster, M., Gallis, C., et al. (eds.), *Forests, Trees and Human Health*. New York: Springer, pp. 127–168.

50. Maggie's Centres (2023). *Maggie's Architecture and Landscape Brief*. https://www.maggies.org/media/filer_public/e0/3e/e03e8b60-ecc7-4ec7-95a1-18d9f9c4e7c9/maggies_architecturalbrief_2015.pdf.

51. An affiliated mental health institution is assumed to provide continued medical oversight of an individual patient who opts to come to the NIC. Ideally, all care and consultation is to be provided on a no-fee basis, and patients are not "sent" to the NIC for treatment. Individuals would come to the NIC voluntarily, strictly by their own accord, like the network of Maggie's Centres.

52. Ranney, M. L., and Jetelina, K. (2023). "Opinion: Trust in science is declining; Here's how we can regain it." CNN, 17 November. https://www.cnn.com/2023/11/17/opinions/public-trust-in-scientists-ranney-jetelina/index.html.

53. Suttie, J. (2019). "Why trees can make you happier." *Greater Good Magazine*, 26 April. https://greatergood.berkeley.edu/article/item/why_trees_can_make_you_happier. Also see Gerstenberg, T., and Hofmann, M. (2016). "Perception and preference of trees: A psychological contribution to tree species selection in urban areas." *Urban Forestry & Urban Greening*, 15(3): 103–111; and Frumkin, H. (2001). "Beyond toxicity: Human health and the natural environment." *American Journal of Preventive Medicine*, 20(2): 234–240.

54. Editorial (2023). "Our views: Trees are our friends, but hurricanes have whacked too many of them." *Nola*, 30 January. https://www.nola.com/opinions/our_views/our-views-trees-are-our-friends-and-we-need-more-of-them/article_e3d16460-9cfe-11ed-a3e6-4bc4a7b7fc9e.html.

55. Ottoson, J., and Grahn, P. (2005). "A comparison of leisure time spent in a garden with leisure time spent indoors: On measures of restoration in residents in geriatric care." *Landscape Research*, 30(4): 23–55. https://doi.org/10.1080/01426390420003

24758. Also see Berto, R. (2014). "The role of nature in coping with physio-physiological stress: A literature review on restorativeness." *Behavioral Sciences*, 4(8): 394–409. https://doi.org/10.3390/bs4040394.

56. Harding, W. (2014). *The Myth of Emptiness and the New American Literature of Place*. Iowa City: University of Iowa Press.

57. Johnson, L. M. (2013). "Plants, places, and the storied landscape: Looking at First Nations perspectives on plants and land." *BC Studies*, 179(3): 85–105.

58. Griggs, D., Stafford-Smith, M., Gaffney, O., et al. (2013). "Sustainable development goals for people and planet." *Nature*, 495: 305–307. Also see Morton, T. (2009). *Ecology without Nature: Rethinking Environmental Aesthetics*. Cambridge, MA: Harvard University Press; Estes, H. (2017). *Anglo-Saxon Literary Landscapes: Eco-theory and the Environmental Imagination*. Amsterdam: Amsterdam University Press; Haskell, D. (2012). *The Forest Unseen: A Year's Watch in Nature*. New York: Penguin Books; and Abbey, E. (2011). *Desert Solitaire: A Season in the Wilderness*. New York: Rosetta Books.

Chapter 5

1. Douthat, R. (2023). "Five rules for an aging world." *New York Times*, 21 January. https://www.nytimes.com/2023/01/21/opinion/aging-climate-change-demographics .html.

2. World Health Organization (2023). "Mental health of older adults." World Health Organization, October. https://www.who.int/news-room/fact-sheets/detail/mental -health-of-older-adults.

3. Bolton, A. (2022). "More older Americans become homeless as inflation rises and housing costs spike." NPR [National Public Radio], 10 November. https://www.npr .org/sections/health-shots/2022/11/10/1135125625/homelessness-elderly-housing -inflation.

4. Spader, J. (2019). *Tenure Projections of Homeowner and Renter Households for 2018–2038*. Cambridge, MA: Joint Center for Housing Studies of Harvard University. https://www.jchs.harvard.edu/sites/default/files/Harvard_JCHS_Spader_Tenure _Projections_2018-2038_1.pdf.

5. Bolton (2022).

6. American Health Care Association / National Center for Assisted Living (2023). *Nursing Home Closures: By the Numbers*. Washington, DC: AHCA/NCAL. https:// www.ahcancal.org/News-and-Communications/Fact-Sheets/FactSheets/SNF -Closures-Report.pdf.

7. Rabheru, K. (2022). "Mental health promotion and risk reduction strategies for mental disorders in older persons: Why should governments and policymakers care?" *Consortium Psychiatricum*, 3(1): 22–28.

8. Temple, J. B., Brijnath, J., Enticott, J., Utomo, A., Williams, R., and Kelaher, M. (2020). "Discrimination reported by older adults living with mental health conditions: Types, contexts and association with healthcare barriers." *Social Psychiatry and Psychiatric Epidemiology*, 56(2): 1003–1004.

9. World Health Organization (2023). "Dementia." World Health Organization, 15 March. https://www.who.int/news-room/fact-sheets/detail/dementia.

10. Dening, T., and Milne, A. (2008). "Mental health in care homes for older people." In Jacoby, R., Oppenheimer, C., and Thomas, A. (eds.), *The Oxford Textbook of Old Age Psychiatry*. Oxford: Oxford University Press.

11. Milne, A. (2010). "The 'D' word: Reflections on the relationship between stigma, discrimination and dementia." *Journal of Mental Health*, 19(3): 227–233.

12. Graham, N., Lindesay, J., Katona, C., et al. (2003). "Reducing stigma and discrimina-

tion against older people with mental disorders: A technical consensus statement." *International Journal of Geriatric Psychiatry*, 18(1): 670–678.

13. Katsumo, T. (2005). "Dementia from the inside: How people with early-stage dementia evaluate their quality of life." *Aging and Society*, 25(2): 197–214.

14. Livingston, G., Huntley, J., Sommerlad, A., et al. (2020). "Dementia prevention, intervention, and care: 2020 report of the *Lancet* Commission." *The Lancet*, 396: 413–446.

15. Engelen, L., Rahmann, M., and de Jong, E. (2022). "Design for healthy ageing— the relationship between design, well-being, and quality of life: A review." *Building Research & Information*, 50(1–2): 19–35. https://doi.org/10.1080/09613218.2021 .1984867.

16. Dreyer, J. (2023). "A giant inland sea is now a desert, and a warning for humanity." *The New York Times*, 28 November. https://www.nytimes.com/2023/11/28/opinion /climate-uzbekistan-water-aral.html.

17. Barsley, E. (2020). *Retrofitting for Flood Resilience*. London: RIBA.

18. Montoro-Ramírez, E. M., Parra-Anguita, L., Álvarez-Nieto, C., Parra, G., and López-Medina, I. (2022). "Effects of climate change in the elderly's health: A scoping review protocol." *BMJ Open*, 12(4): e058063. https://bmjopen.bmj.com/content/12 /4/e058063.

19. Filberto, D., Wethington, E., and Pillemer, K. (2009). "Older people and climate change: Vulnerability and health effects." *Generations*, 33(2): 19–25.

20. Ellis-Petersen, H. (2023). "In India, a growing need for AC could add to global heating." *Mother Jones*, 10 December. https://www.motherjones.com/politics/2023/12 /india-extreme-heat-air-conditioning-global-heating/.

21. Rhodes, J. L., Gruber, J. S., and Horton, B. (2018). "Developing an in-depth understanding of elderly adult's vulnerability to climate change." *The Gerontologist*, 58(3): 567–577.

22. Carter, T. R., Fronzek, S., Lahtinen, A. I., et al. (2016). "Characterizing vulnerability of the elderly to climate change in the Nordic region." *Regional Environmental Change*, 16(1): 43–58.

23. Wang, Z., Xu, N., Wei, W., and Zhao, N. (2020). "Social inequality among elderly individuals caused by climate change: Evidence from a migratory elderly of mainland China." *Journal of Environmental Management*, 272: 111079.

24. Chen, S., Bao, Z., and Lou, V. (2022). "Assessing the impact of the built environment on healthy aging: A gender-oriented Hong Kong study." *Environmental Impact Assessment Review*, 95(2): 21–24. https://doi.org/10.1016/j.eiar.2022.106812.

25. Rosenthal, J. K., Sclasr, E. D., Kinney, P. L., Knowlton, K., Crauderueff, R., and Brandt-Rauf, P. W. (2007). "Links between the built environment, climate and population health: Interdisciplinary environmental change research in New York City." *Annals of the Academy of Medicine Singapore*, 36(10): 834–846.

26. Alves, C. A., Duarte, D. H. S., and Gonçalves, F. L.T. (2016). "Residential buildings' thermal performance and comfort for the elderly under climate changes context in the city of São Paulo, Brazil." *Energy and Buildings*, 114(2): 62–71.

27. Rañeses, M. K., Chang-Richards, A., Wang, K. I. K., and Dirks, K. N. (2022). "Climate-adaptive housing for the elderly: A preliminary study in New Zealand." *World Building Congress 2022: Future-Proof Cities*. IOP Conference Series: Earth and Environmental Science, volume 1101. https://iopscience.iop.org/article/10.1088 /1755-1315/1101/2/022027.

28. White-Newsome, J. L., Sánchez, B. N., Jolliet, O., et al. (2012). "Climate change and health: Indoor heat exposure in vulnerable populations." *Environmental Research*, 112(1): 20–27.

29. Younger, M., Morrow-Almeida, H. R., Vindigni, S. M., and Dannenberg, A. L. (2008). "The built environment, climate change, and health: Opportunities for co-benefits." *American Journal of Preventive Medicine*, 35(5): 517–526.

30. Vince, G. (2022). *Nomad Century: How Climate Migration Will Reshape Our World*. New York: Flatiron Books, p. xi.

31. Roaf, S., Crichton, D., and Nicol, F. (2005). *Adapting Buildings and Cities for Climate Change: A 21st Century Survival Guide*. Amsterdam: Elsevier.

32. Ramirez, R. (2022). "More Americans are moving into harm's way as climate disasters increase." CNN, 8 December. https://www.cnn.com/2022/12/08/us/americans -moving-to-areas-with-high-climate-risk/index.html.

33. Vince (2022), p. 48.

34. de Boer, B., Caljouw, M., Landeweer, E., et al. (2021). "The need to consider relocations within long-term care." *Journal of the American Medical Directors Association*, 21(2): 111–123.

35. Aminzadeh, F., Dalziel, W. B., Molnar, F. J., and Garcia, L. J. (2010). "Meanings, functions, and experiences of living at home for individuals with dementia at the critical point of relocation." *Journal of Gerontological Nursing*, 36(6): 28–35. Also see Wu, C. S., and Rong, J. R. (2020). "Relocation experiences of the elderly to a long-term care facility in Taiwan: A qualitative study." *BMC Geriatrics*, 20(1): 1–11.

36. Kelsey, S., Laditka, S., and Laditka, J. (2009). "Dementia and transitioning from assisted living to memory care units: Perspectives of administrators in three facility types." *The Gerontologist*, 50(2): 192–203.

37. LaMantia, M. A., Scheunemann, L. P., Viera, A. J., Busby-Whitehead, J., and Hanson, L. C. (2010). "Interventions to improve transitional care between nursing homes and hospitals: A systematic review." *Journal of the American Geriatrics Society*, 58(4): 777–782.

38. Falk, H., Wijk, H., and Persson, L-O. (2011). "Frail older persons' experiences of interinstitutional relocation." *Geriatric Nursing*, 32(4): 245–256.

39. Holder, J. M., and Jolley, D. (2012). "Forced relocation between nursing homes: Residents' health outcomes and potential moderators." *Reviews in Clinical Gerontology*, 22(4): 22–25. Also see Jolley, D., Jefferys, P., Katona, C., and Lennon, S. (2011). "Enforced relocation of older people when care homes close: A question of life and death?" *Age and Ageing*, 40(5): 534–537.

40. Cheek, J., Byers, L., Ballantyne, A., and Quan, J. (2006). "Improving the retirement village to residential aged care transition." *Australian Health Review*, 30(3): 344–352. Also see Williams, J., Netten, A., and Ware, P. (2007). "Managing the care home closure process: Care managers' experiences and views." *The British Journal of Social Work*, 37(5): 909–924.

41. Capezuti, E., Boltz, M., Renz, S., Hoffman, D., and Norman, R. G. (2006). "Nursing home involuntary relocation: Clinical outcomes and perceptions of residents and families." *Journal of the American Medical Directors Association*, 7(8): 486–492.

42. McFadden, S. H., and Lunsman, M. (2010). "Continuity in the midst of change: Behaviors of residents relocated from a nursing home environment to small households." *American Journal of Alzheimer's Disease and Other Dementias*, 25(1): 51–57.

43. Yamamoto, K. (2008). "Influences of relocation on well-being of elderly people: A study on city planning and housing considering the adaptation to the town residence of the elderly." *Nihon Kenchiku Gakkai Keikaku-kei Ronbunshu*, 73(628): 1297–1304.

44. Castle, N. G. (2005). "Changes in health status subsequent to nursing home closure." *Ageing International*, 30(3): 263–277.

45. Hagen, B., Esther, C. A., Ikuta, R., Williams, R. J., Le Navenec, C. L., and Aho, M.

(2005). "Antipsychotic drug use in Canadian long-term care facilities: Prevalence, and patterns following resident relocation." *International Psychogeriatrics*, 17(2): 179–193.

46. Castle, N. G., and Engberg, J. B. (2008). "The health consequences for nursing home residents following Hurricane Katrina." *The Gerontologist*, 33(6): 661–687. https://doi.org/10.1177/0164027511412197.

47. Laughlin, A., Parsons, M., Kosloski, K. D., and Bergman-Evans, B. (2021). "Predictors of mortality: Following involuntary interinstitutional relocation." *Journal of Gerontological Nursing*, 33(9): 20–26.

48. Yamada, M., Yamaguchi, K., and Takada, M. (2014). "A study of the process of moving in the housing for the elderly and on the change of life in residents before and after." *Journal of Architecture and Planning*, 79(695): 11–20.

49. Abrahamson, K., Bernard, B., Magnabosco, L., Nazir, A., and Unroe, K. T. (2016). "The experiences of family members in the nursing home to hospital transfer decision." *BMC Geriatrics*, 16(1): 184–184.

50. Cioffi, J. M., Fleming, A., Wilkes, L., Sinfield, M., and Le Miere, J. (2007). "The effect of environmental change on residents with dementia: The perceptions of relatives and staff." *Dementia* (London, England), 6(2): 215–231.

51. Garcia, L. J., Hébert, M., Kozak, J., et al. (2012). "Perceptions of family and staff on the role of the environment in long-term care homes for people with dementia." *International Psychogeriatrics*, 24(5): 753–765. Also see Gaugler, J. E., and Mitchell, L. L. (2021). "Reimagining family involvement in residential long-term care." *Journal of Post-Acute and Long-Term Care Medicine*, 23(2): 235–240.

52. McAuliffe, M., and Oucho, L. A. (2024). *World Migration Report 2024*. Geneva: International Organization for Migration. https://worldmigrationreport.iom.int/msite/wmr-2024-interactive/.

53. Sherriff, L. (2024). "This Louisiana town moved to escape climate-linked disaster." *BBC.com.* 20 January. https://www.bbc.com/future/article/20240130-this-louisiana-town-moved-to-escape-climate-disaster.

54. The Lowlander Center, inclusive of Tribal Leadership, First Peoples' Conservation Council (2022). "Louisiana Tribes adapt to climate change while upholding sovereignty." *Cultural Survival*, 31 August. https://www.culturalsurvival.org/publications/cultural-survival-quarterly/louisiana-tribes-adapt-climate-change-while-upholding.

55. Baurick, T. (2022). "The last days of Isle de Jean Charles: A Louisiana tribe's struggle to escape the rising sea." *Nola*, 28 August. https://www.nola.com/news/environment/the-last-days-of-isle-de-jean-charles-a-louisiana-tribe-s-struggle-to-escape/article_70ac1746-1f22-11ed-bc68-3bde459eba68.html.

56. Panfil, Y. (2020). "The case for 'managed retreat.'" Politico, 14 July. https://www.politico.com/news/agenda/2020/07/14/climate-change-managed-retreat-341753. Challenges associated with buyouts include a loss of local tax base revenue, due to depopulation, and the perpetuation of artificially low hazard insurance premiums, perversely encouraging people to remain in place, which results in repeated rebuilding. Regardless, managed retreat is psychologically, financially, and politically difficult. While it may be politically expedient to elevate homes above their current level and build seawalls, such measures often simply delay the inevitable. Also see Garay, E. (2023). "Environmental disasters and 'dark' tourism: The modern-day ghost towns created by the climate crisis." CNN, 31 October. https://www.cnn.com/travel/modern-day-ghost-towns-climate-crisis-scn/index.html.

57. Cheng, F. (2021). "Is compulsory managed retreat our future?' *New America*, 17 November. https://www.newamerica.org/future-land-housing/briefs/is-compulsory-managed-retreat-our-future. Also see Panfil (2020).

58. Harvison, T., Newman, R., and Judd, B. (2011). *Ageing, The Built Environment and Adaptation to Climate Change*. Canberra: National Climate Change Adaptation Research Network / City Futures Research Centre. https://www.unsw.edu.au/content /dam/pdfs/engineering/civil-environmental/water-research-laboratory/accarnsi /Ageing-the-Built-Environmnet-and-Climate-Change.pdf. In emergencies, several key issues warrant consideration, including the following:

    1. Keep older persons alerted to and fully apprised of their situation, with the freedom and agency to self-prepare with sufficient supplies and medications during the post-move acclimation period, such as knowing the proper dosage required (since access to medical supply lines may be severed in the short term).

    2. To escape immediate danger, provide safe passage to a designated emergency shelter center for persons with physical or cognitive impairments (or both), as well as persons who live alone, have no family, or may accidentally be forgotten or left behind.

    3. Bring along all mobility aids. If the evacuation/relocation is unplanned or needs to be executed quickly, items such as walking aids and wheelchairs may inadvertently be left behind, becoming problematic later.

    4. Consistently monitor older persons, as they may be unable to thermoregulate their body temperature and thus be subject to hypothermia or heat stress, including while in temporary shelters.

    5. Be alert to individuals needing help. They may be reluctant to seek out assistance, or otherwise be incapable of doing so.

Also see Ross, C. E., and Mirowsky, J. (2001). "Neighborhood disadvantage, disorder and health." *Journal of Health and Social Behavior*, 42(1): 258–276.

59. American Association of Retired Persons (2022). "The impact of disasters on older adults," AARP Livable Communities. https://www.aarp.org/livable-communities/tool -kits-resources/info-2022/disaster-risks-to-older-adults.html.

Chapter 6

1. Haraway, D. J. (2016). *Staying With the Trouble: Making Kin in the Chthulucene*. Durham, NC: Duke University Press.

2. Braidotti, R. (2019). "A theoretical framework for the critical posthumanities." *Theory, Culture & Society*, 36(6): 31–61.

3. Jon, I. (2020). "Deciphering posthumanism: Why and how it matters to urban planning in the Anthropocene." *Planning Theory*, 19(4): 392–420.

4. Fox, N. J., and Alldred, P. (2016). "Sociology, environment and health: A materialist approach." *Public Health*, 141(3): 287–293.

5. Rosenberg, C. E. (1979). *Health and History*. New York: Science History. Also see Halpern, D. (2013). *Mental Health and the Built Environment: More Than Bricks and Mortar?* London: Routledge.

6. Lear, J. (2006). *Radical Hope: Ethics in the Face of Cultural Devastation*. Cambridge, MA: Harvard University Press. Also see Lobo, M. (2009). "Affective ecologies: Braiding urban worlds in Darwin, Australia." *Geoforum*, 106(2): 393–401.

7. Kohn, E. (2013). *How Forests Think: Toward an Anthropology beyond the Human*. Berkeley: University of California Press. Also see Tsing, A. (2015). *The Mushroom at the End of the World*. Princeton, NJ, and Oxford: Princeton University Press.

8. Houston, D., Hillier, J., MacCallum, D., Steele, W., and Byrne, J. (2018). "Make kin, not cities!: Multispecies entanglements and 'becoming-world' in planning theory." *Planning Theory*, 17(2): 190–212. Also see Jon (2020), p. 394.

9. Braidotti (2019).

10. Morse, J. M. (2016). *Qualitative Health Research: Creating a New Discipline*. London: Routledge.

11. Sothern, M., and Reid, B. (2018). "Humanism and health geography: Placing the human in health geography." In Crooks, V., Andrews, G. J., and Pearce, J. (eds.), *Routledge Handbook of Health Geography*. London: Routledge.

12. Todres, I., and Wheeler, S. (2001). "The complementarity of phenomenology, hermeneutics and existentialism as a philosophical perspective for nursing research." *International Journal of Nursing Studies*, 38(1): 1–8.

13. Fitzgerald, D., Rose, N., and Singh, I. (2016). "Living well in the neuropolis." *Sociological Review*, 64(Supplement 1): 221–237. Also see Kwan, M. P., and Schwanen, T. (2016). "Geographies of mobility." *Annals of the Association of American Geographers*, 106(2): 243–256. It is important to note that health researchers who have embraced posthumanist perspectives have not advocated a total break from humanist research traditions in the health sciences. Rather, they seek new ways to explore more-than-human materialist interdependencies. Unresolved tensions do remain, however—including lingering questions regarding the nature of subjectivity, agency, and cause and effect—that complicate any tidy break.

14. Guenther, R., and Vittori, G. (2013). *Sustainable Healthcare Architecture*, 2nd edition. New York: Wiley.

15. Jon (2020), p. 394. Also see Head, L. (2016). *Hope and Grief in the Anthropocene: Re-Conceptualizing Human-Nature Relations*. London: Routledge; and Usher, M. (2020). "Territory incognita." *Progress in Human Geography*, 44(6): 1019–1046.

16. Latour, B. (2010). "An attempt at a compositional manifesto." *New Literary History*, 41(3): 471–490. Also see Latour, B. (2015). "Telling friends from foes in the time of the Anthropocene." In Hamilton, C., Bonneuil, C., and Gemenne, F. (eds.), *The Anthropocene and the Global Environmental Crisis*. London: Routledge, pp. 145–155.

17. Rydin, Y. (2014). "The challenges of the 'material turn' for planning studies." *Planning Theory & Practice*, 15(4): 590–595.

18. Jon (2020), p. 396. Also see Marres, N. (2012). *Material Participation: Technology, the Environment and Everyday Publics*. Basingstoke, UK: Palgrave Macmillan; and Beauregard, R. A. (2015). *Planning Matter: Acting with Things*. Chicago: University of Chicago Press.

19. Verderber, S. (2009). "The unbuilding of historic neighborhoods in post-Katrina New Orleans." *Journal of Urban Design*, 14(3): 257–277. Also see Verderber, S. (2012). *Sprawling Cities and Our Endangered Public Health*. London: Routledge, pp. 130–171. This neighborhood recovery workshop was a near-total waste of time (although I did make some new friends). I also attended some of the parallel "district level" meetings in other parts of the city, witnessing firsthand this same thing repeatedly happening, with especially sad, dissonant impacts on the population in the nearly completely devastated suburb of Chalmette. There, a planning team led by the New Urbanist architect-guru Andres Duany led hundreds of downtrodden, highly disoriented, displaced residents through a similarly abstract, hypothetical urban "planning process." Since then, tactical urbanism has emerged as a method for identifying a more materialist approach to enacting positive change in the built environment. It consists of having community members themselves propose specific physical changes they would make in their own neighborhood. In the process of sharing these ideas, all participants can adjust their sights, becoming familiar with one another while coalescing their collective effort. Instead of being passively directed by a professional planner, the workshop participants lead or direct their own proceedings, *facilitated* by, not governed by, professional planners.

20. Webb, D. (2018). "Tactical urbanism: Delineating a critical praxis." *Planning Theory & Practice*, 19(1): 58–73.

21. Beauregard, R. A. (2015). *Planning Matter: Acting with Things*. Chicago: University of Chicago Press.

22. Houston et al. (2018), p. 194.

23. Latour, B. (2004). Politics of Nature. Cambridge, MA: Harvard University Press. Also see Jon (2020) p. 399.

24. Haraway (2016), p. 112.

25. Braidotti, R. (2019). *Posthuman Knowledge*. Medford, MA: Polity, p. 40.

26. Jon (2020), p. 402.

27. Latour, B., and Yaneva, A. (2008). "Give me a gun and I will make all buildings move: An ANT's view of architecture." In Geiser, R. (ed.), *Explorations in Architecture: Teaching, Design, Research*. Basel, Switzerland: Birkhäuser, pp. 80–89.

28. Latour and Yaneva (2008), p. 82. Also see Picon, A., and Ponte, A. (2003). *Architecture and the Sciences: Exchanging Metaphors*. New York: Princeton Architectural Press.

29. See, for example, Venturi, R. (1966). *Complexity and Contradiction in Architecture*. New York: Museum of Modern Art.

30. Andrews, G. J., and Duff, C. (2019). "Matter beginning to matter: On posthumanist understandings of the vital emergence of health." *Social Science & Medicine*, 226: 123–134.

31. Anderson, B., Kearnes, M., McFarlane, C., and Swanton, D. (2012). "On assemblages and geography." *Dialogues in Human Geography*, 2(2): 171–189.

32. Latour, B. (2005). *Reassembling the Social: An Introduction to Actor-Network-Theory*. New York: Oxford University Press.

33. Forlano, L. (2017). "Posthumanism and design." *The Journal of Design, Economics and Innovation*, 3(1): 16–29. Also see Meaney, L. (2013). "Towards posthumanist design: With-water." *FormAkademisk*, 6(2): 1–6. https://doi.org/10.7577/formakademisk.542. Also see Perry. N. (2022). "New Zealand river's personhood status offers hope to Māori." AP [Associated Press], August 14. https://apnews.com/article/religion-sacred-rivers-new-zealand-86d34a78f5fc662ccd554dd7f578d217.

34. Stengers, I. (2015). *In Catastrophic Times: Resisting the Coming Barbarism*. Paris: Open Humanities Press.

35. Keswick, M. (1986). *Chinese Gardens*. London: Academy Editions. Also see Keswick, M., Oberlander, J., and Wai, J. (1990). *In a Chinese Garden: The Art and Architecture of the Dr. Sun Yat-Sen Classical Chinese Garden*. Richmond, British Columbia: Raincoast Books. It is no coincidence that she previously authored or coauthored beautiful books on gardens, their historical origins, and their therapeutic qualities.

36. Verderber, S., and Refuerzo, B. (2020). *Innovations in Hospice Architecture*, 2nd edition. London: Routledge.

37. Andrews, G., and Duff, C. (2019). "Understanding the vital emergence and expression of aging: How matter comes to matter in gerontology's posthumanist turn." *Journal of Aging Studies*, 49(2): 46–55.

38. Verderber, S., Koyabashi, U., Dela Cruz, C., Sadat, A., and Anderson, D. A. (2023). "Residential environments for older persons: A comprehensive literature review (2005–2022)." *Health Environments Research & Design Journal*, 16(3): 291–337.

39. Office of the Premier (2020). "Ontario fast-tracks long-term care home in Toronto." News release, August 11. https://news.ontario.ca/en/release/57958/ontario-fast-tracks-long-term-care-home-in-toronto.

40. Wilson, B. (2023). "Let the post-pandemic city grow wild." *New York Times*, 9 May.

https://www.nytimes.com/2023/05/09/opinion/urban-gardens-rewilding-cities
-biodiversity.html.

41. McFall-Hgai, M. (2017). "Noticing microbial worlds: The postmodern synthesis in biology." In Tsing, A. Bubandt, N., Gan, E., and Bubandt, N. (eds.), *Art of Living on a Damaged Planet*. Minneapolis: University of Minnesota Press: 51–69.

42. Latour, B. (2017). *Facing Gaia: Eight Lectures on the New Climatic Regime*. Hoboken, NJ: Wiley.

43. Jon (2020), p. 415. Also see Serras, M. (1995 [1990]). *The Natural Contract*. Ann Arbor: University of Michigan Press.

44. Anderson, K. (2007). *Race and the Crisis of Humanism*. London: Routledge.

45. DiNovelli-Lang, D. (2013). "The return of the animal: Posthumanism, Indigeneity, and anthropology." *Environment and Society*, 4(2): 137–156.

46. Castañeda, I. (2015). "No aporias allowed: Posthumanism and the humanities." *Symploke*, 23(1–2): 75–90.

47. Raworth, K. (2018). *Doughnut Economics: Seven Ways to Think Like a 21st Century Economist*. London: Random House Business Books.

48. Roaf, S. (2018). "Building resilience in the built environment." In Trogal, K., Bauman, I., Lawrence, R., and Petrescu, D. (eds.), *Architecture and Resilience: Interdisciplinary Dialogues*. London: Routledge, pp. 144–157.

49. Dalziel, M. (2022). "Towards a posthuman practice for architecture and urbanism?" *Nordic Journal of Urban Studies*, 2(1): 90–96.

50. Kotze, L. J., and French, D. (2018). "The anthropocentric ontology of international environmental law and the sustainable development goals: Towards an ecocentric rule of law in the Anthropocene." *Global Journal of Comparative Law*, 7(1): 5–36.

51. Dalziel (2022), p. 92.

52. Braidotti, R. (2019). *Posthuman Knowledge*. Medford, MA: Polity, p. 42.

Chapter 7

1. Verderber, S. (2003). "Architecture for health—2050: An international perspective." *The Journal of Architecture*, 8(3): 281–301.

2. Ulmer, J. (2017). "Posthumanism as research methodology: Inquiry in the Anthropocene." *International Journal of Qualitative Studies in Education*, 30(9): 832–848.

3. Lippert-Rasmussen, K., Thomsen, M. R., and Wamberg, J. (2012). "Posthuman horizons and realities: Introduction." In Lipper-Rasmussen, K., Thomsen, M. R., and Wamberg, J. (eds.), *The Posthuman Condition: Ethics, Aesthetics and Politics of Biotechnological Challenges*. Aarhus, Denmark: Aarhus University Press: 7–14.

4. Lippert-Rasmussen, Thomsen, and Wamberg (2012), p. 8.

5. Lippert-Rasmussen, Thomsen, and Wamberg (2012), p. 10.

6. Gray, C. H. (2012). "Cyborging the posthuman: Participatory evolution." In Lippert-Rasmussen, Thomsen, and Wamberg (eds.), pp. 27–38.

7. See McGee, E. M. (2008). "Bioelectronics and implanted devices." In Gordijn, B., and Chadwick, R. (eds.), *Medical Enhancement and Posthumanity*. New York: Springer, pp. 207–224.

8. Kurzwell, R. (1990). *The Age of Intelligent Machines*. Cambridge, MA: MIT Press.

9. Azagury, J. (2023). "How closing the digital divide can improve the global economic outlook for 2023 and beyond." *Fortune*, 10 January. https://fortune.com/2023/01/10/how-closing-the-digital-divide-can-improve-the-global-economic-outlook-for-2023-and-beyond/.

10. Kichloo, A., Albosta, M., Dettloff, K., et al. (2020). "Telemedicine, the current COVID-19 pandemic and the future: A narrative review and perspectives moving forward in the USA." *Family Medicine and Community Health*, 8(3): 344–363.

11. Verderber, S., and Fine, D. J. (2000). *Healthcare Architecture in an Era of Radical Transformation*. New Haven, CT: Yale University Press. The first building to incorporate the interstitial floor concept was Louis Kahn's Salk Institute of Biological Studies (1965) in La Jolla, California. The mainstream use of the interstitial concept in hospitals commenced with McMaster's Medical Centre (1972) in Hamilton, Ontario.

12. Shubow, J. (2015). "Architecture continues to implode: More insiders admit the profession is failing." *Forbes*, 6 January. https://www.forbes.com/sites/justinshubow /2015/01/06/architecture-continues-to-implode-more-insiders-admit-the-profession -is-failing/?sh=3432ecac4378. The Make it Right Foundation's board is currently bogged down in lawsuits filed by homeowners. A number of the houses have already been demolished, due to their uninhabitability. Architects have failed to grasp the importance of designing *with* nature, rather than in opposition to it.

13. Mercifully, neither proposal was built. Another reason why architecture is verging on ossification is its virtuosos' continued obsession with the "art" of architecture above all else, as if every new building by a leading architect is first and foremost to be assessed as a work of sculpture, as if it were in some museum exhibit. Do the profession's cognoscenti have too little time or interest in addressing the day-to-day nitty gritty? First, the majority of buildings designed by licensed architects still consume too much energy. Second, the COVID-19 pandemic appears to have been another missed opportunity to expand the profession's manifestation of empathic social concern in the name of public interest architecture (see chapter 1).

14. Marsili, L. (2023). "What will life after globalization look like? The Venice Biennale may hold the answer." *The Guardian*, 19 June. https://www.almendron.com/tribuna /what-will-life-after-globalisation-look-like/. In democratic societies, cultural colonialism has rightly been rejected. China's refusal to participate in the 2023 Venice Biennale exhibition illustrates how authoritarianism will threaten the thoughtful reconsideration of Indigenous cultural traditions in the future.

15. Velázquez, L. (2021). "New challenges for ethics: The social impact of posthumanism, robots, and artificial intelligence." *Journal of Healthcare Engineering*, 15(2): 56–72.

16. Kaplan, S., and Kaplan, R. (1982). *Cognition and Environment: Functioning in an Uncertain World*. New York: Praeger.

17. Douglas, E. (2022). "'It's destroying me': Storm after storm, climate change increases strain on Texans' mental health." *Texas Tribune*, 8 September. https://www.houston publicmedia.org/articles/news/health-science/2022/09/08/432466/its-destroying -me-storm-after-storm-climate-change-increases-strain-on-texans-mental-health/.

18. International Society for Traumatic Stress Studies (2021). *Global Climate Change and Trauma. Briefing Paper*. ISTSS. https://istss.org/ISTSS_Main/media/Documents /ISTSS-Briefing-Paper_Climate-Change-Final.pdf.

19. Radke, P. (2023). "In 'Cancer Alley,' US chemical giants mount campaign against grassroots organizers." *The Guardian*, 4 May, https://www.theguardian.com /environment/2023/may/04/cancer-alley-louisiana-environment-oil-industry -opposition. A number of residents in these communities along the river are the descendants of slaves who once worked on the nearby plantations. Many of these plantations were sold off one by one by their owners after the US Civil War (1861–1865), and many of these were then transformed into massive industrial sites.

20. New Orleans' highest ground is the land consisting of silty soil deposits, built up over centuries, that line the east and west banks of the Mississippi River—land locally referred to as the "sliver by the river." These neighborhoods were settled in the eighteenth and nineteenth centuries by Caucasians of comparatively higher socioeconomic status.

21. I-DIEM (2023). "Institute for Diversity and Inclusion in Emergency Management

[overview]." https://i-diem.org. Remnants of Hurricane Katrina's devastation remain visible in the Lower Ninth Ward nineteen years later, with some community hospitals still shuttered. In Katrina's aftermath, Louisiana instituted a Road Home program, giving out rebuilding assistance funds based on an appraised home's value, rather than on its actual rebuilding cost. Unfortunately, after decades of discriminatory economic practices, including redlining, pre-Katrina values for homes in historically White communities typically were appraised far higher than comparable homes in Black neighborhoods. The latter's artificially low property appraisals created dire circumstances, forcing many Black families out of New Orleans permanently.

22. Lee, L. (2023). "Racial disparities are working against disaster recovery for people of color: Climate change could make it worse." CNN, 17 April. https://www.cnn.com /2023/04/14/us/racial-disparities-disaster-recovery-iyw-rd/index. In 2021, the White House acted, issuing an executive order to advance racial equity and disaster aid support for underserved communities through the federal government. Since then, FEMA launched initiatives expanding access to and reducing barriers in its assistance programs. Two years later, FEMA claimed that these changes enabled 124,000 survivors to access over $709 million (USD) in assistance they would have previously been ineligible to receive.

23. Flavelle, C. (2021). "Why does disaster aid often favor white people?" *The New York Times*, updated 27 October. https://www.nytimes.com/2021/06/07/climate/FEMA -race-climate.html.

24. ATSDR [Agency for Toxic Substances and Disease Registry] (2023). "About the Agency for Toxic Substances and Disease Registry." https://www.atsdr.cdc.gov /about/index.html. Also see Elliott, J. R., Brown, P. L., and Loughran, K. (2020). "Racial inequities in the federal buyout of flood-prone homes: A nationwide assessment of environmental adaptation." *Socius*, 6(1): 237802312090543. https://doi.org /10.1177/2378023120905439. The more aid a Caucasian neighborhood received from FEMA, the more this form of inequality grew. See Verderber, S. (2009). "The *un*-building of historic neighborhoods in post-Katrina New Orleans." *Journal of Urban Design*, 14(3): 257–277.

25. Flavelle, C., and Healy, J. (2023). "Arizona limits construction around Phoenix as its water supply dwindles." *The New York Times*, 1 June. https://www.nytimes. com/2023/06/01/climate/arizona-phoenix-permits-housing-water.html.

26. Ajasa, A. (2023). "Carbon dioxide levels in atmosphere mark a near-record surge." *The Washington Post*, 5 June. https://www.washingtonpost.com/climate-environment /2023/06/05/carbon-dioxide-growing-climate-change.

27. Weber, B. (2023). "Research advances date for likely summer ice-free Arctic by a decade." *The Globe and Mail*, 6 June. https://www.theglobeandmail.com/canada /article-research-advances-date-for-likely-summer-ice-free-arctic-by-a-decade-2/.

28. Lu, D., and Flavelle, C. (2019). "Rising seas will erase more cities by 2050, new research shows." *The New York Times*, 29 October. https://www.nytimes.com /interactive/2019/10/29/climate/coastal-cities-underwater.html.

29. Intergovernmental Panel on Climate Change (2022). *Climate Change 2022: Impacts, Adaptation and Vulnerability*. Geneva: IGPCC. https://www.ipcc.ch/report /ar6/wg2/.

30. Reuters (2023). "China provinces and Florida among the most vulnerable regions in the world, analysts find." CNN, updated 20 February. https://www.cnn.com/2023 /02/20/world/regions-climate-risk-extreme-weather-china-florida-xdi-intl/index.html. Also see Kulp, S. A., and Strauss, B. H. (2019). "New elevation data triple estimates of global vulnerability to sea-level rise and coastal flooding." *Nature Communications*, 10(2): article number 4844. https://www.nature.com/articles/s41467-019-12808-z.

31. Milman, O. (2023). "Extreme weather caused 18 disasters in the US last year, costing $165bn." *The Guardian*, 10 January. https://www.theguardian.com/environment/2023/jan/10/extreme-weather-climate-crisis-us-deaths-financial-damage.

32. Lewis, N. (2022). "A floating city in the Maldives begins to take shape." CNN, updated 22 June. https://www.cnn.com/style/article/maldives-floating-city-spc-intl/index.html. In 2019, floods caused nearly 4,500 deaths worldwide, and more than 11,000 deaths were due to all types of natural catastrophes. The article notes that in 2021, flooding cost the global economy more than $82 billion (USD), according to the reinsurance agency Swiss Re, and a report from the World Resources Institute predicts that by 2030, urban property globally worth more than $700 billion (USD) will be destroyed or damaged annually by coastal and river flooding events.

33. Kuntsler, J. H. (2005). *The Long Emergency: Surviving the End of Oil, Climate Change, and Other Converging Catastrophes of the Twenty-First Century*. New York: Grove Press.

> Influenza is an extremely potent threat to populations . . . although its mode of attack is much different from AIDS. . . . The flu can kill in a few days after infection, and it does not rely on a particular form of human behavior to spread. An epidemic requires only large cosmopolitan populations to take off. The flu originated in wild aquatic birds, has spread and mutated in domestic fowl, and tends to jump species upward, first to domestic swine [and] then to humans. . . . Where human populations swell and more people mingle with chickens, ducks, and pigs, the prospects increase dramatically for new brands of flu. This is the case particularly in China, where a peasant population of a billion lives in close quarters with their animals. . . . It travels efficiently in wild birds. . . . Flu mutates continually, like the figures spinning on a slot machine and in about eighty-year cycles hits the jackpot to produce new strains that are violently destructive to human life. . . . The superflu escalates to severe pneumonia, toxic shock, and organ failure, even in the young and healthy. . . . The infamous 1918 influenza, which spun around the planet in the last year of World War I, ended up killing up to 40 million people worldwide, including 675,000 Americans. . . . More people died of that influenza in a single year than in four years of the bubonic plague from 1347 to 1351. The 1918 pandemic affected everyone, with one-quarter of the United States and one-fifth worldwide infected at its height. . . . Bodies piled up as the massive deaths of the epidemic continued. Besides the lack of health care workers and medical supplies there was a shortage of coffins, morticians, and gravediggers. The world is overdue for a new outbreak of supervirus on the order of the 1918 pandemic.

34. Hancock, T. (2016). "Healthcare in the Anthropocene: Challenges and opportunities." *Healthcare Quarterly*, 19(3): 17–22.

35. Verderber, S. (2023). "Pandemical healthcare architecture, social responsibility and health equity." In Tural, E., Ortega-Andeane, P., and Rugger, D. (eds.), *54th Annual Meeting of the Environmental Design Research Association, 2023*. Washington, DC: Environmental Deign Research Association, pp. 54–59. https://www.proceedings.com/content/074/074123webtoc.pdf.

36. Wuebbles, D. J., D. W. Fahey, K. A. Hibbard, D. J. Dokken, B. C. Stewart, and T. K. Maycock, eds. (2018). Fourth National Climate Assessment. Washington, DC: US Global Change Research Program. https://science2017.globalchange.gov/.

37. Goodell, J. (2019). "Can we survive extreme heat?" *Rolling Stone*, 27 August. https://www.rollingstone.com/culture/culture-features/climate-crisis-goodell-survive-extreme-heat-875198.

38. Parshley, L. (2023). "Climate change could happen fast." *The Atlantic*, 20 July. https://www.theatlantic.com/science/archive/2023/07/climate-change-tipping-points/674778/.

39. World Health Organization (2023). "Climate change." World Health Organization, 12 October. https://www.who.int/news-room/fact-sheets/detail/climate-change-and-health.

40. Isai, V., and Bilefsky, D. (2021). "At nearly 116 degrees, heat in Western Canada shatters national record." *The New York Times*, updated 10 July. https://www.nytimes.com/2021/06/28/world/canada/canada-heat-wave-record.html. Also see Ramirez, R. (2023). "Texas's nighttime temperatures are a symptom of a new, more dangerous kind of heat wave." CNN, 27 June. https://www.cnn.com/2023/06/27/weather/texas-heat-wave-nighttime-temperatures-climate/index.html.

41. Diamond, J. (2023). "Like Finland, imagine everything that could go wrong." *The New York Times*, 13 February. https://www.nytimes.com/2023/02/13/opinion/earthquake-natural-disaster.html.

42. Ferrando, F. (2016). "The party of the Anthropocene: Post-humanism, environmentalism and the post-anthropocentric paradigm shift." *Relations*, 4(2): 159–172. https://www.ledonline.it/index.php/Relations/article/view/1073.

Appendix A

1. Wang, X., Rodríguez, D. A., Sarmiento, O. L., and Guaje, O. (2019). "Commute patterns and depression: Evidence from eleven Latin American cities." *Journal of Transport & Health*, 14(4): 100607.

2. Hayward, C. (2016). *Healthcare Facility Planning: Thinking Strategically*, 2nd edition. Washington, DC: Health Administration Press.

3. Maggie's Centres (2023). *Maggie's Architecture and Landscape Brief*. https://www.maggies.org/media/filer_public/e0/3e/e03e8b60-ecc7-4ec7-95a1-18d9f9c4e7c9/maggies_architecturalbrief_2015.pdf.

4. Maggie's Centres (2023).

5. Jencks, C. (2015). *The Architecture of Hope*. London: Frances Lincoln.

6. Aiken, N. E. (1998). *The Biological Origins of Art*. Westport, CT: Praeger.

7. Armstrong, J. (20221). "The healing power of art." *MoMA Magazine*, 17 September. https://www.moma.org/magazine/articles/629.

8. Hathorn, K., and Nanda, U. (2008). *A Guide to Evidence-Based Art*. Hawthorne, CA: The Center for Health Design. https://www.healthdesign.org/chd/knowledge-repository/guide-evidence-based-art.

9. Schumacher, E. F. (1973). *Small is Beautiful: A Study of Economics as if People Mattered*. New York: Vintage Books.

10. Maggie's Centres (2023).

11. Mooventhan, A., and Nivethitha, L. (2014). "Scientific evidence-based effects of hydrotherapy on various systems of the body." *North American Journal of Medical Sciences*, 6(5): 199–209. https://pmc.ncbi.nlm.nih.gov/articles/PMC4049052/.

12. Saleeby, C. W. (1922). "The advance of heliotherapy." *Nature*, 109: 663.

13. Choukroun, J., and Geoffroy, P. A. (2019). "Light therapy in mood disorders: A brief history with psychological insights." *Chronobiological Medicine*, 1(1): 3–8.

14. Getersleben, B., and Andrews, M. (2013). "When walking in nature is not restorative—the role of prospect and refuge." *Health Place*, 20(3): 91–101.

15. Dosen, A., and Ostwald, M. J. (2013). "Prospect and refuge theory: Constructing a critical definition for architecture and design." *The International Journal of Design in Society*, 6(1): 9–23.

16. Loures, L. (2019). "Landscape reclamation as a key factor for sustainable development." In Luís, L (ed.), *Landscape Reclamation—Rising from What's Left*, pp. 1–9. https://www.intechopen.com/books/8295.

17. Kellert, S. R. (2008). "Dimensions, elements, and attributes of biophilic design." In Kellert, S. R., Heerwagen, J. H., and Mador, M. L. (eds.), *Biophilic Design: The Theory, Science and Practice of Bringing Buildings to Life*. New York: John Wiley & Sons.

18. Hahn, J. (2022). "Ten gravity-defying homes that are raised up on stilts." *Dezeen*, 27 May. https://www.dezeen.com/2022/05/27/stilts-homes-architecture-roundup/.

19. Edelstein, L. (1943). *The Hippocratic Oath: Text, Translation and Interpretation*. Baltimore: Johns Hopkins University Press.

20. Verderber, S. (2018). *Innovations in Behavioural Health Architecture*. London: Routledge.

21. Senson, A. (2016) "Virtual reality therapy: Treating the global mental health crisis." *Techcrunch*, 6 January. https://www.techcrunch.com/2016/01/06/virtual-reality -therapy-treating-the-global-mental-health-crisis/.

22. Abraham, A., Sommerhalder, K., and Abel, T. (2010). "Landscape and well-being: A scoping study on the health-promoting impact of outdoor environments." *International Journal of Public Health*, 55(1): 59–69.

23. Zhang, Y. W., Wang, J., and Hong Fang, T. (2022). "The effect of horticultural therapy on depressive symptoms among the elderly: A systematic review and meta-analysis." *Frontiers in Public Health*, 10: article number 4. https://doi.org/10.3389/fpubh.2022 .953363.

24. Poulsen, D. V., Stigsdotter, U. K., Djernis, D., and Sidenius, U. (2016). "Everything just seems much more right in nature: How veterans with post-traumatic stress disorder experience nature-based activities in a forest therapy garden." *Health Psychology Open*, 3(1). https://doi.org/10.1177/2055102916637090.

25. Carrington, D. (2023). "COP28 failed to halt fossil fuels' deadly expansion—so what now?" *The Guardian*, 14 December. https://www.theguardian.com/environment/2023 /dec/14/cop28-fossil-fuels-deadly-expansion-plans-what-now#:~:text=Cop28.html.

Appendix B

1. Verderber, S., Koyabashi, U., Dela Cruz, C., Sadat, A., and Anderson, D. (2023). "Residential environments for older persons: A comprehensive literature review (2005–2022)." *HERD: Health Environments Research & Design Journal*, 16(3): 291–337. https://doi.org/10.1177/19375867231152611.

2. See, for example, Province of Ontario (2023). The Fundamental Principle and the Residents' Bill of Rights under the Fixing Long-Term Care Act, 2021. Publications Ontario, May, with its twenty-nine provisos. https://www.publications.gov.on.ca/store /20170501121/Free_Download_Files/300951.pdf. Also see CLEO (2023). "Residents' Bill of Rights: Your rights if you live in a long-term care home." Community Legal Education Ontario, February. https://www.cleo.on.ca/en/publications/everyres.

3. Van Hoof, J., Verhagen, M. M., Wouters, E. J. M., Marston, H. R., Rijnaard, M. D., and Janssen, B. M. (2015). "Picture your nursing home: Exploring the sense of home of older residents through photography." *Journal of Aging Research*, 15(4): 1–11.

4. Rijnaard, M. D., Van Hoof, J., Janssen, B. M., et al. (2016). "The factors influencing the sense of home in nursing homes: A systematic review from the perspective of residents." *Journal of Aging Research*, 16(1): 6143645.

5. Rodrigue, M. (2022). "Canada's long-term care sector is in crisis: It's time to care for those who care for us." *Toronto Star*, 28 October. https://www.thestar.com/opinion /contributors/2022/10/28/canadas-long-term-care-sector-is-in-crisis-its-time-to-care -for-those-who-care-for-us.html.

6. Craig, C. (2017). "Imagined futures: Designing future environments for the care of older people." *The Design Journal*, 20(Supplement 1): S2336–S2347. https://doi.org /10.1080/14606925.2017.1352749.

7. Lawton, M. P. (1985). "The elderly in context: Perspectives from environmental psychology and gerontology." *Environment and Behavior*, 17(4): 501–519.

8. Orfield, S. (2015). "Dementia environment design in seniors housing: Optimizing

resident perception and cognition." *Seniors Housing and Care Journal*, 23(2): 58–69. https://www.academia.edu/17854834/Dementia_environment_design _optimizing_resident_perception_and_cognition.

9. Chaudhury, H., and Cooke, H. (2014). "Design matters in dementia care: The role of the physical environment in dementia care settings." In Downs, M., and Bowers, B. (eds.), *Excellence in Dementia Care*, 2nd edition. Oxford: Open University Press, pp. 144–158.

10. Aung, M., Koyanagi, Y., Ueno, S., Tiraphat, S., and Yuasa, M. (2021). "A contemporary insight into age-friendly environments contributing to the social network, active ageing and quality of life of community resident seniors in Japan." *Journal of Aging and Environment*, 35(2): 145–160.

11. Verderber, S. (2011). *Innovations in Hospital Architecture*. London: Routledge.

12. Jenkens, R., Thomas, W., and Barber, V. (2012). "Can community-based services thrive in a licensed nursing home?" *Generations: Journal of the American Society on Aging*, 36(1): 125–130. http://www.jstor.org/stable/44875748.

13. Andersson, D., Granath, K., and Nylander, O. (2021). "Aging-in-place: Residents' attitudes and floor plan potential in apartment buildings from 1990 to 2015." *HERD: Health Environments Research & Design Journal*, 14(4): 211–226.

14. Burton, E., and Sheehan, B. (2010). "Care-home environments and well-being: Identifying the design features that most affect older residents." *Journal of Architectural and Planning Research*, 27(3): 241–242.

15. Cerina, V., Fornara, F., and Manica, S. (2017). "Architectural style and green spaces predict older adults' evaluations of residential facilities." *European Journal of Ageing*, 14(3): 207–217. https://www.ncbi.nlm.nih.gov/pmc/articles/PMC5587453/.

16. Boydell, K. (2014). *Best Practice in Housing Design for Seniors' Supportive Housing*. Waterloo, Ontario: Regional Municipality of Waterloo.

17. Wrublowsky, R. (2018). *Design Guide for Long Term Care Homes*. Winnipeg, Manitoba: MMP Architects. https://www.fgiguidelines.org/wp-content/uploads/2018/03 /MMP_DesignGuideLongTermCareHomes_2018.01.pdf.

18. Cohen, L. W., Zimmerman, S., Reed, D., et al. (2016). "The Green House model of nursing home care in design and practice." *Health Services Research*, 51(1): 352–377.

19. Lindheim, R. (1978). "How modern hospitals got that way." *The Co-Evolution Quarterly*, 3(2): 46–54.

20. Cohen et al. (2016).

21. De Rooij, A. H., Luijkx, K. G., Schaafsma, J., Declercq, A. G., Emmerink, P. M., and Schols, J. M. (2012). "Quality of life of residents with dementia in traditional versus small-scale long-term care settings: A quasi-experimental study." *International Journal of Nursing Studies*, 49(8): 931–940. https://doi.org/10.1016/j.ijnurstu.2012.02.007.

22. Anderson, D. C., Grey, T., Kennelly, S., and O'Neill, D. (2020). "Nursing home design and COVID-19: Balancing infection control, quality of life, and resilience." *Journal of the American Medical Directors Association*, 21(11): 1519–1524. https://doi.org /10.1016/j.jamda.2020.09.005.

23. Wrublowsky (2018).

24. Buffel, T., Phillipson, C., and Scharf, T. (2012). "Ageing in urban environments: Developing 'age-friendly' cities." *Critical Social Policy*, 32(4): 597–617. https:// journals.sagepub.com/doi/10.1177/0261018311430457.

25. World Health Organization (2024). "Noncommunicable diseases." World Health Organization, 23 December. https://www.who.int/news-room/fact-sheets/detail /noncommunicable-diseases.

26. Aung, M., Koyanagi, Y., Ueno, S., Tiraphat, S., and Yuasa, M. (2021) "A contemporary insight into an age-friendly environment contributing to the social network, active

aging and quality of life of community resident seniors in Japan." *Journal of Aging and Environment*, 35(2): 145–160. https://doi.org/10.1080/26892618.2020.1813232.

27. Alley, D., Liebig, P., Pynoos, J., Banerjee, T., and Choi, I. H. (2007). "Creating elder-friendly communities: Preparations for an aging society." *Journal of Gerontological Social Work*, 49(1–2): 1–18. https://doi.org/10.1300/J083v49n01_01.

28. Anderson et al. (2020).

29. Söderberg, M., Ståhl, A., and Emilsson, U. M. (2012). "Family members' strategies when their elderly relatives consider relocation to a residential home—adapting, representing and avoiding." *Journal of Aging Studies*, 26(4): 495–503. https://doi.org/10.1016/j.jaging.2012.07.002.

30. Steele, L., Carr, R., Swaffer, K., Phillipson, L., and Fleming, R. (2020). "Human rights and the confinement of people living with dementia in care homes." *Health and Human Rights*, 22(1): 7–19.

31. Innes, A., Kelly, F., and Dincarslan, O. (2011). "Care home design for people with dementia: What do people with dementia and their family carers value?" *Aging & Mental Health*, 15(5): 548–556. https://doi.org/10.1080/13607863.2011.556601.

32. Steele et al. (2020). Also see Wang, C., and Kuo, N. (2006). "Zeitgeists and development trends in long-term care facility design." *The Journal of Nursing Research*, 14(2): 123–132. https://doi.org/10.1097/01.JNR.0000387570.43727.12.

33. Healthwatch, Bradford and District (2017). "The big conversation: Engagement report." Bradford and District, UK, 25 November. https://www.healthwatchbradford.co.uk/report/2017-11-25/big-conversation.

34. Anderson et al. (2020). Also see Calkins, M., and Cassella, C. (2007). "Exploring the cost and value of private versus shared bedrooms in nursing homes." *The Gerontologist*, 47(2): 169–183. https://doi.org/10.1093/geront/47.2.169.

35. Agarwal, M., Stone, P. W., and Dick, A. (2019). "Evaluation of nursing home infection control programs: A pre- and post-study." *American Journal of Infection Control*, 47(6, Supplement): S34. https://doi.org/10.1016/j.ajic.2019.04.075.

36. Stone, P. W., Herzig, C. T., Pogorzelska-Maziarz, M., et al. (2015). "Understanding infection prevention and control in nursing homes: A qualitative study." *Geriatric Nursing* (New York), 36(4): 267–272. https://doi.org/10.1016/j.gerinurse.2015.02.023.

37. Brown, K. A., Jones, A., Daneman, N., et al. (2021). "Association between nursing home crowding and COVID-19 infection and mortality in Ontario, Canada." *JAMA Internal Medicine*, 181(2): 229–236. https://doi.org/10.1001/jamainternmed.2020.6466.

38. Gordon, A., Goodman, C., Achterberg, W., et al. (2020). "Commentary: COVID in care homes—challenges and dilemmas in healthcare delivery." *Age and Ageing*, 49(5): 701–705. https://doi.org/10.1093/ageing/afaa113.

39. Bengtsson, A., Hägerhäll, C., Englund, J.-E., and Grahn, P. (2015). "Outdoor environments at three nursing homes: Semantic environmental descriptions." *Journal of Housing for the Elderly*, 29(1–2): 53–76. https://doi.org/10.1080/02763893.2014.987863.

40. Rijnaard et al. (2016).

41. Vecellio, D. J., Bardenhagen, E. K., Lerman, B., and Brown, R. D. (2021). "The role of outdoor microclimatic features at long-term care facilities in advancing the health of its residents: An integrative review and future strategies." *Environmental Research*, 20(1): 111583–111583. https://doi.org/10.1016/j.envres.2021.111583.

42. Chu, C. H., Donato-Woodger, S., and Dainton, C. J. (2020). "Competing crises: COVID-19 countermeasures and social isolation among older adults in long-term care." *Journal of Advanced Nursing*, 76(10): 2456–2459. https://doi.org/10.1111/jan.14467.

43. Van Hoof, J., Janssen, M. L., Heesakkers, C. M. C., et al. (2016). "The importance of personal possessions for the development of a sense of home in nursing home residents." *Journal of Housing for the Elderly*, 30(1): 35–51. https://doi.org/10.1080/02763893.2015.1129381.

44. Chaudhury, H., Cooke, H. A., Cowie, H., and Razaghi, L. (2018). "The influence of the physical environment on residents with dementia in long-term care settings: A review of the empirical literature." *The Gerontologist*, 58(5): 325–337. https://doi.org/10.1093/geront/gnw259.

45. Steeves, J. (2005). "Examination of universal design in kitchens and bathrooms of the Housing and Urban Development demonstration program: Elderly cottage housing opportunity." PhD diss., Virginia Polytechnic Institute and State University. http://hdl.handle.net/10919/77131.

46. Wrublowsky (2018).

47. Boge, J., Callewaert, S., and Petersen, K. A. (2017). "The impact of bathroom design on privacy for users with special needs." *Ageing International*, 44(3): 300–317. https://doi.org/10.1007/s12126-017-9311-9.

48. Chu et al. (2020).

49. Brown et al. (2021).

50. Castle, N. G., Wagner, L. M., Perera, S., Ferguson, J. C., and Handler, S. M. (2010). "Assessing resident safety culture in nursing homes: Using the nursing home survey on resident safety." *Journal of Patient Safety*, 6(2): 59–67. https://doi.org/10.1097/PTS.0b013e3181bc05fc.

51. Calkins, M. P. (2009). "Evidence-based long term care design." *NeuroRehabilitation*, 25(3): 151–152.

52. Chaudhury, H., Hung, L., & Badger, M. (2013). "The role of physical environment in supporting person-centered dining in long-term care: A review of the literature." *American Journal of Alzheimer's Disease and Other Dementias*, 28(2): 492–500.

53. Chaudhury, H., Hung, L., Rust, T., and Wu, S. (2016). "Do physical environmental changes make a difference? Supporting person-centered care at mealtimes in nursing homes." *Dementia: The International Journal of Social Research and Practice*, 14(2): 879–896.

54. Verbeek, H., van Rossum, E., Zwakhalen, S. M., Kempen, G. I., and Hamers, J. P. (2009). "Small, homelike care environments for older people with dementia: A literature review." *International Psychogeriatrics*, 21(3): 252–264.

55. Van Hoof, J., Wetzels, M., Dooremalen, A. M., et al. (2014). "Technological and architectural solutions for Dutch nursing homes: Results of a multidisciplinary mind mapping session with professional stakeholders." *Technology in Society*, 36(1): 1–12.

56. Ferdous, F. (2021). "Redesigning memory care in the COVID-19 era: Interdisciplinary spatial design interventions to minimize social isolation in older adults." *Journal of Aging & Social Policy*, 33(4–5): 555–569. https://doi.org/10.1080/08959420.2021.1924345.

57. Campo, M., and Chaudhury, H. (2012). "Informal social interaction among residents with dementia in special care units: Exploring the role of the physical and social environments." *Dementia: The International Journal of Social Research and Practice*, 11(2): 401–423.

58. Verbeek et al. (2009).

59. Campo and Chaudhury (2012).

60. Nasrallah, E., and Pati, D. (2021). "Can physical design help reduce loneliness in the elderly? A theoretical exploration." *HERD: Health Environments Research & Design Journal*, 14(3): 374–385.

61. Stevens, R., Petermans, A., Vanrie, J., and Van Cleempoel, K. (2013). "Well-being from the perspective of interior architecture: Expected experience about residing in residential care centers." *IASDR 2013: Consilience and Innovation in Design*. International Association of Societies of Design Research Conference, Tokyo, pp. 26–30.

62. Boydell (2014).

63. Rijnaard et al. (2016).

64. Hsieh, C.-H., Chen, C.-M., Yang, J.-Y., Lin, Y.-J., Liao, M.-L., and Chueh, K.-H. (2021). "The effects of immersive garden experience on the health care of elderly residents with mild-to-moderate cognitive impairment living in nursing homes after the COVID-19 pandemic." *Landscape and Ecological Engineering*, 18(1): 45–56.

65. Chi, P., Gutberg, J., and Berta, W. (2020). "The conceptualization of the natural environment in healthcare facilities: A scoping review." *HERD: Health Environments Research & Design Journal*, 13(1): 30–47.

66. Peters, T., and Verderber, S. (2022). "Biophilic design strategies in long-term residential care environments for persons with dementia." *Journal of Aging and Environment*, 36(3): 227–255. https://doi.org/10.1080/26892618.2021.1918815.

67. Browning, W. D., Ryan, C. O., and Clancy, J. O. (2014). *14 Patterns of Biophilic Design*. New York: Terrapin Bright Green. https://www.terrapinbrightgreen.com/reports /14-patterns/. Also see Ryan, C. O., Browning, W. D., Clancy, J. O., Andrews, S. L., and Kallianpurkar, N. B. (2014). "Biophilic design patterns: Emerging nature-based parameters for health and well-being in the built environment." Archnet—International Journal of Architectural Research, 8(2): 62–76. https://earthwise.education/wp -content/uploads/2019/10/Biophilicdesign-patterns.pdf.

68. Goldin, G. (1994). *Work of Mercy: A Picture History of Hospitals*. Boston: Boston Mills Press.

69. Xie, Q., and Yuan, X. (2021). "Functioning and environment: Exploring outdoor activity-friendly environments for older adults with disabilities in a Chinese long-term care facility." *Building Research and Information: International Journal of Research, Development and Demonstration*, 50(1–2): 1–17.

70. Rijnaard et al. (2016).

71. Engelen, L., Rahmann, M., and de Jong, E. (2022). "Design for healthy ageing—the relationship between design, well-being, and quality of life: A review." *Building Research & Information*, 50(1–2): 19–35.

72. Connell, B. R., Sanford, J. A., and Lewis, D. (2007). "Therapeutic effects of an outdoor activity program on nursing home residents with dementia." *Journal of Housing for the Elderly*, 21(3–4): 194–209. https://doi.org/10.1300/J081v21n03_10.

73. Center for Maximum Potential Building Systems (n.d.). "Green Guide for Health Care." CMPBS. https://www.cmpbs.org/projects/green-guide-health-care.

74. Sun, K., Specian, M., and Hong, T. (2020). "Nexus of thermal resilience and energy efficiency in buildings: A case study of a nursing home." *Buildings and Environment*, 17(2): 1–25.

75. Stone et al. (2015).

76. Bentayeb, M., Norback, D., Bednarek, M., et al. (2015). "Indoor air quality, ventilation and respiratory health in elderly residents living in nursing homes in Europe." *The European Respiratory Journal*, 45(5): 1228–1238. https://doi.org/10.1183/09031936 .00082414.

77. Tartarini, F., Cooper, P., Fleming, R., and Batterham, M. (2017). "Indoor air temperature and agitation of nursing home residents with dementia." *American Journal of Alzheimer's Disease and Other Dementias*, 32(5): 272–281. https://doi.org/10.1177/1533317 517704898.

78. Jo, H., Song, C., and Miyazaki, Y. (2019). "Physiological benefits of viewing nature:

A systematic review of indoor experiments." *International Journal of Environmental Research and Public Health*, 16(23): 4739.

79. Barrick, A. L., Sloane, P. D., Williams, C. S., et al. (2010). "Impact of ambient bright light on agitation in dementia." *International Journal of Geriatric Psychiatry*, 25(10): 1013–1021. https://doi.org/10.1002/gps.2453.

80. WWF [World Wildlife Fund] (2023). *Living Planet Report 2024: A System in Peril*. Gland, Switzerland: World Wildlife Fund. https://www.worldwildlife.org/publications /2024-living-planet-report.

81. Baldwin, R. F., Powell, R. B., and Kellert, S. R. (2011). "Habitat as architecture: Integrating conservation planning and human health." *Ambio*, 40(3): 322–327. https://doi.org/10.1007/s13280-010-0103-7.

82. Alzheimer's Association (2022). "2022 Alzheimer's disease facts and figures." *Alzheimer's & Dementia*, 18(4): 700–789. https://doi.org/10.1002/alz.12638.

83. World Health Organization (2023). "Dementia." World Health Organization, 15 March. https://www.who.int/news-room/fact-sheets/detail/dementia.

84. Caspi, E. (2014). "Wayfinding difficulties among elders with dementia in an assisted living residence." *Dementia*, 13(4): 429–450. https://doi.org/10.1177/14713012145 35134.

85. Marquardt, G., and Schmieg, P. (2009). "Dementia-friendly architecture: Environments that facilitate wayfinding in nursing homes." *American Journal of Alzheimer's Disease and Other Dementias*, 24(4): 333–340.

86. Marquardt, G. (2011). "Wayfinding for people with dementia: A review of the role of architectural design." *HERD: Health Environments Research & Design Journal*, 4(2): 75–90. https://doi.org/10.1177/193758671100400207.

87. Algase, D. L., Beattie, E. R., Antonakos, C., Beel-Bates, C. A., and Yao, L. (2010). "Wandering and the physical environment." *American Journal of Alzheimer's Disease and Other Dementias*, 25(4): 340–346. https://doi.org/10.1177/1533317510365342.

84. Detweiler, M. B., Murphy, P. F., Myers, L. C., and Kim, K. Y. (2008). "Does a wander garden influence inappropriate behaviors in dementia residents?" *American Journal of Alzheimer's Disease and Other Dementias*, 23(1): 31–45. https://doi.org/10.1177 /1533317507309799.

89. Detweiler, M. B., Murphy, P. F., Kim, K. Y., Myers, L. C., and Ashai, A. (2009). "Scheduled medications and falls in dementia patients utilizing a wander garden." *American Journal of Alzheimer's Disease and Other Dementias*, 24(4): 322–332. https://doi .org/10.1177/1533317509334036.

90. Chaudhury et al. (2018).

91. De Rooij, A. H., Luijkx, K. G., Schaafsma, J., Declercq, A. G., Emmerink, P. M., and Schols, J. M. (2012). "Quality of life of residents with dementia in traditional versus small-scale long-term care settings: A quasi-experimental study." *International Journal of Nursing Studies*, 49(8): 931–940. https://doi.org/10.1016/j.ijnurstu.2012.02.007.

92. de Boer, B., Bozdemir, B., Jansen, J., Hermans, M., Hamers, J. P., and Verbeek, H. (2021). "The Homestead: Developing a conceptual framework through co-creation for innovating long-term dementia care environments." *International Journal of Environmental Research and Public Health*, 18(1): 57–74. https://doi.org/10.3390 /ijerph18010057.

93. Orfield (2015).

94. Verderber, S. (2014). "Exploring healthcare architecture through the medium of film: Motives and techniques." *International Journal of Architectural Research*, 8(1): 29–49.

95. Burton and Sheehan (2010).

96. Preiser, W. F. E., and Smith, K., eds. (2010). *Universal Design Handbook*, 2nd edition. New York: McGraw-Hill.

97. Carr, K., Weir, P. L., and Azar, N. R. (2013). "Universal design: A step toward successful aging." *Journal of Aging Research*, 12 (2): 44–58. https://doi.org/10.1155/2013/324624.

98. Brown, P. B., Hudak, S. L., Horn, S. D., Cohen, L. W., Reed, D. A., and Zimmerman, S. (2016). "Workforce characteristics, perceptions, stress, and satisfaction among staff in Green House and other nursing homes." *Health Services Research*, 51(Supplement 1): 418–432. https://doi.org/10.1111/1475-6773.12431.

99. Verbeek, H., Zwakhalen, S. M., van Rossum, E., Ambergen, T., Kempen, G. I., and Hamers, J. P. (2010). "Dementia care redesigned: Effects of small-scale living facilities on residents, their family caregivers, and staff." *Journal of the American Medical Directors Association*, 11(9): 662–670. https://doi.org/10.1016/j.jamda.2010.08.001.

100. Ben Natan, M. (2008). "Perceptions of nurses, families, and residents in nursing homes concerning residents' needs." *International Journal of Nursing Practice*, 14(3): 195–199. https://doi.org/10.1111/j.1440-172X.2008.00687.x.

101. Goldfarb, A., and Teodorisis, F. (2022)."Why is AI adoption in health care lagging?" The Brookings Institution, 9 March. https://www.brookings.edu/research/why-is-ai-adoption-in-health-care-lagging/.

102. Tsigkari, M., Tarabishy, S., and Kosicki, M. (2022). "Towards artificial intelligence in architecture: How machine learning can change the way we approach design." *Foster + Partners*, 29 March. https://www.fosterandpartners.com/insights/plus-journal/towards-artificial-intelligence-in-architecture-how-machine-learning-can-change-the-way-we-approach-design.

103. Suleman, R., and Bhatia, F. (2021). "Intergenerational housing as a model for improving older-adult health." *BC Medical Journal*, 63(4): 171–173.

104. Poole, A. (2019). "B.C. Company helps seniors find young people to share a home, expenses." *CBC News*, 13 August. http://www.cbc.ca/news/canada/british-columbia/roomies-happipad-intergenerational housing-1.5244021.

105. Tan, J. Y., Tam, W. S., Goh, H. S., Ow, C. C., and Wu, X. V. (2021). "Impact of sense of coherence, resilience and loneliness on quality of life amongst older adults in long-term care: A correlational study using the salutogenic model." *Journal of Advanced Nursing*, 77(11): 4471–4489.

106. Tsai, F. J., Motamed, S., and Rougemont, A. (2013). "The protective effect of taking care of grandchildren on elders' mental health? Associations between changing patterns of intergenerational exchanges and the reduction of elders' loneliness and depression between 1993 and 2007 in Taiwan." *BMC Public Health*, 13(2): 567.

107. Young, T. K., Chatwood, S., and Marchildon, J. D. (2016). "Healthcare in Canada's Far North: Are we getting value for the money?" *Healthcare Policy*, 12(1): 59–70.

108. Wilson, K. (2003). "Therapeutic landscapes and First Nations peoples: An exploration of culture, health and place." *Health & Place*, 9(2): 83–93.

109. Government of Canada (2009). *Canada's Northern Strategy: Our North, Our Heritage, Our Future*. Ottawa: Ministry of Public Works and Government Services Canada. https://library.arcticportal.org/1885/1/canada.pdf.

110. Verderber, S., Wolf, J. P., and Skouris, E. (2020). "Indigenous ecohumanist architecture for health in Canada's Far North." *HERD: Health Environments Research & Design Journal*, 13(3): 41–56. https://journals.sagepub.com/doi/10.1177/1937586720933176.

111. Howlett, K., and Chambers, S. (2023). "Ontario to lose nursing homes as owners, facing mandatory upgrades, opt to sell to housing developers." *The Globe and Mail*, 12 April. https://www.theglobeandmail.com/canada/article-ontario-toronto-for-profit-nursing-homes/.

112. Holder, J. M., and Jolley, D. (2012). "Forced relocation between nursing homes: Residents' health outcomes and potential moderators." *Reviews in Clinical Gerontology*, 22(4): 301–319.

113. Kelsey, S., Laditka, S., and Laditka, J. (2009). "Dementia and transitioning from assisted living to memory care units: Perspectives of administrators in three facility types." *The Gerontologist*, 50(2): 192–203. https://doi.org/10.1093/geront/gnp115.

114. Elizarova, O., and Dowd, K. (2017). "Participatory design in practice." *UX Magazine*, 14 December. https://uxmag.com/articles/participatory-design-in-practice.

115. Jiang, Y., Xia, Q., Zhou, P., Jiang, S., Diwan, V. K., and Xu, B. (2021). "Environmental hazards increase the fall risk among residents of long-term care facilities: A prospective study in Shanghai, China." *Age and Ageing*, 50(3): 875–881. https://doi.org/10.1093/ageing/afaa218.

116. Castle et al. (2010).

117. Van Steenwinkel, I., Baumers, S., and Heylighen, A. (2012). "Home in later life: A framework for the architecture of home environments." *Home Cultures*, 9(2): 195–217. https://doi.org/10.2752/175174212X13325123562304.

118. Cater, D., Tunalilar, O., White, D. L., Hasworth, S., and Winfree, J. (2021). "*Home is home*: Exploring the meaning of home across long-term care settings." *Journal of Aging and Environment*, 12(3): 1–18. https://doi.org/10.1080/26892618.2021.1932012.

119. Ferdous (2021).

120. Giggins, O., Doyle, J., Hogan, K., and George, M. (2019). "The impact of a cycled lighting intervention on nursing home residents: A pilot study." *Gerontological Geriatric Medicine*, 5(1): 141–162. https://doi.org/10.1177/2333721419897453.

121. Dowling, G. A., Mastick, J., Hubbard, E. M., Luxenberg, J. S., and Burr, R. L. (2005). "Effect of timed bright light treatment for rest-activity disruption in institutionalized patients with Alzheimer's disease." *International Journal of Geriatric Psychiatry*, 20(8): 738–743. http://doi.org/10.1002/gps.1352.

122. Barrick, A. L., Sloane, P. D., Williams, C. S., et al. (2010). "Impact of ambient bright light on agitation in dementia." *International Journal of Geriatric Psychiatry*, 25(10): 1013–1021. https://doi.org/10.1002/gps.2453.

123. De Lepeleire, J., Bouwen, A., De Coninck, L., and Buntinx, F. (2007). "Insufficient lighting in nursing homes." *Journal of the American Medical Directors Association*, 8(3): 314–317. https://doi.org/10.1016/j.jamda.2007.01.003.

124. Kovach, C. R., Taneli, Y., Neiman, T., Dyer, E. M., Arzaga, A. J. A., and Kelber, S. T. (2017). "Evaluation of an ultraviolet room disinfection protocol to decrease nursing home microbial burden, infection and hospitalization rates." *BMC Infectious Diseases*, 17(1): 186–186. https://doi.org/10.1186/s12879-017-2275-2.

125. Bharathan, T., Glodan, D., Ramesh, A., et al. (2007). "What do patterns of noise in a teaching hospital and nursing home suggest?" *Noise & Health*, 9(35), 31–34. https://journals.lww.com/nohe/fulltext/2007/09350/what_do_patterns_of_noise_in_a_teaching_hospital.1.aspx.

126. Graham, M. E. (2019). "Long-term care as contested acoustical space: Exploring resident relationships and identities in sound." *Building Acoustics*, 27(1): 61–73. Also see Joosse, L. L. (2011). "Sound levels in nursing homes." *Journal of Gerontological Nursing*, 37(8): 30–35. https://doi.org/10.3928/00989134-20110329-01.

127. Aletta, F., Botteldooren, D., Thomas, P., et al. (2017). "Exploring the soundscape quality of five nursing homes in Flanders (Belgium): Preliminary results from the AcustiCare project." *Inter.Noise Conference Proceedings*, 27–30 August, Hong Kong. https://www.acusticare.be/files/43_Aletta_Botteldooren_Thomas_Vander%20Mynsbrugge_%20De%20Vriendt_Van%20de%20Velde_Devos_2017.pdf.

128. Joosse, L. L. (2012). "Do sound levels and space contribute to agitation in nursing home residents with dementia?" *Research in Gerontological Nursing*, 5(3): 174–184. https://doi.org/10.3928/19404921-20120605-02.

129. Bentayeb et al. (2015).

130. ASHRAE (2025). *Standard 55—Thermal Environmental Conditions for Human*

Occupancy. Atlanta: American National Standards Institute. https://www.ashrae.org
/technical-resources/bookstore/standard-55-thermal-environmental-conditions-for
-human-occupancy#compliancehtml.

131. Tartarini et al. (2017).

132. Lynch, R. M., and Goring, R. (2020). "Practical steps to improve air flow in long-term
care resident rooms to reduce COVID-19 infection risk." *Journal of the American
Medical Directors Association*, 21(7): 893–894. https://doi.org/10.1016/j.jamda.2020
.04.001.

133. Wang, Z. (2021). "Use the environment to prevent and control COVID-19 in senior
-living facilities: An analysis of the guidelines used in China." *HERD: Health Environments Research & Design Journal*, 14(1): 130–140. https://doi.org/10.1177/19375
86720953519.

134. Gallant, S. (2017). "Multisensory stimulation improves quality of life for long-term care
patients." Alberta Health Services, 6 November. https://www.albertahealthservices
.ca/news/features/2017/Page14155.aspx.

135. Banerjee, S., and Ford, C. (2018). *Sensory Rooms for Patients with Dementia in
Long-Term Care: Clinical and Cost-Effectiveness, and Guidelines*. Ottawa: Canadian
Agency for Drugs and Technologies in Health.

136. Lundstedt, R., Håkansson, C., Lõhmus, M., and Wallergård, M. (2021). "Designing
virtual natural environments for older adults in residential care facilities." *Technology
and Disability*, 33(4): 305–318. https://doi.org/10.3233/TAD-210344.

137. Smith, R. E., and Quale J. D. (2017). *Offsite Architecture: Constructing the Future*.
London: Routledge.

138. Verderber, S. (2016). *Innovations in Transportable Healthcare Architecture*. London:
Routledge.

139. Suchomel, J. L. (2018). "Ready to assemble: Implementing prefabrication in health
facility projects." *Health Facilities Management*, 31(6): 45. Also see Peters, A. (2019).
"These flat-pack homes can be fully assembled in less than three months." *Fast
Company*, 26 July. http://www.fastcompany.com/90381454/these-flatpackhomes
-can-be-fully-assembled-in-less-than-three months.

140. Lulo, L. D. (2009). "Hybrid prefabrication: Prototypes for green residential construc-
tion." In Clouston, P., Mann, R. K., and Schreiber, S. (eds.), *Without A Hitch—New
Directions in Prefabricated Architecture*. Proceedings of the 2008 Northeast Fall
Conference of the Association of Collegiate Schools of Architecture. Amherst: MA:
University of Massachusetts, pp. 44–51.

141. Chatwood, S., Paulette, F., Baker, G. R., et al. (2017). "Indigenous values and health
systems stewardship in circumpolar countries." *International Journal of Environmental Research and Public Health*, 14(2): 1462–1482.

142. Verderber et al. (2020). Also see Martin, C. (2014). "Exhibition: Arctic health-care
architecture." *The Lancet*, 384(6): 845.

143. Collinge, T. S. (2018). "Indigenous perspectives on the notions of architecture."
The Site Magazine, 4(6): 14–31. https://www.thesitemagazine.com/read/indigenous
-perspectives.

144. Demirkan, H. (2007). "Housing for the aging population." *European Review of Aging
and Physical Activity*, 4(1): 33–38.

145. Abramsson, M., and Andersson, E. (2016). "Changing preferences with ageing—
housing choices and housing plans of older people." *Housing, Theory, and Society*,
33(2): 217–241.

146. Stevens et al. (2013).

147. Halloway, K. (2019). "The building of a net-zero hospital." *Health Facilities*, 26 June,
pp. 44–48. https://www.hfmmagazine.com/articles/3671-the-building-of-a-net-zero
-hospital.

148. Global Development Research Center (n.d.). *Defining Life Cycle Assessment*. https://gdrc.org/uem/lca/lca-define.html.

149. Brownell, E. (2016). "Understanding embodied energy in design." *Architect*, 29 April. https://www.architectmagazine.com/technology/understanding-embodied-energy-in-design_o.

150. Zimring, C., Godfried, L., Augenbroe, E., Malone, B., and Sadler, B. L. (2008). "Implementing healthcare excellence: The vital role of the CEO in evidence-based design." *HERD: Health Environments Research & Design Journal*, 1(3): 7–21.

151. National Academies of Sciences, Engineering, and Medicine (2022). *The National Imperative to Improve Nursing Home Quality: Honoring Our Commitment to Residents, Families, and Staff*. Washington, DC: The National Academies Press. https://doi.org/10.17226/26526. Also see Institute of Medicine Committee on Quality of Health Care in America (1999). To Err Is Human: Building a Safer Health System. Washington, DC: National Academies Press.

152. Preiser, W. F. E., Hardy, A., and Schramm, U., eds. (2018). *Building Performance Evaluation: From Delivery Process to Life Cycle Phases*. New York: Springer.

153. Cutler, L. J., and Kane, R. A. (2009). "Post occupancy evaluation of a transformed nursing home: The first four Green House® settings." *Journal of Housing for the Elderly*, 23(4): 304–334. Also see Zimmerman, S., Bowers, B. J., Cohen, L. W., Grabowski, D. C., Horn, S. D., and Kemper, P. (2016). "New evidence on the Green House model of nursing home care: Synthesis of findings and implications for policy, practice, and research." *Health Services Research*, 51(Special Issue): 475–496. https://doi.org/10.1111/1475-6773.12430.

154. Associated Press (2007). "Jury acquits nursing home owners in Katrina deaths." CBC News/World, 7 September. https://www.cbc.ca/news/world/jury-acquits-nursing-home-owners-in-katrina-deaths-1.680280. Also see Engberg, J. B., and Castle, N. (2008). "Health outcomes of nursing home residents following post-Katrina relocation." *The Gerontologist*, 33(6): 661–687. https://doi.org/10.1177/0164027511412197.

155. Robinson, K. (2013). "Eight years after Katrina: St. Rita's owners still feel the stigma." ABC News, 29 August. https://www.abcnews.go.com/US/years-katrina-st-ritas-owners-feel-stigma/story?id=20110312.html.

156. Peters, T., and Verderber, S. (2017). "Territories of engagement in the design of ecohumanist healthcare environments." HERD: Health Environments Research & Design Journal, 10(2): 104–123. https://doi.org/10.1177/1937586716668635.

157. Grunden, N., and Hagood, C. (2012). *Lean-Led Hospital Design: Creating the Efficient Hospital of the Future*. Boca Raton: CRC Press/Taylor & Francis.

158. International Facilities Management Association (2017). *Operations and Maintenance Benchmarks Survey for Healthcare Facilities*. London: IFMA.

159. Lahtinen, M., Sirola, P., Peltokorpi, A., et al. (2020). "Possibilities for user-centric and participatory design in modular healthcare facilities." *Intelligent Buildings International*, 12(2): 100–114.

160. Suchomel, J. L. (2018). "Prefabrication and healthcare construction." *Health Facilities Management*, 6 July. https://www.hfmmagazine.com/articles/3411-prefabrication-and-health-care-construction.

161. Schwarz, K. (2015). "Can salutogenic outcomes be achieved through public-private partnerships?" World Health Design, 8(6): 68–77; and Craig (2017).

Index